MR Neurography

Editor

AVNEESH CHHABRA

NEUROIMAGING CLINICS
OF NORTH AMERICA

www.neuroimaging.theclinics.com

Consulting Editor

SURESH K. MUKHERJI

February 2014 • Volume 24 • Number 1

ELSEVIER

1600 John F. Kennedy Boulevard • Suite 1800 • Philadelphia, Pennsylvania, 19103-2899

http://www.neuroimaging.theclinics.com

NEUROIMAGING CLINICS OF NORTH AMERICA Volume 24, Number 1
February 2014 ISSN 1052-5149, ISBN 13: 978-0-323-26668-0

Editor: John Vassallo (j.vassallo@elsevier.com)
Developmental Editor: Yonah Korngold

Neuroimaging Clinics of North America (ISSN 1052-5149) is published quarterly by Elsevier Inc., 360 Park Avenue South, New York, NY 10010-1710. Months of issue are February, May, August, and November. Business and editorial offices: 1600 John F. Kennedy Blvd., Suite 1800, Philadelphia, PA 19103-2899. Business and editorial offices: 6277 Sea Harbor Drive, Orlando, FL 32887-4800. Periodicals postage paid at New York, NY, and additional mailing offices. Subscription prices are USD 360 per year for US individuals, USD 514 per year for US institutions, USD 180 per year for US students and residents, USD 415 per year for Canadian individuals, USD 655 per year for Canadian institutions, USD 525 per year for international individuals, USD 655 per year for international institutions and USD 260 per year for Canadian and foreign students and residents. To receive student/resident rate, orders must be accompanied by name of affiliated institution, date of term, and the *signature* of program/residency coordinator on institution letterhead. Orders will be billed at individual rate until proof of status is received. Foreign air speed delivery is included in all *Clinics* subscription prices. All prices are subject to change without notice. POSTMASTER: Send address changes to *Neuroimaging Clinics of North America*, Elsevier Health Sciences Division, Subscription Customer Service, 3251 Riverport Lane, Maryland Heights, MO 63043. Telephone: 1-800-654-2452 (U.S. and Canada); 314-447-8871 (outside U.S. and Canada). Fax: 314-447-8029. E-mail: journalscustomerservice-usa@ elsevier.com (for print support); journalsonlinesupport-usa@elsevier.com (for online support).

Reprints. For copies of 100 or more of articles in this publication, please contact the Commercial Reprints Department, Elsevier Inc., 360 Park Avenue South, New York, NY 10010-1710. Tel.: 212-633-3874; Fax: 212-633-3820; E-mail: reprints@elsevier.com.

Neuroimaging Clinics of North America is covered by *Excerpta Medical/EMBASE,* the RSNA Index of Imaging Literature, *MEDLINE/PubMed (Index Medicus),* MEDLINE/MEDLARS, SciSearch, Research Alert, and Neuroscience Citation Index.

Printed and bound by CPI Group (UK) Ltd, Croydon, CR0 4YY

Transferred to digital print 2012

PROGRAM OBJECTIVE

The goal of Neuroimaging Clinics of North America is to keep practicing radiologists and radiology residents up to date with current clinical practice in radiology by providing timely articles reviewing the state of the art in patient care.

TARGET AUDIENCE

Practicing radiologists, radiology residents, and other healthcare professionals who utilize neuroimaging findings to provide patient care.

LEARNING OBJECTIVES

Upon completion of this activity, participants will be able to:
1. Review the technical considerations of MR neurography.
2. Describe the effectiveness of MR neurography research.
3. Discuss anatomical considerations and techniques in MRI of upper, central, and lower cranial nerves.

ACCREDITATION

The Elsevier Office of Continuing Medical Education (EOCME) is accredited by the Accreditation Council for Continuing Medical Education (ACCME) to provide continuing medical education for physicians.

The EOCME designates this enduring material for a maximum of 15 *AMA PRA Category 1 Credit*(s)™. Physicians should claim only the credit commensurate with the extent of their participation in the activity.

All other health care professionals requesting continuing education credit for this enduring material will be issued a certificate of participation.

DISCLOSURE OF CONFLICTS OF INTEREST

The EOCME assesses conflict of interest with its instructors, faculty, planners, and other individuals who are in a position to control the content of CME activities. All relevant conflicts of interest that are identified are thoroughly vetted by EOCME for fair balance, scientific objectivity, and patient care recommendations. EOCME is committed to providing its learners with CME activities that promote improvements or quality in healthcare and not a specific proprietary business or a commercial interest.

The planning committee, staff, authors and editors listed below have identified no financial relationships or relationships to products or devices they or their spouse/life partner have with commercial interest related to the content of this CME activity:

Shivani Ahlawat, MD; Gustav Andreisek, MD; Nafi Aygun, MD; Pablo A. Baltodano, MD; Kiran Batra, MD; Christopher Beaulieu, MD, PhD; Ashkan Heshmatzadeh Behzadi, MD; Allan J. Belzberg, MD; Jenny Bencardino, MD; Ari M. Blitz, MD; Alissa J. Burge, MD; Majid Chalian, MD; Zachary D. Chonka, MD; Asim F. Choudhri, MD; Tae Chung; Holly Delaney, MB BCh; John Eng, MD; Patrick Eppenberger, MD; Jan Fritz, MD; Gary L. Gallia, MD, PhD; Stephanie L. Gold, BA; Brynne Hunter; Ahmet T. Ilica, MD; Sharon Kuong, MD; Sandy Lavery; Thomas E. Lloyd, MD, PhD; Amelie M. Lutz, MD; Leonardo L. Macedo, MD; Jill McNair; Suresh K. Mukherji, MD, FACR; Lindsay Parnell; Jonathan Pindrik, MD; Kalpana Prasad, MBBS; Zehava Sadka Rosenberg, MD; Gedge D. Rosson, MD; Jaimie T. Shores, MD; Theodoros Soldatos, MD, PhD; Karthikeyan Subramaniam; Gaurav K. Thawait, MD; Anne J.W. Tong, MBBS; John Vassallo; Eric H. Williams, MD.

The planning committee, staff, authors and editors listed below have identified financial relationships or relationships to products or devices they or their spouse/life partner have with commercial interest related to the content of this CME activity:

Jaishri Blakely, MD has research grants from Children's Tumor Foundation, NIH, Ninds, CTEP and NCI.
John A. Carrino, MD, MPH is a consultant/advisor and has a research grant from Siemens Medical Systems.
Avneesh Chhabra, MD is a consultant/advisor for Siemens Medical Solutions, and has research grants from Siemens Medical Solutions, Integra Life Sciences and GE-AUR.
Aaron Flammang, MBA has stock ownership and an employment affiliation with Siemens Healthcare.
Garry Gold, MD, MS is a consultant/advisor for GE Healthcare, Itso, Inc., Zimmer, Inc., and Boston Scientific, Inc.; has research grants with GE Healthcare.
Abraham Padua Jr, RT has an employment affiliation with Siemens Healthcare and MR R&D Application Specialist.
Hollis Potter, MD has a research grant from GE Healthcare.
Kenneth C. Wang, MD, PhD is co-founder of Dex-Note, LLC.

UNAPPROVED/OFF-LABEL USE DISCLOSURE

The EOCME requires CME faculty to disclose to the participants:
1. When products or procedures being discussed are off-label, unlabelled, experimental, and/or investigational (not US Food and Drug Administration (FDA) approved); and
2. Any limitations on the information presented, such as data that are preliminary or that represent ongoing research, interim analyses, and/or unsupported opinions. Faculty may discuss information about pharmaceutical agents that is outside of FDA-approved labelling. This information is intended solely for CME and is not intended to promote off-label use of these medications. If you have any questions, contact the medical affairs department of the manufacturer for the most recent prescribing information.

TO ENROLL

To enroll in the *Neuroimaging Clinics of North America* Continuing Medical Education program, call customer service at 1-800-654-2452 or sign up online at http://www.theclinics.com/home/cme. The CME program is available to subscribers for an additional annual fee of $212 USD.

METHOD OF PARTICIPATION

In order to claim credit, participants must complete the following:
1. Complete enrolment as indicated above.
2. Read the activity.
3. Complete the CME Test and Evaluation. Participants must achieve a score of 70% on the test. All CME Tests and Evaluations must be completed online.

CME INQUIRIES/SPECIAL NEEDS

For all CME inquiries or special needs, please contact elsevierCME@elsevier.com.

NEUROIMAGING CLINICS OF NORTH AMERICA

RELATED INTEREST

Magnetic Resonance Imaging Clinics, Vol. 21, No. 2, May 2013
Modern Imaging Evaluation of the Brain, Body and Spine
Lara A. Brandão, *Editor*

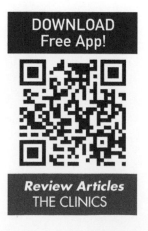

DOWNLOAD Free App!

Review Articles
THE CLINICS

NOW AVAILABLE FOR YOUR iPhone and iPad

NEUROIMAGING CLINICS OF NORTH AMERICA

Contributors

CONSULTING EDITOR

SURESH K. MUKHERJI, MD, FACR
Professor and Chairman; W.F. Patenge
Endowed Chair, Department of Radiology,
Michigan State University, East Lansing,
Michigan

EDITOR

AVNEESH CHHABRA, MD
Adjunct Professor, The Russell H. Morgan
Department of Radiology and Radiological
Science, The Johns Hopkins Hospital,
Baltimore, Maryland; Division Chief,
Musculoskeletal Radiology; Associate
Professor of Radiology and Orthopedic
Surgery, University of Texas Southwestern,
Dallas, Texas

AUTHORS

SHIVANI AHLAWAT, MD
Clinical Instructor, The Russell H. Morgan
Department of Radiology and Radiological
Science, The Johns Hopkins Hospital,
Baltimore, Maryland

GUSTAV ANDREISEK, MD
Department of Radiology, University Hospital
Zurich, Zurich, Switzerland

NAFI AYGUN, MD
Associate Professor, Division of
Neuroradiology, The Russell H. Morgan
Department of Radiology and Radiologic
Science, The Johns Hopkins Hospital,
Baltimore, Maryland

PABLO A. BALTODANO, MD
Postdoctoral Research Fellow, Department of
Plastic and Reconstructive Surgery, The Johns
Hopkins Hospital, Baltimore, Maryland

KIRAN BATRA, MD
The Russell H. Morgan Department of
Radiology and Radiological Science, The
Johns Hopkins Hospital, Baltimore, Maryland

CHRISTOPHER BEAULIEU, MD, PhD
Professor of Radiology, Department of
Orthopedic Surgery (by Courtesy); Department
of Radiology, Stanford University School of
Medicine, Stanford, California

ASHKAN HESHMATZADEH BEHZADI, MD
Johns Hopkins University, Baltimore, Maryland

ALLAN J. BELZBERG, MD
Associate Professor, Department of
Neurosurgery, Johns Hopkins University
School of Medicine, Baltimore, Maryland

JENNY BENCARDINO, MD
Associate Professor of Radiology, Department
of Radiology, New York University Hospital for
Joint Diseases, New York, New York

JAISHRI BLAKELY, MD
Assistant Professor of Neurology, Oncology
and Neurosurgery, Department of Neurology;
Director, The Johns Hopkins Hospital
Comprehensive Neurofibromatosis Center,
The Johns Hopkins Hospital, Baltimore,
Maryland

ARI M. BLITZ, MD
Director, Skull Base Imaging; Assistant
Professor, Division of Neuroradiology, The
Russell H. Morgan Department of Radiology
and Radiologic Science, The Johns Hopkins
Hospital, Baltimore, Maryland

ALISSA J. BURGE, MD
Department of Radiology and Imaging,
Hospital for Special Surgery, New York,
New York

JOHN A. CARRINO, MD, MPH
Associate Professor of Radiology and
Orthopedic Surgery and Section Chief,
Musculoskeletal Radiology Section, The
Russell H. Morgan Department of Radiology
and Radiological Science, The Johns Hopkins
Hospital, Baltimore, Maryland

MAJID CHALIAN, MD
Johns Hopkins University, Baltimore, Maryland

AVNEESH CHHABRA, MD
Adjunct Professor, The Russell H. Morgan
Department of Radiology and Radiological
Science, The Johns Hopkins Hospital,
Baltimore, Maryland; Division Chief,
Musculoskeletal Radiology; Associate
Professor of Radiology and Orthopedic
Surgery, University of Texas Southwestern,
Dallas, Texas

ZACHARY D. CHONKA, MD
Clinical Fellow, Division of Neuroradiology, The
Russell H. Morgan Department of Radiology
and Radiologic Science, The Johns Hopkins
Hospital, Baltimore, Maryland

ASIM F. CHOUDHRI, MD
Assistant Professor of Radiology,
Ophthalmology, and Neurosurgery; Director
of Neuroradiology, Le Bonheur Neuroscience
Institute; Assistant Chair, Research Affairs,
Department of Radiology, Le Bonheur
Children's Hospital, University of Tennessee
Health Science Center, Memphis, Tennessee

TAE CHUNG, MD
Neuromuscular Fellow, Department of
Neurology, The Johns Hopkins Hospital,
Baltimore, Maryland

HOLLY DELANEY, MB BCh
Department of Radiology, New York University
Hospital for Joint Diseases, New York,
New York

JOHN ENG, MD
Associate Professor of Radiology, The Russell
H. Morgan Department of Radiology and
Radiological Science, The Johns Hopkins
Hospital, Baltimore, Maryland

PATRICK EPPENBERGER, MD
Department of Radiology, University Hospital
Zurich, Zurich, Switzerland

AARON FLAMMANG, MBA
Siemens AG, Healthcare sector- MRI,
Erlangen, Germany

JAN FRITZ, MD
Radiologist, Musculoskeletal Radiology, The
Russell H. Morgan Department of Radiology
and Radiological Science, The Johns Hopkins
Hospital, Baltimore, Maryland

GARY L. GALLIA, MD, PhD
Assistant Professor of Neurosurgery,
Oncology, Otolaryngology and Head and Neck
Surgery; Director of Endoscopic and Minimally
Invasive Neurosurgery; Director, Neurosurgery
Skull Base Surgery Center, Department of
Neurosurgery, The Johns Hopkins Hospital,
Baltimore, Maryland

GARRY GOLD, MD, MS
Professor of Radiology, Department of
Radiology, Lucas Center; Department of
Orthopedic Surgery (by Courtesy), Stanford
University School of Medicine; School of
Bioengineering, Stanford University, Stanford,
California

STEPHANIE L. GOLD, BA
Department of Radiology and Imaging,
Hospital for Special Surgery, New York,
New York

AHMET T. ILICA, MD
Research Fellow, Division of Neuroradiology,
The Russell H. Morgan Department of
Radiology and Radiologic Science, The Johns
Hopkins Hospital, Baltimore, Maryland

SHARON KUONG, MD
Department of Radiology, Precision Medical Imaging, Fallon Clinic, Worcester, Massachusetts

THOMAS E. LLOYD, MD, PhD
Assistant Professor, Department of Neurology; Department of Neuroscience, The Johns Hopkins Hospital, Baltimore, Maryland

AMELIE M. LUTZ, MD
Assistant Professor of Radiology, Department of Radiology, Stanford University School of Medicine, Stanford, California

LEONARDO L. MACEDO, MD
Staff Neuroradiologist, Cedimagem/Alliar Diagnostic Center, Juiz de Fora, Minas Gerais, Brazil

ABRAHAM PADUA Jr, RT
Siemens Healthcare, Malvern, Pennsylvania

JONATHAN PINDRIK, MD
Assistant Resident/Housestaff, Department of Neurosurgery, The Johns Hopkins Hospital, Baltimore, Maryland

HOLLIS G. POTTER, MD
Department of Radiology and Imaging, Hospital for Special Surgery, Weill Cornell Medical College of Cornell University, New York, New York

KALPANA PRASAD, MBBS
Neuromuscular Fellow, Department of Neurology, The Johns Hopkins Hospital, Baltimore, Maryland

ZEHAVA SADKA ROSENBERG, MD
Professor of Radiology and Orthopedic Surgery, Department of Radiology, New York University Hospital for Joint Diseases, New York, New York

GEDGE D. ROSSON, MD
Associate Professor, Department of Plastic and Reconstructive Surgery, The Johns Hopkins Hospital, Baltimore, Maryland

JAIMIE T. SHORES, MD
Johns Hopkins University, Baltimore, Maryland

THEODOROS SOLDATOS, MD, PhD
The Russell H. Morgan Department of Radiology and Radiological Science, The Johns Hopkins Hospital, Baltimore, Maryland

GAURAV K. THAWAIT, MD
Research Fellow, Musculoskeletal Radiology Section, The Russell H. Morgan Department of Radiology and Radiological Science, The Johns Hopkins Hospital, Baltimore, Maryland

ANNE J.W. TONG, MBBS
Postdoctoral Research Fellow, Department of Plastic and Reconstructive Surgery, The Johns Hopkins Hospital, Baltimore, Maryland

KENNETH C. WANG, MD, PhD
Radiologist, Musculoskeletal Radiology, The Russell H. Morgan Department of Radiology and Radiological Science, The Johns Hopkins Hospital, Baltimore, Maryland

ERIC H. WILLIAMS, MD
Johns Hopkins University, Baltimore, Maryland

Contents

> Various methods of cross-sectional imaging are used for visualization of the cranial
> nerves, relying heavily on MR imaging. The success of the MR imaging sequences
> for visualization of cranial nerves depends on their anatomic context at the point
> of evaluation. The heterogeneity of opinion regarding optimal evaluation of the cra-
> nial nerves is partly a function of the complexity of cranial nerve anatomy. A variety of
> approaches are advocated and variations in equipment and terminology cloud the
> field. This article proposes a segmental classification and corresponding nomencla-
> ture for imaging evaluation of the cranial nerves and reviews technical consider-
> ations and applicable literature.

> The authors review the course and appearance of the major segments of the upper
> cranial nerves from their apparent origin at the brainstem through the proximal
> extraforaminal region, focusing on the imaging and anatomic features of particular
> relevance to high-resolution magnetic resonance imaging evaluation. Selected path-
> ologic entities are included in the discussion of the corresponding cranial nerve
> segments for illustrative purposes.

> Imaging evaluation of cranial neuropathies requires thorough knowledge of the
> anatomic, physiologic, and pathologic features of the cranial nerves, as well as
> detailed clinical information, which is necessary for tailoring the examinations,
> locating the abnormalities, and interpreting the imaging findings. This article
> provides clinical, anatomic, and radiological information on lower (7th to 12th)
> cranial nerves, along with high-resolution magnetic resonance images as a
> guide for optimal imaging technique, so as to improve the diagnosis of cranial
> neuropathy.

article reviews the normal 3-T MR neurographic appearance of the upper extremity nerves, and abnormal findings related to injury, entrapment, and other pathologic conditions.

Recent advances in magnetic resonance (MR) imaging have revolutionized peripheral nerve imaging and made high-resolution acquisitions a clinical reality. High-resolution dedicated MR neurography techniques can show pathologic changes within the peripheral nerves as well as elucidate the underlying disorder or cause. Neurogenic pain arising from the nerves of the pelvis and lumbosacral plexus poses a particular diagnostic challenge for the clinician and radiologist alike. This article reviews the advances in MR imaging that have allowed state-of-the-art high-resolution imaging to become a reality in clinical practice.

Magnetic resonance (MR) imaging of the nerves, commonly known as MR neurography is increasingly being used as a noninvasive means of diagnosing peripheral nerve disease. High-resolution imaging protocols aimed at imaging the nerves of the hip, thigh, knee, leg, ankle, and foot can demonstrate traumatic or iatrogenic injury, tumorlike lesions, or entrapment of the nerves, causing a potential loss of motor and sensory function in the affected area. A thorough understanding of normal MR imaging and gross anatomy, as well as MR findings in the presence of peripheral neuropathies will aid in accurate diagnosis and ultimately help guide clinical management.

Peripheral nerve enlargement may be seen in multiple conditions including hereditary or inflammatory neuropathies, sporadic or syndromic peripheral nerve sheath tumors, perineurioma, posttraumatic neuroma, and intraneural ganglion. Malignancies such as neurolymphoma, intraneural metastases, or sarcomas may also affect the peripheral nervous system and result in nerve enlargement. The imaging appearance and differentiating factors become especially relevant in the setting of tumor syndromes such as neurofibromatosis type 1, neurofibromatosis type 2, and schwannomatosis. This article reviews the typical magnetic resonance neurography imaging appearances of neurogenic as well as nonneurogenic neoplasms and tumorlike lesions of peripheral nerves, with emphasis on distinguishing factors.

Peripheral nerve surgery represents a broad field of pathologic conditions, medical specialties, and anatomic regions of the body. Anatomic understanding of hierarchical nerve structure and the peripheral nervous system aids diagnosis and management of nerve lesions. Many peripheral nerves coalesce into organized arrays, including the cervical, brachial, and lumbosacral plexuses, controlling motor and sensory functions of the trunk and extremities. Individual or groups of nerves may be affected by various pathologic conditions, including trauma, entrapment, tumor, or iatrogenic damage. Current research efforts focus on enhancing the peripheral nerve regenerative process by targeting Schwann cells, nerve growth factors, and nerve allografts.

Magnetic resonance (MR) neurography–guided nerve blocks and injections describe techniques for selective percutaneous drug delivery, in which limited MR neurography and interventional MR imaging are used jointly to map and target specific pelvic nerves or muscles, navigate needles to the target, visualize the injected drug and detect spread to confounding structures. The procedures described, specifically include nerve blocks of the obturator nerve, lateral femoral cutaneous nerve, pudendal nerve, posterior femoral cutaneous nerve, sciatic nerve, ganglion impar, sacral spinal nerve, and injection into the piriformis muscle.

Diagnostic limitations exist in the assessment of postoperative nerve regeneration. This article describes the role of available methods, such as clinical assessment, electrophysiologic studies, and magnetic resonance neurography in the postoperative evaluation of peripheral nerve repairs.

Magnetic resonance (MR) neurography has progressed in the past 2 decades because of rapid technological developments in both hardware and software. In addition to improvements in high-resolution anatomic pulse sequences, functional techniques are becoming feasible. This article presents the current state-of-the-art three-dimensional anatomic techniques, discusses the advantages of functional techniques being exploited, and portrays novel contrast types and molecular techniques that are under development and promise a bright future for this rapidly evolving technique.

Magnetic resonance neurography (MRN) is a specialized technique that is rapidly becoming part of the diagnostic algorithm of peripheral nerve pathology. However, in order for this modality to be considered appropriate, its value compared with current methods of diagnosis should be established. Therefore, radiologists involved in MRN research should use appropriate methodology to evaluate MRN's effectiveness with a multidisciplinary approach. This article reviews the various tiers of research available to assess the clinical value of a diagnostic modality with an emphasis on how to evaluate the impact of MRN on diagnostic thinking and therapeutic decisions.

Foreword
MR Neurography

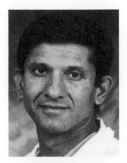

Suresh K. Mukherji, MD, FACR
Consulting Editor

In this issue, Dr Avneesh Chhabra discusses the growing area of magnetic resonance neurography (MRN). This has always been a perplexing but expanding area. An example is a patient presenting with radicular pain or "sciatica." Historically, such a patient would undergo a lumbar spine MRI. However, advances in MR now permit us to evaluate individual nerves and there is a changing paradigm that permits MR studies to be focused on the "painful" nerve as opposed to the body parts the nerve traverses.

This unique and comprehensive edition contains state-of-the-art articles that describe nerve anatomy, pathophysiology, approach to MRN imaging, and interpretation. This issue is "image-rich" with numerous examples of pathology involving the brachial plexus, lower extremity, and lumbosacral plexus. Other articles focus on MR-guided perineural interventions, peripheral nerve surgery approaches, and postoperative imaging.

I wish to thank Dr Chhabra for accepting this challenging topic and all of the contributors for their outstanding contributions. This is truly a unique edition that will be a valuable resource for many years to come!

Suresh K. Mukherji, MD, FACR
Department of Radiology
Michigan State University
East Lansing, MI 48824, USA

E-mail address:
Mukherji@rad.msu.edu

http://dx.doi.org/10.1016/j.nic.2013.09.003
1052-5149/14/$ – see front matter © 2014 Published by Elsevier Inc.

Preface
MR Neurography

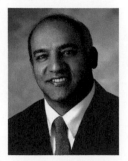

Avneesh Chhabra, MD
Editor

Magnetic resonance neurography (MRN) is becoming a popular technique for the evaluation of peripheral nerves. It was my pleasure and honor to guest edit this issue of *Neuroimaging Clinics* focused on this subject. The issue has three main objectives: first, to stress the immense potential of MRN for imaging the peripheral nerves; second, to provide the readers with an updated, convenient and practical reference guide to utilize the technique effectively and interpret the findings more critically; and finally, to solicit contributions from experts from multiple related specialties in this domain to bring out a whole body of knowledge on this subject.

This issue contains articles that describe state-of-the-art high-resolution MR imaging techniques performed for both cranial and peripheral nerve imaging. The comprehensive text covers nerve anatomy, pathophysiology, approach to MRN image interpretation, and imaging depiction of a variety of nerve lesions of upper extremity, brachial plexus, lower extremity, lumbosacral plexus, nerve tumor, and tumor-like conditions. Other articles focus on MR-guided perineural interventions, peripheral nerve surgery approaches, postoperative imaging, as well as research techniques to assess the impact of this technique. Lots of figures and tables have been used to help the discussion, as well as a clarification of the differential diagnoses and gamuts of peripheral nerve disorders.

I thank all the contributors and the whole team of *Neuroimaging Clinics* who worked really hard in making this issue possible and putting out an excellent piece of knowledge that will serve as a reference for many years to come. I am grateful to my family for allowing me to set aside considerable time to finish the project in a timely manner.

In summary, this issue will assist radiologists, technologists, and referring clinicians to use MRN technique confidently and enable an educated interpretation of the examination.

Avneesh Chhabra, MD
University of Texas Southwestern
Dallas, TX 75390, USA

The Russell H. Morgan Department of Radiology
and Radiological Science
The Johns Hopkins Hospital
Baltimore, MD 21287, USA

E-mail address:
avneesh.chhabra@utsouthwestern.edu

Neuroimag Clin N Am 24 (2014) xvii
http://dx.doi.org/10.1016/j.nic.2013.09.002
1052-5149/14/$ – see front matter © 2014 Published by Elsevier Inc.

Anatomic Considerations, Nomenclature, and Advanced Cross-sectional Imaging Techniques for Visualization of the Cranial Nerve Segments by MR Imaging

Ari M. Blitz, MD[a],*, Asim F. Choudhri, MD[b],
Zachary D. Chonka, MD[a], Ahmet T. Ilica, MD[a],
Leonardo L. Macedo, MD[c], Avneesh Chhabra, MD[d],
Gary L. Gallia, MD, PhD[e], Nafi Aygun, MD[a]

KEYWORDS

- Cranial nerve segments • Cross-sectional imaging • MR imaging

KEY POINTS

- The cranial nerves (CNs) pursue a complex course through tissues with widely varying MR imaging signal characteristics as they extend from brainstem nuclei into the fluid-filled subarachnoid spaces and ultimately pass through the skull base to exit the cranium.
- In turn, the reported success of the variety of available MR imaging sequences for visualization of the CNs depends largely on their anatomic context at the point of evaluation.
- Consideration of the general segmental architecture of the CNs aids in evaluation of patients with pathologic conditions affecting or adjoining their course.

INTRODUCTION

The 12 pairs of cranial nerves (CNs) arise directly from the brain within the cranial vault (with the exception of spinal rootlets of CN XI, which arises from the rostral cervical spine). The CNs serve a variety of highly specialized functions, including those necessary for vision, movement of the eyes and face, and identification and consumption of food. The branching patterns and/or proximity of CNs to each other at points along their course may allow localization of pathology on clinical grounds.[1] MR imaging plays an important role in the localization and identification of pathology as well as presurgical planning. A variety of modalities have been used in the imaging evaluation of CNs. Clinically, the first cross-sectional imaging study to directly demonstrate the CNs was pneumoencephalography. During pneumoencephalography, the introduction of subarachnoid air surrounding the CNs allowed for visualization of the optic, oculomotor, trigeminal, and hypoglossal nerves within the basal cisterns.[2] The

[a] Division of Neuroradiology, The Russell H. Morgan Department of Radiology and Radiologic Science, The Johns Hopkins Hospital, Phipps B-100, 600 North Wolfe Street, Baltimore, MD 21287, USA; [b] Department of Radiology, University of Tennessee Health Science Center, Le Bonheur Neuroscience Institute, Le Bonheur Children's Hospital, 848 Adams Avenue-G216, Memphis, TN 38103, USA; [c] Cedimagem/Alliar, Diagnostic Center, 150 Centro, Juiz de Fora, Minas Gerais 36010-600, Brazil; [d] The University of Texas Southwestern, 5323 Harry Hines Blvd, Dallas, TX 75390-9178, USA; [e] Department of Neurosurgery, Neurosurgery Skull Base Surgery Center, The Johns Hopkins Hospital, Phipps 101, 600 North Wolfe Street, Baltimore, MD 21287, USA
* Corresponding author.
E-mail address: Ablitz1@jhmi.edu

Neuroimag Clin N Am 24 (2014) 1–15
http://dx.doi.org/10.1016/j.nic.2013.03.020
1052-5149/14/$ – see front matter © 2014 Elsevier Inc. All rights reserved.

advent of CT enabled visualization of the region of the CNs with a greater degree of detail and with injection of intrathecal contrast; the CNs were visualized as linear filling defects within the subarachnoid space.[3] In both pneumoencephalography and CT cisternography, visualization was principally limited to the cisternal/subarachnoid course of the CNs and pathology was implied by alterations in the adjacent osseous structures. With the advent of MR imaging, cross-sectional examination of the structures of the head and neck without ionizing radiation became possible, with the ability to acquire images in any arbitrary plane allowing for the examination to be tailored to the CN in question. MR imaging is now the standard mode of imaging of the CNs and is the focus of this article.

TECHNICAL CONSIDERATIONS FOR MR IMAGING ACQUISITION FIELD STRENGTH

Fischbach and colleagues[4] studied T2-weighted spin-echo imaging of the CNs at 1.5T and 3T, the two most commonly available field strengths of clinical MR imaging units, and found that images acquired at higher spatial resolution on the 3T scanner nonetheless also had higher clarity and signal-to-noise ratio. The detection of perineural spread of neoplastic disease in the face initially not detected on 1.5T evaluation was possible on repeat examination at 3T.[5] Such results are not generally surprising because the tissue discrimination generally improved with higher field strengths.[6] Although 3T evaluation is generally preferred over 1.5T evaluation, diagnostic images may be obtained at either field strength, in particular when 3T MR imaging is not available, of questionable safety, or otherwise deemed inappropriate.

COIL CHOICE

Various approaches to coil choice and combination have been advocated[7] although phased-array head coils are typically used in the clinical setting and are adequate for most applications.

VOXEL SIZE AND COVERAGE

Thin-section imaging significantly improves detection of the CNs[8] although visualization of the cisternal trochlear (CN IV), abducens (CN VI), and accessory (CN XI) nerves may remain challenging. Due to its small caliber and proximity to multiple vascular structures, visualization of CN IV is particularly dependent on the spatial resolution of the sequences acquired. Choi and colleagues[9] compared conventional resolution (0.67 mm × 0.45 mm × 1.4 mm) to high-resolution (0.3 mm × 0.3 mm × 0.25 mm) imaging for detection of the cisternal trochlear nerve and found that the rate at which the nerve could probably or definitely be identified rose significantly from approximately 23% to 100%. **Fig. 1** demonstrates visualization of the trochlear nerve on 0.4-mm, 0.5-mm, and 0.6-mm isotropic constructive interference in the steady-state (CISS) images. Although increasing spatial resolution may improve visualization of small structures, the trade-off with respect to length of acquisition, reduced coverage, and/or decreased signal-to-noise ratio renders optimal coverage in all cases difficult. In the authors' practice, multiple 3-D sequences are typically used and include CISS imaging for the highest spatial resolution acquisition. The typical CISS acquisition includes 0.6-mm isotropic voxels with coverage of the entirety of the posterior fossa, skull base, and upper face. In select cases where CN IV palsy has been clinically diagnosed, a higher spatial resolution is often used.

2-D VERSUS 3-D IMAGING

Initially, MR imaging tailored to the CNs required careful attention to 2-D slice angulation to best demonstrate the CN in question.[10] Modern MR imaging equipment allows 3-D acquisition from

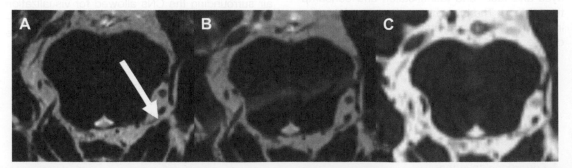

Fig. 1. Axial CISS images through the lower midbrain acquired at (*A*) 0.4-mm, (*B*) 0.5-mm, and (*C*) 0.6-mm isotropic resolution. The proximal cisternal CN IV, the obliquely oriented structure marked with an arrow (*A*), is progressively less well visualized as voxel size increases.

which post hoc reconstruction in multiple planes can be created, often better demonstrating the CNs.[8,11,12] One study of the cisternal components of the CNs in the cerebellopontine angle cistern with fast spin-echo technique found that 3-D imaging was superior to 2-D imaging due to suppression of flow artifacts and thinner sections and suggested that MR imaging evaluation of the cisterns be performed with 3-D technique.[13] When isotropic 3-D images are acquired, post hoc reconstructions can be made in any arbitrary plane, which is often useful in evaluating the complex anatomy of the CNs and surrounding structures.

INJECTION OF INTRAVENOUS CONTRAST AGENTS

The central nervous system (CNS) components of the CNs (including the entirety of the ophthalmic (CN I) and optic (CN II) nerves, which are properly tracts of the CNS rather than nerves per se) are at least partly isolated from the contents of the bloodstream by the blood-brain barrier and do not normally demonstrate visible contrast enhancement. The components of the CNs in the peripheral nervous system (PNS) are likewise separated by the blood-nerve barrier. When there is disruption of the blood-nerve barrier or blood-brain barrier, it is detected by the presence of an increase in intensity on postcontrast MR images with T1 weighting. Perhaps owing to lack of a similar barrier mechanism or increased blood flow, enhancement of the ganglia of the CNs may be detected as a physiologic finding.[14] Additionally, a circumneural arteriovenous plexus surrounds portions of the CNs in the interdural and foraminal regions of the skull base. Enhancement of the arteriovenous plexus may be seen, for instance, in the region of the tympanic and mastoid segments of the facial nerve (CN VII) in addition to the region of the geniculate ganglion.[15] Enhancement in the other CN components is pathologic. When present pathologic enhancement aids in the detection/localization of pathologic conditions of the CNs such as neoplastic, infectious, or inflammatory diseases.[16]

NOMENCLATURE

International consensus on anatomic nomenclature has been established in the *Terminologia Anatomica*.[17] The accepted terms for the CNs are olfactory nerve (CN I), optic nerve (CN II), oculomotor nerve (CN III), trochlear nerve (CN IV), trigeminal nerve (CN V), abducens or abducent nerve (CN VI), facial nerve (CN VII), vestibulocochlear nerve (CN VIII), glossopharyngeal nerve (CN IX), vagus nerve (CN X), accessory nerve (CN XI), and hypoglossal

nerve (CN XII). The system defines multiple named subcomponents of the CNs by function. Structures with a single function and without branches, such as CN VI, receive no further subclassification. The international nomenclature incompletely serves the needs of a radiologist or clinician. For instance, lesions in various locations along the course of CN VI, although presenting with a similar clinical deficit of abduction of the globe, may have vastly differing differential diagnostic and clinical implications. Therefore, the authors propose a systematic method of segmental imaging evaluation of the CNs.

ANATOMIC SEGMENTS

After emerging from the brain, each of the CNs courses through the cerebral spinal fluid (CSF) before it traverses the meninges, extending through an associated skull base foramen to emerge into the head and neck. Along this path, the nerves are surrounded by CSF in the subarachnoid space, venous blood in the interdural compartment, bone within the skull base foramina, and various soft tissues after exiting from the skull. Although the anatomic course of each of the CNs is different, some fundamental anatomic considerations are sufficiently similar to allow a systematic classification of different segments, which share similar imaging properties (**Fig. 2**). General anatomic and imaging considerations for each segment follow. Selected information on pathology is included for illustrative purposes, although a comprehensive description of pathology affecting each segment is beyond the scope of this article.

a. Nuclear Segment

Anatomic considerations
The CN nuclei contain the cell bodies of neurons that either give rise to the efferent fibers, which

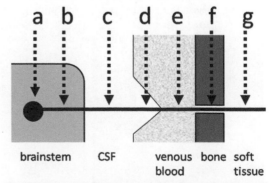

Fig. 2. Anatomic segments of the CNs with surrounding tissue (a, nuclear; b, parenchymal fascicular; c, cisternal; d, dural cave; e, interdural; f, foraminal; and g, extraforaminal).

exit the brainstem or receive afferent input. The CN nuclei extend from the midbrain (CN III) cranially into the rostral cervical spine caudally (CN XI).[18,19] The afferent nuclei generally rest lateral and dorsal to their efferent counterparts. Nuclei are further separated by their functional and evolutionary relationships from the somatic, branchial, and visceral (autonomic) motor nuclei. The visceral, somatic, and special sensory nuclei are arranged in columns approximately medial to lateral.[20]

Imaging approaches
In the fetal and neonatal brain, MR imaging allows direct identification of several CN nuclei, because the nucleus and proximal fibers myelinate earlier than the surrounding mesencephalic and rhombencephalic white matter tracts, best seen on T2-weighted imaging (**Fig. 3**).[21] Direct visualization of CN nuclei in the mature brain is difficult, and identification of pathology that has an impact on the nuclei requires knowledge of the location and function of the nuclei. The location of CN II.a, the lateral geniculate nuclei, can be directly seen as a focal protrusion on the posterolateral thalamus. The location of CN VI.a within the dorsal pons can be deduced when the facial colliculus is visualized (a name earned due to the traversing motor fibers of CN VII.b). The locations of components of CN V.a are reported as visible using diffusion tensor imaging (DTI) in the research setting.[22]

Selected pathologic entities
Most acquired pathologic conditions that have an impact on CN nuclei are related to regional abnormalities as opposed to abnormalities specific to the nucleus itself; thus, any process that has an impact on the adjacent brain parenchyma can have an impact on the nucleus of the CNs. Stroke, inflammatory processes, infection, tumor, and metabolic disorders, for instance, can result in nuclear-based cranial neuropathies.

b. Parenchymal Fascicular Segment

Anatomic considerations
The parenchymal fascicular segment runs from the point fibers exit the nuclei through the parenchyma to the point of separation from the brainstem at the apparent origin (AO). With the exception of CN IV.b, which alone exits the brainstem along the dorsal surface (see **Fig. 1**), the parenchymal fascicles of the CNs (also known as the CN tracts) pursue an anterior and lateral course through the brainstem to exit its ventral surface. Before separating from the brainstem to enter the cisternal segment, the CN fascicles may course along the surface of the brainstem. The point at which a discrete fascicle emerges from the parenchyma is known as the root exit point and the fascicular component, which may then course on the surface of the brainstem, is known anatomically as the attached segment (AS).[23,24] Studies in mammals demonstrate that these emergent fibers largely retain central myelination by oligodendrocytes before separating from the brainstem within the cisternal segment[25]; there are similar findings in humans.[23]

Imaging approaches
T2-weighted imaging The normal course of the fascicles of CN fibers extending from the nuclei toward the surface of the brainstem can sometimes be seen (see **Fig. 3**B) during the process of myelination in fetal or neonatal life using T2-weighted

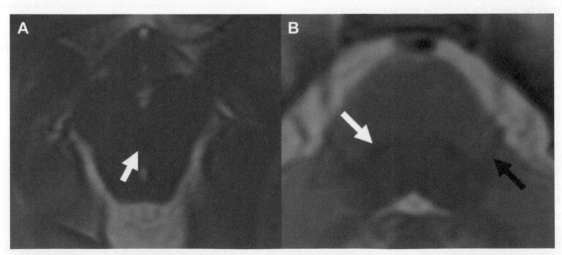

Fig. 3. (*A*) Axial T2-weighted image through the midbrain in a 5-week-old girl born at 25 weeks' gestation (corrected gestational age 30 weeks) demonstrates hypointensity in the region of CN III.a (*arrow*). (*B*) In the same patient, at the level of the pons, CN VII.a (*white arrow*) and a component of CN V.b (*black arrow*) are noted.

imaging, because the tightly packed layers of mature myelin around the nerve fibers have a decreased water content compared with the surrounding incompletely myelinated parenchyma.[21] The fascicles are not typically visualized on standard anatomic imaging in patients who are maturely myelinated but may be outlined by pathologic conditions. In the research realm, advances in high-resolution imaging shows promise for more clear depiction of the fascicular segments at higher field strengths than those currently used clinically.[26] Likewise, the root exit point and AS are not readily appreciated on modern clinical imaging and must be inferred by comparison to anatomic references.

Diffusion tensor imaging DTI is a technique that allows identification of fiber tracts within the brain parenchyma by virtue of the manner in which they constrain water diffusion. The technique has been used with limited success for visualization of the CN fascicles, largely due to their small size. The tracts associated with CN II and CN III.b are visualized with success.[27] In one patient with CN III palsy, abnormal signal in the region of CN III.b not well seen on standard imaging was demonstrated with thin-section DTI.[28] In the research setting, multishot diffusion-weighted imaging with periodically rotated overlapping parallel lines with enhanced reconstruction (PROPELLER) has been suggested to improve visualization of the visualization of the fascicular component of the

CNs in normal volunteers but with insufficient signal-to-noise ratio for routine clinical use.[29]

Selected pathologic entities
The fascicular segment of the CNs may be interrupted by any pathologic condition within the brainstem, including demyelinating disease and neoplastic processes, such as those arising from the glial support cells found in the CNS or other masses. Surgical data on patients treated for hemifacial spasm suggest that the neurovascular compression occurs in the terminal fascicular component of the CN VII.b in many cases, often with compression of the brainstem rather than the cisternal segment itself as generally assumed[24] (discussed later).

c. Cisternal Segment

Anatomic considerations
The end of the parenchymal fascicular segment and beginning of the cisternal segment is known anatomically as the root detachment point,[23,24] corresponding approximately to the AO, where the CN can be visualized surrounded by CSF on imaging (**Fig. 4**B). As described previously, the root exit point is not synonymous with the AO for at least some of the CNs. The term, *root exit zone*, is considered ambiguous[23] and its use is discouraged. Occasionally, multiple small free rootlets are visible (see **Fig. 4**) that converge on a root or several individual roots.[25,30,31]

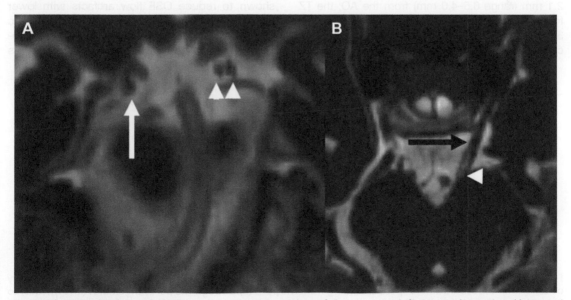

Fig. 4. (*A*) Coronal reformatted CISS demonstrates 2 rootlets of the proximal left CN III.c (*arrowheads*). Typical anatomy with a single root of CN III.c is seen on the right (*arrow*). (*B*) Axial CISS demonstrates the proximal rootlets joining (*arrow*) to form a single left CN III.c root within the midcisternal segment. The point of AO of the left CN III.c is marked with an arrowhead.

The proximal nerves in this segment are covered by pia mater[32] and surrounded by CSF within the subarachnoid space. In the cisternal segment, the CNs may adjoin arterial or venous structures as well as the arachnoidal septae. Arterial or venous structures may directly abut, surround, or even divide the cisternal components of the CNs.[33] The cisternal nerve roots extend toward the porus of the dural cave segment (described later) (Fig. 5).

The zone of transition between the oligodendrocyte-myelinated CNS and the Schwann cell–myelinated PNS is called the CNS-PNS transitional zone (TZ) (sometimes given the eponym Obersteiner-Redlich zone). The TZ was initially described as a thinning of the myelin sheaths of spinal nerves just before the junction of the dorsal root and the cord,[34] and the CNS component of the nerve proximal to this point is thought more prone to irritation. This point of transition is visible to the neurosurgeon through the operating microscope, because pia mater can be seen covering the centrally myelinated CNS component.[32]

The length of the centrally myelinated portion of the cisternal segment and, therefore, the site of the TZ varies between the CNs. Among CNs III–XII (as reported by Lang[32]) the TZ is approximately 1 mm or less from the AO at the surface of the brainstem for CNs IV, V (motor root only), VI, IX, X, and XI. The other CNs vary significantly in the length of the CNS component/location of the TZ. The TZ of CN III.c is typically located 1.9 mm (range 1.0–4.0 mm) from the AO; the TZ of CN VII.c is located 2.1 mm (range 0.5–4.0 mm) from the AO; the TZ for the sensory root of CN V.c is located on average 3.6 mm (range 2.0–6.0 mm) from the AO. The longest centrally myelinated cisternal component of a CN is that of CN VIII.c, with the TZ located most often at or near the porus acousticus, approximately 10.0 mm from the brainstem (range 6.0–15.0 mm).[32]

Imaging approaches

CN evaluation in the cisternal segment most often depends on negative contrast with a heavily T2-weighted appearance of CSF, an approach sometimes termed, *magnetic resonance cisternography*.

Although the cisternal CNs are generally well visualized, reports of visualization of CN IV.c have been variously reported as inconsistent[35] to excellent,[9] depending on technique and owing to its small size. Visualization is significantly improved with voxel sizes less than the diameter of the nerve.[9] The site of the TZ, although visible to neurosurgeons through the operating microscope,[32] is not readily identifiable through imaging alone, and its approximate location must be inferred through knowledge of the relevant CN anatomy.

Spin-echo T2-weighted imaging Early MR imaging experience with imaging of the cisternal CNs with 2-D heavily T2-weighted turbo spin-echo imaging using peripheral pulse gating to minimize CSF flow artifacts was successful, particularly in visualizing CNs I, II, III, VII, and VIII.[36] Subsequent studies demonstrated a significant advantage in detection of the CNs with 3-D compared with 2-D fast spin-echo sequences.[13] The addition of driven equilibrium radiofrequency reset pulse (DRIVE) to turbo spin-echo 3-D imaging has been shown to reduce CSF flow artifacts with lower scan times.[37] Comparison of 3-D fast asymmetric spin-echo and 3-D CISS imaging of the cerebellopontine angle cistern by one group of investigators

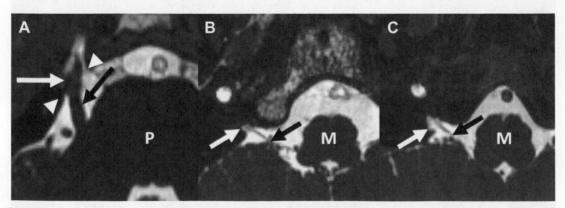

Fig. 5. (*A*) Axial CISS image demonstrates CN V.c (*black arrow*) as a filling defect surrounded by T2 hyperintensity of CSF within the subarachnoid space extending from the pons (P) through the porus trigeminus (*arrowheads*) to enter the trigeminal cistern within the Meckel cave as CN V.d (*white arrow*). (*B*) At the level of the medulla (M) CN IX.c (*black arrow*) extends through the jugular porus into a small dural cave (*white arrow*) of the right jugular foramen on precontrast CISS. (*C*) Significant variation is seen from patient to patient in the size of the dural cave segment; compare the extent of CSF evagination to that seen in (*B*).

favored 3-D fast asymmetric spin-echo due to "more prominent flow ghosts and magnetic susceptibility artifacts" on CISS.[38]

Steady-state free precession imaging High-resolution steady-state free precession (SSFP) sequences with a heavily T2-weighted appearance have become the mainstay of visualization of the cisternal component of the CNs[39] since their introduction by Casselman and colleagues.[40] Several studies have assessed visualization of the CNs in the cisternal segment.[35,41] 3-D CISS[11,35] and the analogous 3-D fast imaging using steady-state acquisition (FIESTA)[12] have been shown to be superior to 2-D T2-weighted images for the cisternal CNs. Additionally, comparison of CISS to 3-D magnetization-prepared rapid gradient echo (MP-RAGE), a T1-weighted 3-D technique, has favored CISS.[11] In patients undergoing surgery for neurovascular compression of CN V.c, comparison of CISS to magnetic resonance angiography (MRA) suggested that CISS more accurately predicts intraoperative findings with respect to the relationship of vascular structures to the CN.[42]

Although commonly thought of as a T2-weighted technique, CISS and FIESTA-C are fully refocused (balanced) steady-state sequences that demonstrate both T2 and T1 components.[43] This combination of weightings is ideal for the evaluation of the CNs because it allows both high spatial resolution with suppression of CSF flow artifacts and the use of contrast agents (Fig. 6). The use of contrast-enhanced CISS images for evaluation of cisternal masses has been proposed by Shigematsu and colleagues,[44] who suggested that the technique could reveal the accurate location of CN VII.c and CN VIII.c relative to cerebellopontine angle masses.

Diffusion tensor imaging Hodaie and colleagues[27] assessed visualization of the CNs, finding that evaluation of the lower cisternal CNs was particularly challenging. DTI has been used to determine the location of CN VII.c and CN VIII.c adjacent to large vestibular schwannomas in the cerebellopontine angle cistern.[45,46] In addition to information on the location of the cisternal components of the CNs, DTI reveals alterations in the coherence of water diffusion (fractional anisotropy) and has been shown to demonstrate significantly decreased fractional anisotropy in CN V.c on the side affected by trigeminal neuralgia[47] due to neurovascular compression.

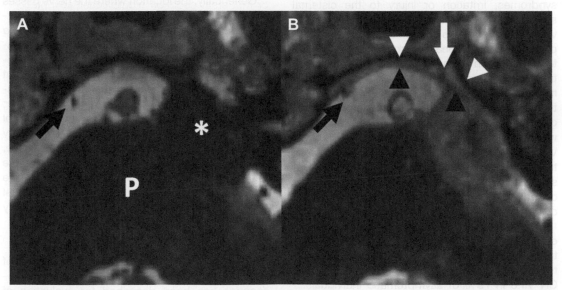

Fig. 6. (A) On axial precontrast CISS, the right CN VI.c (*black arrow*) is noted. A mass (*asterisk*) fills the left prepontine cistern indenting the left ventral pons (P). The location of the left CN VI.c is ambiguous. (B) After the administration of intravenous contrast, the left CN VI.e (*white arrow*) is clearly seen in the petroclival venous confluence. As seen in the precontrast image, right CN VI.c (*black arrow*) has not yet pierced the dura at this level, reflecting slight physiologic asymmetry in the cranial-caudal location of CN VI.d. The relationship of the mass to the inner layer of dura (*black arrowheads*) is now clear, without evidence of extension of the presumed meningioma into the interdural space adjacent to CN VI.e. The inner table of the skull (*white arrowheads*) to which the outer periostial layer of dura is applied, denoting the outer margin of the interdural space, is also noted. The patient presented with left-sided facial pain and decreased facial sensation due to compression of the left CN V.c (not shown). Extraocular movements were intact.

Selected pathologic entities

There are several clinical implications of the location of the TZ within the cisternal segment for most of the CNs. CN injuries distal to the TZ (ie, within the PNS) have different clinical implications from proximal CNS injuries. The PNS may regenerate with near-normal function, unlike the CNS, where a gliotic response to injury and persistent loss of axons is normal.[48] Because glial cells differ between the CNS and PNS pathology, the TZ forms a boundary for differential diagnostic considerations as well. Because Schwann cells are found only in the PNS, schwannomas likewise are found only distal to the TZ. In cases of vestibular schwannomas, for instance,[49] because the TZ for CN VIII is often found at or near the porus acousticus, the diagnosis of vestibular schwannoma is unlikely for masses located within the cerebellopontine angle cistern without involvement of the internal auditory canal.

The basal cisterns contain numerous arterial and venous structures. Since it was first demonstrated by Janetta[50] that neurovascular compression could cause trigeminal neuralgia and that neurosurgical decompression could result in relief from pain, several similar syndromes of neurovascular conflict have been identified. In these syndromes, grouped together as the hyperactive dysfunctional syndromes, irritation or injury to the cisternal segment of the CNs from direct contact with vascular structures is hypothesized. Although hyperactive dysfunctional syndromes may arise due to compression of any segment of a CN, the centrally myelinated components of the nerve are more vulnerable to such syndromes. In particular, trigeminal neuralgia, hemifacial spasm, and vagoglossopharyngeal neuralgia have been associated with neurovascular compression of CN V.c, CN VII.c, and CN IX/CN X.c, respectively. The susceptibility of these nerves to neurovascular compression is thought proportionate to the length of the centrally myelinated component within the cistern.[51]

Readers should be aware that neurovascular contact is common in the absence of the symptoms discussed previously. One study found neurovascular contact with CN V.c is seen in 49% and CN VII.c in 79% of asymptomatic individuals.[52] Additionally, a surgical series of microvascular decompression of CN VII for hemifacial spasm demonstrated compression in the 74% of cases not in CN VII.c but rather the attached segment distal segment of CN VII.b.[24] Although imaging may predict the intraoperative findings in many patients,[42] false-negative and false-positive cases are common.[53] As discussed previously, the measurement of fractional anisotropy with DTI has been reported as abnormal in trigeminal neuralgia and may increase specificity when neurovascular compression of CN V.c is suspected.[47] Such an approach is less likely to be helpful for CNs of smaller diameter due to spatial resolution and current system limitations.

d. Dural Cave Segment

Anatomic considerations

As the CNs leave the intracranial compartment, they transit several complex anatomic spaces. The dural cave segment is surrounded by an evagination of the arachnoid membrane within the inner (variously known as the lamina propria, cerebral, or meningeal) layer of the dura and its opening is called the porus (see Fig. 5). The dural cave forms the region of transition from the cisternal segment centrally to the interdural segment distally. The segment is variable from CN to CN and may also vary in prominence from individual to individual (see Fig. 5). In this regard, CN V.d that resides within the Meckel cave is the most familiar and provides an archetype of the relevant anatomic considerations. Each of the CNs makes a similar transition, with the dural cave of CN VI, for instance, also formed by an evagination of the inner layer of dura lined by arachnoid membrane.[54]

Generically, the location where the nerve passes out of the subarachnoid space and is no longer surrounded by CSF is termed, *the subarachnoid angle*.[55] For CN V.d, the arachnoid membrane typically terminates as perineurium distal to the posterior margin of the gasserian ganglion.[56] The point at which the arachnoid becomes adherent to the ganglion and its distal divisions is variable, however; thus, the volume and extent of the trigeminal cistern are variable. Although this cistern closely approximates the dimensions of the Meckel cave, and for the purposes of imaging is defined as the region with visible CSF surrounding the CN V, the two are not formally synonymous, with the Meckel cave slightly larger and extending farther anteriorly than the trigeminal cistern proper.[57]

Imaging approaches

Spin-echo–based T2-weighted imaging The use of 3-D fast asymmetric spin-echo magnetic resonance has been described for evaluation of CN VI.d (although not described as such) in volunteers.[58]

Steady-state free precession imaging CSF within the dural caves is well visualized with high-resolution T2-weighted SSFP imaging. The use of noncontrast CISS imaging for evaluation of CN III.d[59] as well as CN VI.d[60] have been described. Yousry and colleagues[61] also reported the use of postcontrast CISS for visualization of the gasserian (trigeminal) ganglion within the Meckel cave.

Selected pathologic entities

Although dural-based masses, such as meningioma, may become sufficiently large to compress a CN anywhere in the cisternal segment, small masses may become symptomatic at an earlier point if strategically positioned within the region of the dural interface (**Fig. 7**). Schwannoma may affect the CNs at any point distal to the TZ but seems to predilect the dural cave segment.

e. Interdural Segment

Anatomic considerations

The dura mater is composed of two layers.[56] The outer (periosteal) layer is closely adherent to the underlying bone and is continuous with the outer periosteum of the skull through sutures and neural foramina. The inner layer of dura (also known as lamina propria or meningeal or cerebral layer) is typically fused with the outer dural layer. There are interdural spaces, however, where the two are not closely opposed, such as in the region of the dural venous sinuses,[62] and the space between the inner and outer layers of dura contains an extensive venous plexus.[63] Several of the CNs exit the inner layer of dura and course between the inner and outer dural layers in the interdural compartment[64] before exiting the cranial vault through the skull base foramina. The prototypical space in this regard is the cavernous sinus, in which CNs III.e, IV.e, V.1.e, V.2.e and VI.e are surrounded by venous blood.

Imaging approaches

Postcontrast SSFP Although high-resolution 3-D imaging has traditionally principally been used without contrast for the evaluation of the cisternal segments of the CNs (described previously), administration of contrast and use of mixed-weighting SSFP or reversed fast imaging with steady-state precession (PSIF) (described later) sequences allows simultaneous high spatial resolution and evaluation of contrast enhancement. For this reason, the CNs, which do not normally enhance, can be well visualized inside the cavernous sinuses surrounded by contrast-enhanced venous blood (**Fig. 8**).[65] The petroclival CN VI.e is also well seen on CISS after the administration of intravenous contrast (see, for instance, **Fig. 6B** and the accompanying article by Blitz and colleagues in this issue).

Contrast-enhanced magnetic resonance angiography Linn and colleagues[66] described the application of contrast-enhanced MRA (CE-MRA) for evaluation of the cavernous segments of the CNs. Much like the approach taken with postcontrast CISS, CE-MRA relies on contrast enhancement of the venous plexus surrounding the cavernous CNs. The authors used a CE-MRA technique on a 3-T MR imaging lasting greater than 7 minutes' duration. The authors were able to produce multiplanar reconstructed images that depict the cavernous segments of the CNs in relation to sellar and cavernous masses extremely well.

Selected pathologic entities

The interdural space sits at the intersection of the osseous structures of the skull base and the intracranial compartment. Neoplastic processes arising from the meninges (see **Fig. 6**) or nerve root sheaths as well as inflammatory processes

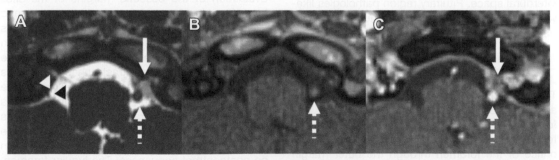

Fig. 7. A 57-year-old woman presented with denervation of her left tongue of uncertain cause. Standard MR imaging had been unrevealing. (*A*) Axial noncontrast CISS demonstrates the right CN XII.c (*black arrowhead*) extending toward a small dural cave (*white arrowhead*, continued for reference in following frames). On the left side an approximately 6 mm mass (*white arrow*) is noted extending from the region of the left CN XII.d into the cistern just anterolateral to the V4 segment of the left vertebral artery (*dashed arrow*). The mass was not visualized on noncontrast axial volumetric interpolated breath-hold examination (VIBE), a T1-weighted technique. (Please note that breath holds are not typically employed with this technique when employed in neuroradiology despite the acronymn.) (*B*) but demonstrated enhancement (*white arrow*) on postcontrast fat saturated VIBE (*C*).

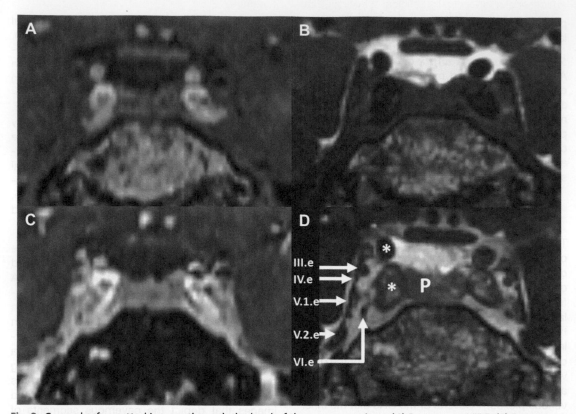

Fig. 8. Coronal reformatted images through the level of the cavernous sinus. (A) Precontrast VIBE. (B) Precontrast CISS. (C) Postcontrast VIBE demonstrates enhancement of the cavernous sinus. (D) Postcontrast CISS best demonstrates the normal appearance of the interdural oculomotor (III.e), trochlear (IV.e), ophthalmic (V.1.e), maxillary (V.2.e), and abducens (VI.e) nerves. The internal carotid artery (*asterisk*) and pituitary (P) are labeled for orientation purposes.

may be seen in this region. Additionally, intraosseous abnormalities may gain access to the interdural space if they pierce the outer layer of dura. Perineural spread of disease passing intracranially through the foraminal regions may also affect the interdural space. Pituitary region pathologies likewise may spread into the interdural space, in particular, the cavernous sinus.

f. Foraminal Segment

Anatomic considerations

The passage of the CNs through the skull is accomplished via the skull base foramina. The foraminal segment of each CN is defined as extending from the inner margin of the internal orifice of the foramen through the outer margin of the outer table of the skull at the external orifice. CN VIII alone among the CNs does not have a component that exits the skull base. The foramina are lined by the outer (periostial) layer of dura, which is continuous at the outer margin of the foramina with the periosteum as well as the epineurium.[56] The CNs are typically surrounded in their foraminal segments by a circumneural venous plexus, the enhancement of which allows visualization of the normally nonenhancing CN.[14]

Imaging approaches

Evaluation of the osseous margins of the skull base foramina is most frequently accomplished clinically with CT; however, MR imaging has the added advantage of allowing visualization of the CN with contrast-enhanced technique (Fig. 9A, B). Just as contrast-enhanced venous blood allows visualization of the CNs in the cavernous sinus, the presence of cortical bones lining the skull base foramina and venous plexus surrounding the foraminal components of the CNs allows similar high-resolution 3-D evaluation on postcontrast sequences. The jugular foramen, given its complexity, is an excellent example of the potential visualization of the CNs as they pass through the foraminal segment.

Postcontrast SSFP After the administration of intravenous contrast, CN IX.f, CN X.f, and CN XI.f are well visualized within the jugular foramen due to surrounding venous enhancement on FIESTA.[67]

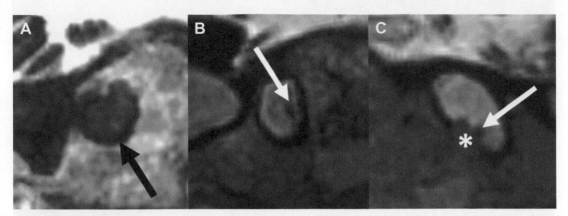

Fig. 9. (A) Precontrast CISS in a patient without osseous pathology of the skull base. Multiplanar reformat perpendicular to the hypoglossal canal demonstrating the cortical margin (*arrow*). (B) Postcontrast CISS demonstrates CN XII.f (*arrow*) surrounded by enhancement of the venous plexus. The cortical margin of the foramen is intact. (C) On the contralateral side, a component of a large chordoma (*asterisk*) involving the posterior skull base interrupts the cortical margin of the foramen and minimally extends into the hypoglossal canal to abut CN XII.f (*arrow*).

Contrast-enhanced magnetic resonance angiograph Linn and colleagues[68] have described the use of CE-MRA in the jugular foramen and reported overall improved visualization of the CNs compared with contrast-enhanced FIESTA although some structures were better visualized with contrast-enhanced FIESTA. The investigators were careful to match time of acquisition; however, CE-MRA was performed before contrast-enhanced FIESTA. It is not clear to what extent the greater than 7-minute delay for performance of CE-MRA may have had on comparison with the subsequently performed FIESTA. The investigators suggest performance of CE-MRA if pathology of the foramen itself is suspected and FIESTA imaging for cases when lower CN pathology is suspected but the timing is less clear.

Selected pathologic entities

When encountered in isolation, pathologic conditions of the foraminal segment of the CNs are most commonly the result of extension of an abnormality from within the adjacent bone (eg, see **Fig. 9**C).

g. Extraforaminal Segment

Anatomic considerations

The extraforaminal segment (g) begins at the plane that passes through the outer cortex of the outer margin of the appropriate foramen. The proximal extraforaminal segment typically passes at least initially through fat before coming into contact with the vascular structures, glands, and muscles of the head and neck. Among the CNs, CN X.g has the most extensive extraforaminal course (implied by the name of CN X, *vagus* [wanderer]) and reaches as far as the abdomen.

Imaging approaches

CISS with and without contrast Both fat and fluid return high signal on balanced SSFP sequences, such as CISS, due to their high T2/T1 ratios.[43] The environment of the extraforaminal CNs consists of fat, muscle, bone, and vascular structures, which can be readily distinguished on CISS. Despite the course of multiple extraforaminal components of the CNs near the air-containing paranasal sinuses and aerodigestive tract, perhaps because of the reduced T2* sensitivity of balanced SSFP sequences[43] as well as the small voxels used, resultant artifacts tend not to significantly limit such evaluations. The use of CISS imaging in the extraforaminal regions of the suprahyoid neck allows exquisite anatomic definition of structures that have not been typically well visualized with prior techniques (**Fig. 10**) and has been extensively used at the authors' institution for this purpose. The addition of intravenous contrast heightens the distinction between the extraforaminal CNs and adjacent structures. In conjunction with 3-D T1 and short tau inversion recovery (STIR) sequences, comparison of precontrast and postcontrast CISS imaging allows evaluation of small regions of pathologic enhancement, such as might be encountered in perineural spread of neoplasm or in highlighting the relationship of the CN to an enhancing mass (see **Fig. 10**C).

Reverse FISP/Neurography 3-D PSIF with diffusion weighting has been reported by Zhang and colleagues[69] as demonstrating the course of the CNs. The investigators evaluated the results of an approximately 10-minute PSIF acquisition with a diffusion moment of 20 mT/m*ms and concluded the technique "cannot be used as a

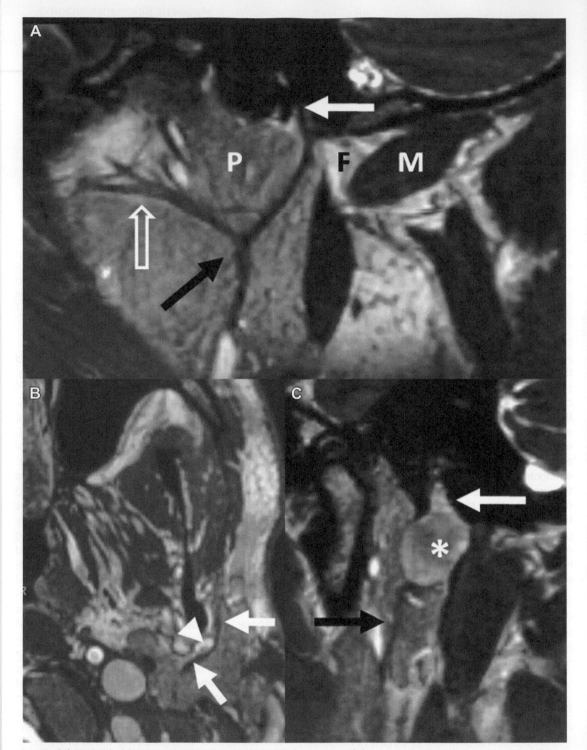

Fig. 10. (*A*) Sagittal oblique postcontrast CISS through the region of the parotid. CN VII.g is seen exiting the sty-lomastoid foramen (*white closed arrow*) and coursing inferiorly to enter the parotid gland (P). The primary intra-parotid branch point (*black arrow*) into the temporofacial branch (superiorly) and cervicofacial branch (inferiorly) are seen. Secondary (*open white arrow*) intraparotid branch points are also well visualized as the nerve extends anteriorly. High-resolution imaging of the CNs in the extraforaminal compartment relies on differential signal characteristics of the CNs surrounded by fat (F), muscle (M), and organs, such as the parotid (P). (*B*) Axial postcon-trast CISS demonstrates the relationship of the intraparotid CN VII.g (*arrows*) to the retromandibular vein (*arrow-head*). (*C*) Sagittal postcontrast CISS in a different patient demonstrates an enhancing mass (*asterisk*) extending from the stylomastoid foramen (*white arrow*) into the parotid gland. The distal intraparotid CN VII.g (*black arrow*) can be seen emanating from the caudal aspect of the mass, a presumed schwannoma.

substitute for other standard sequences such as 3D-CISS sequence or the 3-D fast spin echo (FSE) sequence" but may be most useful for evaluation of CNs outside of the cranial compartment. This technique may be most useful in regions, such as the carotid sheath, where visualization of the CNs is inconstant.

Diffusion tensor imaging DTI using fat saturation at 3T with tractography has been reported by Akter and colleagues[70] for imaging of the CNs within the head and neck; they describe at least partial correlation between DTI and operative findings in 4 of the 5 patients studied.

SUMMARY

Imaging of the CNs presents a challenge due to their small size and course. This article proposes a segmental classification system for radiologic evaluation of the CNs, which the authors hope proves useful in clinical practice while providing a framework for future high-resolution CN imaging research. MR imaging is currently the gold standard technique and a variety of pulse sequences are available to demonstrate the CNs. The optimal imaging approach depends largely on which sequence is best suited to demonstrating the CN in the segment of interest. Within the nuclear and fascicular segments, the CNs are often difficult to distinguish from surrounding brain parenchyma. Cisternal and dural cave segments are best visualized on T2-weighted sequences and SSFP sequences. The interdural segments are best seen with techniques that allow enhancement of the surrounding venous blood, such as contrast-enhanced MRA or contrast-enhanced SSFP sequences; a similar approach is helpful for visualization within the skull base foramina. Within the extraforaminal segment, the CNs adjoin vascular structures, fat, muscle, and/or bone as they pass through the head and neck and may be visualized with a variety of techniques with SSFP sequences, such as CISS and PSIF, providing excellent anatomic detail. DTI has also been used for visualization of the CNs in the fascicular, cisternal, and extraforaminal segments.

The heterogeneity of anatomic context presents significant challenges for images. Given advantages and pitfalls of various imaging pulse sequences, a fully refocused SSFP technique, such as CISS, allows visualization of much of the CN course when precontrast and postcontrast techniques are used. The accompanying article by Blitz and colleagues elsewhere in this issue describes the relevant anatomy and imaging appearance of the upper CNs on high-resolution CISS imaging, using the segmental approach advocated in this article.

REFERENCES

1. Brazis PW, Masdeu JC, Biller J. Localization in Clinical Neurology. Philadelphia: Lippincott Williams & Wilkins; 2011.
2. Di Chiro G. An Atlas of Detailed Normal Pneumoencephalographic Anatomy, 2e. Springfield: Charles C. Thomas Publisher; 1971.
3. de Slegte R, Valk J, Lohman A, et al. Cisternographic Anatomy of the Poster Cranial Fossa: High Resolution CT and MRI Study. Wolfeboro: Vam Gorcum; 1986.
4. Fischbach F, Müller M, Bruhn H. Magnetic resonance imaging of the cranial nerves in the posterior fossa: a comparative study of t2-weighted spin-echo sequences at 1.5 and 3.0 tesla. Acta Radiol 2008;49(3):358–63.
5. Penn R, Abemayor E, Nabili V, et al. Perineural invasion detected by high-field 3.0-T magnetic resonance imaging. Am J Otolaryngol 2010;31(6): 482–4.
6. Hart H, Bottomley P, Edelstein W, et al. Nuclear magnetic resonance imaging: contrast-to-noise ratio as a function of strength of magnetic field. Am J Roentgenol 1983;141(6):1195–201.
7. Casselman J, Mermuys K, Delanote J, et al. MRI of the cranial nerves—more than meets the eye: technical considerations and advanced anatomy. Neuroimaging Clin N Am 2008;18(2):197–231.
8. Fischbach F, Müller M, Bruhn H. High-resolution depiction of the cranial nerves in the posterior fossa (N III–N XII) with 2D fast spin echo and 3D gradient echo sequences at 3.0 T. Clin Imaging 2009;33(3):169–74.
9. Choi B, Kim J, Jung C, et al. High-resolution 3D MR imaging of the trochlear nerve. AJNR Am J Neuroradiol 2010;31(6):1076–9.
10. Leblanc A. The Cranial Nerves: Anatomy, Imaging, Vascularisation. New York: Springer-Verlag; 1995.
11. Held P, Nitz W, Seitz J, et al. Comparison of 2D and 3D MRI of the optic and oculomotor nerve anatomy. Clin Imaging 2000;24(6):337–43.
12. Hatipoğlu HG, Durakoğlugil T, Ciliz D, et al. Comparison of FSE T2W and 3D FIESTA sequences in the evaluation of posterior fossa cranial nerves with MR cisternography. Diagn Interv Radiol 2007;13(2):56–60.
13. Iwayama E, Naganawa S, Ito T, et al. High-resolution MR cisternography of the cerebellopontine angle: 2D versus 3D fast spin-echo sequences. AJNR Am J Neuroradiol 1999;20(5):889–95.
14. Williams LS, Schmalfuss IM, Sistrom CL, et al. MR imaging of the trigeminal ganglion, nerve, and the perineural vascular plexus: normal appearance

and variants with correlation to cadaver specimens. AJNR Am J Neuroradiol 2003;24(7):1317–23.

15. Gebarski S, Telian S, Niparko J. Enhancement along the normal facial nerve in the facial canal: MR imaging and anatomic correlation. Radiology 1992;183(2):391–4.

16. Saremi F, Helmy M, Farzin S, et al. MRI of cranial nerve enhancement. Am J Roentgenol 2005; 185(6):1487–97.

17. Whitmore I. Terminologia Anatomica: International Anatomical terminology; FIPAT, Federative international Programme on Anatomical Terminologies. New York: Thieme; 2011.

18. Nieuwenhuys R, Voogd J, Voogd J, et al. The Human Central Nervous System, 4e. Springer Verlag; 2008.

19. Wilson-Pauwels L, Akesson EJ, Stewart PA. Cranial Nerves. Hamilton, Canada: Decker; 1988.

20. Nolte J. The Human Brain: An Introduction to its Functional Anatomy, 5e. St. Louis: Mosby; 2002.

21. Barkovich AJ. MR of the normal neonatal brain: assessment of deep structures. AJNR Am J Neuroradiol 1998;19(8):1397–403.

22. Nagae-Poetscher LM, Jiang H, Wakana S, et al. High-resolution diffusion tensor imaging of the brain stem at 3 T. AJNR Am J Neuroradiol 2004; 25(8):1325–30.

23. Tomii M, Onoue H, Yasue M, et al. Microscopic measurement of the facial nerve root exit zone from central glial myelin to peripheral Schwann cell myelin. J Neurosurg 2003;99(1):121–4.

24. Campos-Benitez M, Kaufmann AM. Neurovascular compression findings in hemifacial spasm. J Neurosurg 2008;109(3):416–20.

25. Fraher J, Smiddy P, O'Sullivan V. The central-peripheral transitional regions of cranial nerves. Oculomotor nerve. J Anat 1988;161:103–13.

26. Naidich TP, Duvernoy HM, Delman BN, et al. Duvernoy's Atlas of the Human Brain Stem and Cerebellum. Vienna (Austria): Springer-Verlag; 2009.

27. Hodaie M, Quan J, Chen DQ. In vivo visualization of cranial nerve pathways in humans using diffusion-based tractography. Neurosurgery 2010;66(4): 788–96.

28. Yamada K, Shiga K, Kizu O, et al. Oculomotor nerve palsy evaluated by diffusion-tensor tractography. Neuroradiology 2006;48(6):434–7.

29. Adachi M, Kabasawa H, Kawaguchi E. Depiction of the cranial nerves within the brain stem with use of PROPELLER multishot diffusion-weighted imaging. AJNR Am J Neuroradiol 2008;29(5):911–2.

30. Nathan H, Ouaknine G, Kosary IZ. The abducens nerve. J Neurosurg 1974;41(5):561–6.

31. Fraher J, Smiddy P, O'Sullivan V. The central-peripheral transitional regions of cranial nerves. Trochlear and abducent nerves. J Anat 1988;161: 115–23.

32. Lang J. Clinical Anatomy of the Head. Berlin: Springer-Verlag; 1983.

33. Marinkovic SV, Gibo H, Stimec B. The neurovascular relationships and the blood supply of the abducent nerve: surgical anatomy of its cisternal segment. Neurosurgery 1994;34(6):1017–26.

34. Obersteiner H, Redlich E. Ueber Wesen Und Pathogenese Der Tabischen Hinterstrangdegeneration. Arb Neurol Inst Univ Wien 1894;1(3):152–72.

35. Yousry I, Camelio S, Schmid U, et al. Visualization of cranial nerves I–XII: value of 3D CISS and T2-weighted FSE sequences. Eur Radiol 2000; 10(7):1061–7.

36. Mamata Y, Muro I, Matsumae M, et al. Magnetic resonance cisternography for visualization of intracisternal fine structures. J Neurosurg 1998;88(4): 670–8.

37. Ciftci E, Anik Y, Arslan A, et al. Driven equilibrium (drive) MR imaging of the cranial nerves V–VIII: comparison with the T2-weighted 3D TSE sequence. Eur J Radiol 2004;51(3):234–40.

38. Naganawa S, Koshikawa T, Fukatsu H, et al. MR cisternography of the cerebellopontine angle: comparison of three-dimensional fast asymmetrical spin-echo and three-dimensional constructive interference in the steady-state sequences. AJNR Am J Neuroradiol 2001;22(6):1179–85.

39. Sheth S, Branstetter BF IV, Escott EJ. Appearance of normal cranial nerves on steady-state free precession MR images1. Radiographics 2009;29(4): 1045–55.

40. Casselman J, Kuhweide R, Deimling M, et al. Constructive interference in steady state-3DFT MR imaging of the inner ear and cerebellopontine angle. AJNR Am J Neuroradiol 1993;14(1):47–57.

41. Seitz J, Held P, Fründ R, et al. Visualization of the IXth to XIIth cranial nerves using 3-dimensional constructive interference in steady state, 3-dimensional magnetization-prepared rapid gradient echo and T2-weighted 2-dimensional turbo spin echo magnetic resonance imaging sequences. J Neuroimaging 2001;11(2):160–4.

42. Yoshino N, Akimoto H, Yamada I, et al. Trigeminal neuralgia: evaluation of neuralgic manifestation and site of neurovascular compression with 3D CISS MR imaging and MR angiography1. Radiology 2003;228(2):539–45.

43. Chavhan GB, Babyn PS, Jankharia BG, et al. Steady-state MR imaging sequences: physics, classification, and clinical applications. Radiographics 2008;28(4):1147–60.

44. Shigematsu Y, Korogi Y, Hirai T, et al. Contrast-enhanced CISS MRI of vestibular schwannomas: phantom and clinical studies. J Comput Assist Tomogr 1999;23(2):224–31.

45. Taoka T, Hirabayashi H, Nakagawa H, et al. Displacement of the facial nerve course by

vestibular schwannoma: preoperative visualization using diffusion tensor tractography. J Magn Reson Imaging 2006;24(5):1005–10.

46. Chen DQ, Quan J, Guha A, et al. Three-dimensional in vivo modeling of vestibular schwannomas and surrounding cranial nerves with diffusion imaging tractography. Neurosurgery 2011;68(4):1077–83.

47. Lutz J, Linn J, Mehrkens JH, et al. Trigeminal neuralgia due to neurovascular compression: high-spatial-resolution diffusion-tensor imaging reveals microstructural neural changes. Radiology 2011; 258(2):524–30.

48. Fraher JP. The transitional zone and CNS regeneration. J Anat 1999;194(2):161–82.

49. Xenellis JE, Linthicum FH Jr. On the myth of the glial/schwann junction (Obersteiner-Redlich zone): origin of vestibular nerve schwannomas. Otol Neurotol 2003;24(1):1.

50. Jannetta PJ. Arterial compression of the trigeminal nerve at the pons in patients with trigeminal neuralgia. J Neurosurg 1967;26(Suppl 1):159–62.

51. Guclu B, Sindou M, Meyronet D, et al. Cranial nerve vascular compression syndromes of the trigeminal, facial and vago-glossopharyngeal nerves: comparative anatomical study of the central myelin portion and transitional zone; correlations with incidences of corresponding hyperactive dysfunctional syndromes. Acta Neurochir 2011;153(12):2365–75.

52. Kakizawa Y, Seguchi T, Kodama K, et al. Anatomical study of the trigeminal and facial cranial nerves with the aid of 3.0-tesla magnetic resonance imaging. J Neurosurg 2008;108(3):483–90.

53. Benes L, Shiratori K, Gurschi M, et al. Is preoperative high-resolution magnetic resonance imaging accurate in predicting neurovascular compression in patients with trigeminal neuralgia? Neurosurg Rev 2005;28(2):131–6.

54. Joo W, Yoshioka F, Funaki T, et al. Microsurgical anatomy of the abducens nerve. Clin Anat 2012; 25(8):1030–42.

55. McCabe JS, Low FN. The subarachnoid angle: an area of transition in peripheral nerve. Anat Rec 1969;164(1):15–33.

56. Janjua RM, Al-Mefty O, Densler DW, et al. Dural relationships of Meckel cave and lateral wall of the cavernous sinus. Neurosurg Focus 2008;25(6):1–12.

57. Kaufman B, Bellon EM. The trigeminal nerve cistern. Radiology 1973;108(3):597–602.

58. Ono K, Arai H, Endo T, et al. Detailed MR imaging anatomy of the abducent nerve: evagination of CSF into Dorello canal. AJNR Am J Neuroradiol 2004; 25(4):623–6.

59. Everton K, Rassner U, Osborn A, et al. The oculomotor cistern: anatomy and high-resolution imaging. AJNR Am J Neuroradiol 2008;29(7):1344–8.

60. Yousry I, Camelio S, Wiesmann M, et al. Detailed magnetic resonance imaging anatomy of the cisternal segment of the abducent nerve: Dorello's canal and neurovascular relationships and landmarks. J Neurosurg 1999;91(2):276–83.

61. Yousry I, Moriggl B, Schmid UD, et al. Trigeminal ganglion and its divisions: detailed anatomic MR imaging with contrast-enhanced 3D constructive interference in the steady state sequences. AJNR Am J Neuroradiol 2005;26(5):1128–35.

62. Yasuda A, Campero A, Martins C, et al. The medial wall of the cavernous sinus: microsurgical anatomy. Neurosurgery 2004;55(1):179–90.

63. Parkinson D. Extradural neural axis compartment. J Neurosurg 2000;92(4):585–8.

64. Umansky F, Valarezo A, Elidan J. The microsurgical anatomy of the abducens nerve in its intracranial course. Laryngoscope 1992;102(11): 1285–92.

65. Yagi A, Sato N, Taketomi A, et al. Normal cranial nerves in the cavernous sinuses: contrast-enhanced three-dimensional constructive interference in the steady state MR imaging. AJNR Am J Neuroradiol 2005;26(4):946–50.

66. Linn J, Peters F, Lummel N, et al. Detailed imaging of the normal anatomy and pathologic conditions of the cavernous region at 3 Tesla using a contrast-enhanced MR angiography. Neuroradiology 2011; 53(12):947–54.

67. Davagnanam I, Chavda S. Identification of the normal jugular foramen and lower cranial nerve anatomy: contrast-enhanced 3D fast imaging employing steady-state acquisition MR imaging. AJNR Am J Neuroradiol 2008;29(3):574–6.

68. Linn J, Peters F, Moriggl B, et al. The jugular foramen: imaging strategy and detailed anatomy at 3T. AJNR Am J Neuroradiol 2009;30(1):34–41.

69. Zhang Z, Meng Q, Chen Y, et al. 3-T imaging of the cranial nerves using three-dimensional reversed FISP with diffusion-weighted MR sequence. J Magn Reson Imaging 2008;27(3):454–8.

70. Akter M, Hirai T, Minoda R, et al. Diffusion tensor tractography in the head-and-neck region using a clinical 3-T MR scanner. Acad Radiol 2009;16(7): 858–65.

High-Resolution CISS MR Imaging With and Without Contrast for Evaluation of the Upper Cranial Nerves

Segmental Anatomy and Selected Pathologic Conditions of the Cisternal Through Extraforaminal Segments

Ari M. Blitz, MD[a],*, Leonardo L. Macedo, MD[b],
Zachary D. Chonka, MD[a], Ahmet T. Ilica, MD[a],
Asim F. Choudhri, MD[c], Gary L. Gallia, MD, PhD[d],
Nafi Aygun, MD[a]

KEYWORDS

- High-resolution MR imaging • Cranial nerves • Segmental classification • CISS
- Upper cranial nerves

KEY POINTS

- High-resolution isotropic three-dimensional (3D) magnetic resonance imaging acquisition relying heavily on constructive interference in the steady state (CISS) with and without contrast has largely replaced 2D techniques previously used for the evaluation of the cranial nerves (CNs) at the authors' institution and allows for high-contrast evaluation of the CNs along a greater portion of their extent than was previously possible.
- The cisternal and dural cave segments of the upper CNs, with the possible exception of the fourth cranial nerve, are well evaluated with noncontrast CISS.
- The interdural and foraminal segments of the CNs are revealed after the administration of intravenous contrast.
- The proximal extraforaminal segments of the CNs are often well visualized on 3D high-resolution imaging with CISS.
- Evaluation for pathologic contrast enhancement in segments of the upper CNs which were previously not well seen, and on a scale previously not well depicted, is now possible with high-resolution 3D technique.

[a] Division of Neuroradiology, The Russell H. Morgan Department of Radiology and Radiologic Science, The Johns Hopkins Hospital, Phipps B-100, 600 North Wolfe Street, Baltimore, MD 21287, USA; [b] Cedimagem/Alliar Diagnostic Center, 150- Centro, Juiz de Fora, Minas Gerais 36010-600, Brazil; [c] Department of Radiology, University of Tennessee Health Science Center, Le Bonheur Neuroscience Institute, Le Bonheur Children's Hospital, 848 Adams Avenue-G216, Memphis, TN 38103, USA; [d] Department of Neurosurgery, Neurosurgery Skull Base Surgery Center, The Johns Hopkins Hospital, Phipps 101, 600 North Wolfe Street, Baltimore, MD 21287, USA
* Corresponding author.
E-mail address: Ablitz1@jhmi.edu

Neuroimag Clin N Am 24 (2014) 17–34
http://dx.doi.org/10.1016/j.nic.2013.03.021

INTRODUCTION

Although long used for the evaluation of the course of the cranial nerves (CNs) within the subarachnoid space,[1] the recognition of the utility of enhancement on postcontrast constructive interference in the steady state (CISS) imaging allows for the evaluation of the remainder of the extended course of the CNs once they exit the subarachnoid space.[2] In this article, the authors review the recent literature on the evaluation of the CNs with CISS and analogous sequences and describe the use of such techniques for the evaluation through the extraforaminal segments. In many instances, such techniques enable visualization of nearly the entire course of many of the upper CNs, and the relevant anatomy is described here following the segmental classification suggested in the article by Blitz, Choudhri, Chonka and colleagues within this issue (**Box 1**).

CISS imaging combines true and reversed fast imaging in steady state precession (FISP) imaging to allow for high-signal, high-spatial resolution imaging with suppression of banding artifacts caused by unbalanced imaging gradients and field inhomogeneities. CISS is a gradient echo technique, and images acquired have the appearance of strong T2 weighting but, in fact, demonstrate some degree of mixed weighting, which allows for the visualization of enhancement.[3]

The application of precontrast and postcontrast CISS imaging has several significant advantages over other techniques used for cranial nerve evaluation. CISS imaging allows for the acquisition of high spatial resolution isotropic 3-dimensional (3D) imaging in a clinically acceptable time period, allowing for the evaluation of the entirety of the skull base and posterior fossa at 0.6-mm isotropic resolution in less than 6 minutes. The addition of contrast allows for the depiction of the CNs in most segments with a single sequence, and it is simultaneously possible to assess for pathologic contrast enhancement. Unless otherwise noted, the images in this article were acquired on a 3T

Siemens Verio (Ehrlangen, Germany) with 0.6-mm isotropic resolution.

Although for the purposes of this discussion the authors use the nomenclature established in the article by Blitz, Choudhri, Chonka and colleagues within this issue for CN I to VI, CN I and CN II are properly considered tracts of the central nervous system (CNS) rather than true cranial nerves passing into the peripheral nervous system (PNS) and do not entirely conform to the same anatomic outline as CN III to VI. Although classically anatomists describe nerves from their point of origination to their destination, the mixed afferent and efferent components of several cranial nerves makes this challenging and potentially confusing. For the sake of simplicity, descriptions are given here following the nerve from their point of apparent origin at the brainstem peripherally into the extraforaminal components.

CN dysfunction may arise from pathologic conditions interrupting fiber bundles at any point from the CN nuclei to the end organ innervated by the nerve or often even from lesions within pathways that themselves innervate the CN nuclei. Lesions within the brain, cranial nerve nuclei, or fiber tracts, as they course to exit the brain and give rise to the CNs, are often associated with other signs of damage to the CNS[4]; such lesions are discoverable on imaging of the brain. Imaging of the cranial nerve nuclei and course of fibers within the substance of the brainstem itself is beyond the scope of this discussion, which focuses on imaging the CNs from their apparent origin at the surface of the brainstem through their exit from the skull base foramina. The interested reader will find excellent information on the location and course of the nuclear and fascicular segments, for instance, in the recent text by Naidich and colleagues.[5] Additionally, it is important to note that the entirety of the extraforaminal course of the upper CNs is complex and limited space precludes treatment of the entirety of the topic beyond some introductory remarks within this article.

CN I: OLFACTORY NERVE

The olfactory nerve provides the sense of smell. The portions of the olfactory nerve visible on magnetic resonance (MR) imaging, namely, the olfactory bulb (OB) and olfactory tract (OT), are not components of a cranial nerve in the formal sense but rather a forward extension of the telencephalon,[6] more properly a tract of the CNS. As such, CN I does not follow the typical segmental pattern of CNs III to XII. For the purposes of this discussion, the authors define cisternal, foraminal, and extraforaminal segments. The olfactory tracts

---

Box 1
Anatomic segments of the cranial nerves
a. Nuclear
b. Parenchymal fascicular
c. Cisternal
d. Dural cave
e. Interdural
f. Foraminal
g. Extraforaminal

carry information on smell from the cisternal segment into the olfactory stria to the primary olfactory cortex located in the inferomedial aspect of the temporal lobe.

CN I.c (Cisternal): Anatomy

CN I.c consists of the OB and the OT (**Fig. 1**). The OB sits above the cribriform plate and receives input from primary sensory neurons. The CNS-PNS transitional zone (TZ), located in the OB, is histologically distinct from that of the other CNs with a cell type, the ensheathing cell, not found in other CNs.[7] The OB is uniformly well visualized with CISS.[8] The neurons of the OB project posteriorly into the OT, which in turn extends posteriorly toward the brain. The OT is distinguished from the OB by a change in caliber, although the lack of a constant landmark has led to variability in identification between subjects and readers, hampering clinical evaluation and research. Some investigators advocate spin echo imaging rather than CISS for the evaluation of CN I.c to avoid artifacts in this region caused by air tissue inferface.[9] In the authors' experience, diagnostic images of the anterior cranial fossa and paranasal sinuses can be obtained with CISS, with the significant advantage of also allowing for the assessment of contrast enhancement at a high spatial resolution. The quantitative size evaluation of OB and OT has demonstrated a correlation between OB/OT volume and olfactory function and an age-related decrease in OT volume.[10,11]

CN I.c: Selected Pathologic Conditions

The congenital absence of CN I.c may be detected in patients as a component of Kallmann syndrome.[12,13] Idiopathic olfactory loss is common, and patients with idiopathic olfactory loss demonstrate decreased OB volumes compared with normal controls.[14] Idiopathic anosmia can be a harbinger of Parkinson disease or Alzheimer disease.[15–17] Intra-axial and extra-axial tumors, most frequently meningioma, arising from the anterior skull base can result in anosmia. The vulnerability of the CN I.c to head trauma and post-traumatic olfactory dysfunction is well documented and also correlates with OB/OT size.[18]

CN I.f (Foraminal): Anatomy

Up to 100 unmyelinated axons of the olfactory neuroepithelium form bundles (olfactory fila, the olfactory nerves proper) (see **Fig. 1**B white arrows) that extend intracranially through the openings of the cribriform plate before penetrating the dura. The numerous fila and the foramina in the cribriform plate are not reliably visualized with the current imaging resolution.

CN I.f: Selected Pathologic Conditions

Traumatic injury to the cribriform plate resulting in loss of olfaction or cerebrospinal fluid (CSF) leak (CSF rhinorrhea) may occur in this region.

CN I.g (Extraforaminal): Anatomy

The primary olfactory neurons are located in the neuroepithelium lining the superior nasal cavity.

CN I.g: Selected Pathologic Conditions

The most common cause of anosmia involving the CN I.f is rhinosinusitis. The prototypical tumor of the CN I.g is esthesioneuroblastoma (olfactory

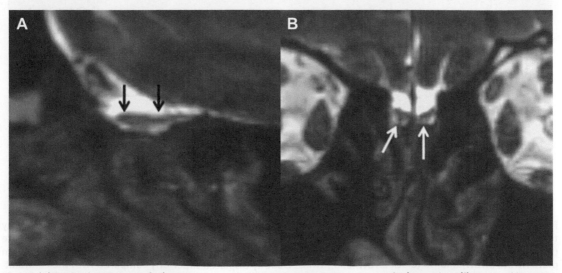

Fig. 1. (*A*) Sagittal CISS through the anterior cranial fossa demonstrates CN I.c with change in caliber noted between the OB and OT (*black arrows*). (*B*) On the coronal CISS image the olfactory fila (*white arrows*) joining the OB can be seen.

neuroblastoma), a rare lesion arising from the olfactory epithelium. A variety of tumors typically arise at the anterior skull base and in the region of CN I.g that commonly extend superiorly toward CN I.f. One of the main surgical considerations for malignant sinonasal tumors, including esthesioneuroblastomas, is whether the tumor has extended intracranially, which has an impact on the surgical approach as well as the prognosis.[19] CISS imaging provides a very accurate identification of the intracranial extension of disease and may allow the radiologist to detect the possibility of even a very small amount of intracranial tumor (**Fig. 2**).

CN II: OPTIC NERVE

The optic nerve carries visual information from the globes into the intracranial compartment with a partial decussation of fibers at the optic chiasm and synapses at the lateral geniculate nucleus of the thalamus. As noted earlier, CN II is not a cranial nerve by the strict definition and does not conform to the segmental classification described. For the purposes of this discussion, the authors divide the nerve into cisternal, dural cave, foraminal, and extraforaminal segments. All of these CN II segments are intradural; however, the surrounding tissue signal varies from CSF to bone and fat. For

the purposes of this discussion, the authors define the attached component of CN II, the optic chiasm and optic tracts, as the fascicular component extending toward the lateral geniculate nucleus posterolaterally. As with the other CNs, the cisternal segment is limited to the component surrounded by the subarachnoid space on all sides. High-resolution CISS imaging provides superb anatomic detail regarding the location of CN II and its relationship to surrounding structures; postcontrast CISS imaging may also demonstrate subtle contrast enhancement within the nerve. For the assessment of intrinsic T2 signal abnormality, such as seen in optic neuritis, reliance on CISS technique alone is not advised, and imaging can be supplemented with spin echo–based T2 techniques.[20]

CN II.c (Cisternal): Anatomy

For the purposes of this article, the cisternal anatomy of the optic nerves is limited to the portion of the prechiasmatic optic nerve, which extends from the posterior margin of the anterior clinoid process posteromedially to the optic chiasm (**Fig. 3**).

CN II.c: Selected Pathologic Conditions

The most commonly encountered pathologic condition of CN II.c in adults is caused by extrinsic

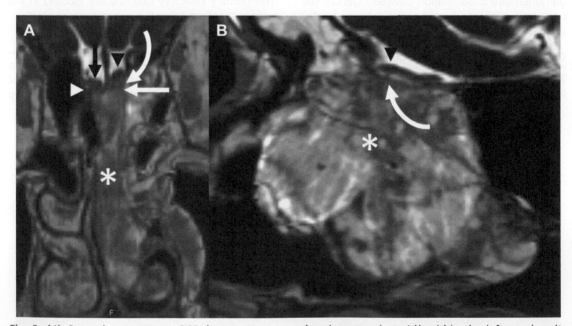

Fig. 2. (*A*) Coronal postcontrast CISS demonstrates an enhancing mass (*asterisk*) within the left nasal cavity traversing the nasal septum superiorly and extending to the level of the undersurface of the right cribriform plate (*white arrowhead*). On the left side, there is minimal soft tissue (*curved arrow*) interposed between the cribriform plate (*white arrow*) and OB (*black arrowhead*), which is subtly displaced superiorly compared with the contralateral side (*black arrow*). (*B*) Sagittal reformat again demonstrates 2 mm of extension across the left cribriform plate displacing the OB. Focal extension of esthesioneuroblastoma was noted in this location at the time of surgery.

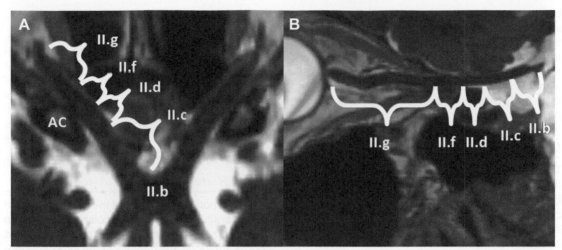

Fig. 3. (A) Axial postcontrast CISS demonstrates the posterior aspect of CN II.g within the orbital apex extending into the optic canals (CN II.f) and then passing intracranially as CN II.d medial to the anterior clinoid process (AC). CN II.c passes posteriorly to join the contralateral nerve as the first attached segment, the optic chiasm (II.b above). (B) In sagittal multi-planar reformat, the entirety of the nerve can be visualized from the orbit (II.g) through the optic chiasm (II.b).

compression by masses, such as pituitary macroadenoma, meningioma, or craniopharyngioma. The location of CN II.c in relation to the mass (**Fig. 4**) is of critical importance for procedural planning and is often clarified with the use of high-resolution imaging, such as CISS or fast imaging employing steady-state acquisition.[21] Intrinsic masses of the nerve, such as optic nerve gliomas, are most commonly encountered in the pediatric population. Because the entirety of CN II is within the CNS, no Schwann cells exist to give rise to schwannomas.

CN II.d (Dural Cave): Anatomy

The definition of the dural cave segment of CN II is somewhat arbitrary, but it does exist and may

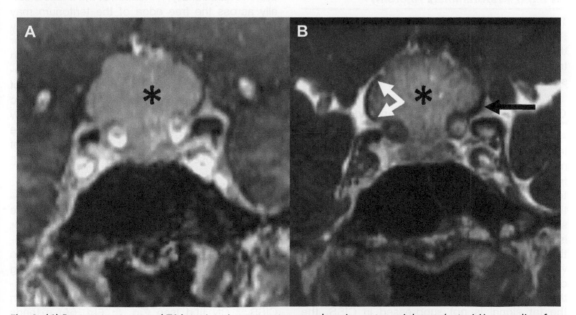

Fig. 4. (A) Postcontrast coronal T1 imaging demonstrates an enhancing extra-axial mass (*asterisk*) extending from the planum sphenoidale into the suprasellar cistern. (B) The relationship of the mass to the right CN II.c (*white arrows*) as well as the left CN II.c (*black arrow*) is best appreciated on postcontrast CISS. On postcontrast CISS, the mass extended along and deformed the CN II.d and proximal CN II.f segments while compressing the optic chiasm (CN II.b) (not shown). Meningioma was proven pathologically after debulking.

be seen as a CSF-filled recess partially surrounding the optic nerve before it emerges from the optic canal. The anterior border of CN II.d is difficult to define anatomically but may be construed on MR imaging as the point beyond which no CSF signal is visible. The posterior border of CN II.d is at the posterior margin of the anterior clinoid process.

CN II.f (Foraminal): Anatomy

The optic nerves pass through the skull base via the optic canals (see **Fig. 3**), which are bounded by the anterior clinoid processes laterally and the orbital plates of the ethmoid bones medially. CN II.f may at times be difficult to evaluate on CISS because of susceptibility artifacts created by bone and air in the adjacent paranasal sinuses and sometimes pneumatized anterior clinoid process.

CN II.f: Selected Pathologic Conditions

Masses in this region are often small and comparatively difficult to visualize. Meningioma is the most common mass lesion affecting CN II.f. Primary and secondary bony processes involving the anterior clinoid process and inflammatory and neoplastic processes involving the paranasal sinuses may also secondarily affect CN II.f.

CN II.g (Extraforaminal): Anatomy

The optic nerve is visible within the orbit (see **Fig. 3**B) and is separated from the orbital fat by the optic nerve sheath, which contains fluid similar to CSF and variably communicates with the subarachnoid space.[22]

CN II.g: Selected Pathologic Conditions

A myriad of neoplastic and non-neoplastic mass lesions may affect CN II.g. In case of intraorbital masses associated with the CN II.g, it is crucial for differential diagnosis and surgical planning to know whether the mass is originating from the optic nerve itself, the optic nerve sheath, or surrounding structures; whether the optic nerve is encased or displaced by tumor; and what the relative position of the nerve is compared with the mass. Postcontrast CISS imaging is often helpful in this regard because it shows the nerve against the enhancing tumor. Because the fat signal is not suppressed in CISS, the addition of high-resolution, postcontrast, fat-suppressed, T1-weighted images can be helpful in demonstrating enhancing tumor/orbital fat interface.

CN III: OCULOMOTOR NERVE

The oculomotor nerve has both a motor function, innervating most of the muscles associated with the orbit, as well as a parasympathetic component that functions to constrict the pupil. The nuclei of the oculomotor nerve are located in the dorsal aspect of the midbrain just ventral to the cerebral aqueduct at the midline. From the nuclei, fibers course anteriorly and slightly laterally to exit the ventral aspect of the brainstem.

CN III.c (Cisternal Course): Anatomy

The oculomotor nerve arises at the ventral aspect of the midbrain in the interpeduncular cistern. Within the cisternal segment, the oculomotor nerves course anteriorly and laterally in the interpeduncular cistern. The nerve passes between the posterior cerebral artery (PCA) superiorly and the superiorly cerebellar artery (SCA) inferiorly (**Fig. 5**A). The nerve then passes medial to the uncus of the temporal lobes (see **Fig. 5**B). The TZ of CN III.c is located, on average, approximately 1.9 mm from the apparent origin (range 1.0–4.0 mm).[23]

CN III.c: Selected Pathologic Conditions

As the parasympathetic fibers of the nerve pass within its periphery, uncal herniation with CN III.c impingement will result in pupillary dilation caused by unopposed action of the sympathetic nervous system. Additionally, herniation of the uncus medially across the free edge of the tentorium may impinge on the nerve. Oculomotor palsy may result from compression of CN III.c by tumors or neurovascular compression, with findings on CISS correlating well with those at surgery.[24] Isolated reversible enhancement and thickening of CN III.c has been reported in ophthalmoplegic migraine by standard imaging[25]; one recent review of ophthalmoplegic migraine found that nerve thickening and enhancement is seen in 75% of cases diagnosed clinically.[26]

CN III.d (Dural Cave): Anatomy

The dural cave of the CN III is a segment of variable length and is given the name of the oculomotor cistern. The length of the oculomotor cistern is reported on anatomic studies as ranging from 3.0 to 11.0 mm, averaging 6.5 mm,[27] and on MR imaging averaging 4.2 mm with a range of ± 3.2 mm, visualized in 75% of screening MR imaging with CISS.[28] CN III.d (see **Fig. 5**; **Fig. 6**A) extends from the oculomotor porus at the posterior margin of the oculomotor cistern to exit anteriorly into the lateral wall of the cavernous sinus at its superior extent (see **Fig. 6**B).

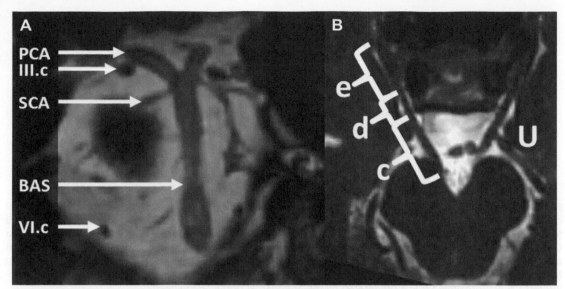

Fig. 5. (*A*) Coronal contrast-enhanced CISS demonstrates CN III.c (c) passing below the proximal PCA and above the SCA. The basilar artery (BAS) is also shown. (*B*) Axial oblique reformatted CISS with contrast demonstrating CN III.c as it arises from the midbrain within the interpeduncular cistern. The nerve extends anterolaterally coursing medial to the uncus (U). The CN III.d (d) segment is visible before the nerve pierces the dura to enter the cavernous sinus as CN III.e (e).

CN III.e (Interdural): Anatomy

CN III.e is entirely contained within the lateral wall of the cavernous sinus, with CN III entering the posterior aspect lateral to the posterior clinoid process and exiting the anterior aspect into the superior orbital fissure below the anterior clinoid process.[29] CN III.e is the most superior of the CNs within the cavernous sinus.

CN III.e: Selected Pathologic Conditions

Because the CN III.e is the most superior of the intracavernous cranial nerves, compressive lesions expanding from above, such as aneurysms arising from the posterior communicating artery (PCOM) origin or superior hypophyseal aneurysms, may lead to compression in this region (Fig. 7).

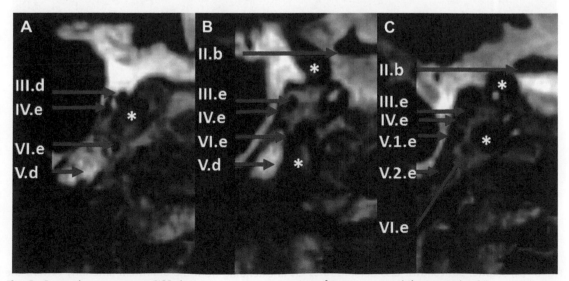

Fig. 6. Coronal postcontrast CISS through the cavernous sinus from posterior (*A*) to anterior (*C*). Cranial nerve segments as noted. The internal carotid artery is marked with an asterisk.

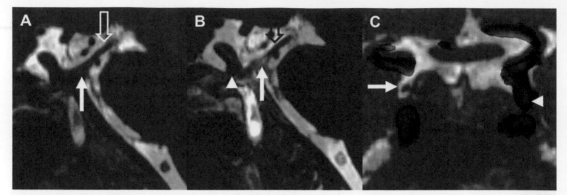

Fig. 7. A 38-year-old woman with left third nerve palsy. (*A*) Sagittal noncontrast CISS demonstrates a normal caliber of the midcisternal left CN III.c (*open arrow*) passing anteriorly between the PCA superiorly and the SCA inferiorly. The distal CN III.c is significantly thickened (*closed arrow*). (*B*) On the corresponding postcontrast CISS image, enhancement of the distal left CN III.c is seen (*closed arrow*) and the dome of a large PCOM origin aneurysm can be seen (*arrowhead*) overlying the cavernous sinus. (*C*) Coronal color-mapped fused time-of-flight MR angiography precontrast CISS demonstrates a normal right CN III.d (*arrow*) with the region of the corresponding left CN III.d/proximal CN III.e obliterated by the aneurysmal dome (*arrowhead*).

CN III.f (Foraminal): Anatomy

CN III enters the superior orbital fissure from the superior aspect of the cavernous sinus where it courses superiorly.[23,30] As the oculomotor nerve passes anteriorly in the superior orbital fissure, it assumes an inferior position[31] within the central sector.[32] The nerve can be seen as a distinct structure at the posterior margin of the superior orbital fissure/anterior cavernous sinus (**Fig. 8**), although as the space narrows toward the orbital apex, typically, individual nerves are difficult to distinguish.

CN III.g (Extraforaminal): Anatomy

On exiting from the superior orbital fissure, CN III.g passes anteriorly through the annulus of Zinn into the intraconal compartment of the orbit. The nerve then divides into a superior and inferior division. The superior division innervates the superior rectus muscle and continues medial to the superior rectus to innervate the levator palpebrae superioris muscle. The inferior division travels below the optic nerve and divides to innervate the inferior and medial recti as well as the inferior oblique

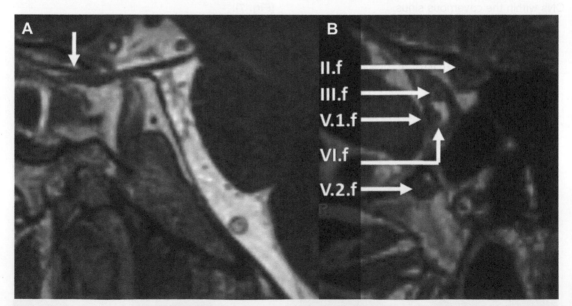

Fig. 8. (*A*) Sagittal postcontrast CISS demonstrates CN III extending from the brainstem anteriorly toward the superior orbital fissure (*arrow*). (*B*) Coronal postcontrast CISS through the level of the posterior aspect of the superior orbital fissure and optic canal.

and also carries parasympathetic fibers to the ciliary ganglion. The distal CN III.g branches destined for the extraocular muscles innervate their targets at the junction along the inner aspect of the muscle at the division between the posterior one-third and anterior two-thirds.[33]

CN III.g: Selected Pathologic Conditions

(Fig. 9).

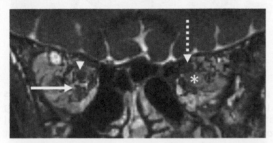

Fig. 9. A 42-year-old woman with atypical neurofibromatosis was initially diagnosed with a lesion of the left optic nerve at the orbital apex at an outside institution. Coronal postcontrast CISS on a 1.5-T magnet demonstrates a normal right CN II.g (*arrowhead*). The inferior division of the right CN III.g is also seen (*arrow*). On the left, an enhancing mass (*asterisk*) displaces the left CN II.g (*dashed arrow*) superiorly rather than arising from it and was thought to likely reflect a neurofibroma of the left inferior division of CN III.g.

CN IV: TROCHLEAR NERVE

The trochlear nerve (CN IV) has the smallest diameter of the upper cranial nerves and innervates the superior oblique muscle. The nucleus of CN IV can be found in the caudal and dorsal midbrain and is exceptional in its location on the contralateral side of the brainstem from the muscle it innervates. The trochlear nerve is also unusual because it is the only cranial nerve to emerge from the dorsal aspect of the brainstem.

CN IV.c (Cisternal): Anatomy

The trochlear nerve emerges from the dorsal aspect of the caudal midbrain just below the inferior colliculi and on either side of the frenulum of the superior medullary velum[34] within the quadrigeminal cistern (Fig. 10) and courses laterally and then anteriorly into the ambient cistern along the lateral aspect of the midbrain.[35] Yousry and colleagues[36] found that the apparent origin varied from 3 to 9 mm from the midline on CISS imaging. Because of its small size, even the proximal cisternal segment is not always routinely visualized; however,

Choi and colleagues,[37] using 3D-balanced turbo-field echo (bFTE) in healthy research subjects undergoing acquisitions lasting in excess of 7 minutes, have reported that with voxels smaller than the nerve diameter, CN IV.c may be visualized 100% of the time. The investigators suggest with sufficient spatial resolution, the nerve could be differentiated from the small adjacent vasculature structures that might otherwise be mistakenly identified as the nerve itself and measured a mean diameter of 0.54 mm (range 0.35–0.96 mm).[37] In its distal component, CN IV.c passes under the free edge of the tentorium cerebelli where it is potentially vulnerable during operative approaches to this region[38] and is not typically well visualized on imaging.[36] Although CN IV.c is seen as a single root when it is visualized on MR imaging, 2 rootlets may arise from the brainstem on anatomic studies; this was seen 31% of the time in one study with the rootlets arising up to 4 mm apart.[39] Given the small size and consequent challenge of visualization of even a solitary root of the CN IV.c, it is possible that such variant anatomy could partly account for the significant variation in diameter and detection of the trochlear nerve reported on imaging. The TZ is located, on average, 0.3 mm from the apparent origin (range 0–1.0 mm).[23]

CN IV.c: Selected Pathologic Conditions

As with the other CNs (except CN I and II), peripheral nerve sheath tumors may arise from CN IV.c. In addition, CN IV.c passes just below the tentorium cerebelli and may be compressed by masses in this region. Fig. 10 demonstrates a small mass arising from the left CN IV.c or adjacent tentorium in a patient presenting with left superior oblique palsy. Myokymia of the superior oblique caused by neurovascular conflict has been reported.[36] Congenital absence of the fourth cranial nerve has been demonstrated via lack of visualization of CN IV.c in congenital superior oblique palsy with superior oblique hypoplasia with voxel size of 0.3 × 0.3 × 0.25 mm.[40]

CN IV.d (Dural Cave)

CN IV is not typically associated with a visible dural cave. The nerve pierces the lamina propria of the dura caudal to the intersection of the free and attached segments of the tentorium cerebelli.[38]

CN IV.e (Interdural)

The interdural course of CN IV is entirely contained within the lateral wall of the cavernous sinus, entering posterolateral to CN III.e.[29]

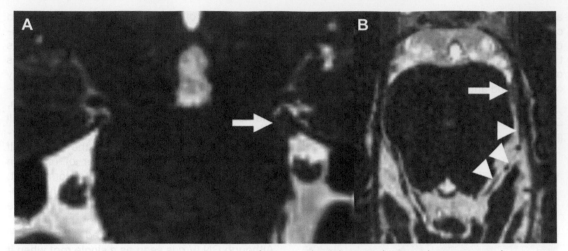

Fig. 10. A 38-year-old woman presenting with a left CN IV palsy. (*A*) Coronal CISS without contrast demonstrates an asymmetric filling defect within the subarachnoid space (*arrow*) caused by a mass measuring up to 5 mm along the undersurface of the free edge of left aspect of the tentorium cerebelli. (*B*) On postcontrast CISS in the axial plane (3T, 0.5 mm isotropic resolution), the left CN IV.c (*arrowheads*) can be seen extending through the ambient cistern into the region of the mass, which demonstrates enhancement (*arrow*).

CN IV.f (Foraminal)

CN IV.f passes through the superior aspect of the superior orbital fissure[31] in the lateral sector[32] and is hard to detect in this region.

CN IV.g (Extraforaminal)

CN IV.g enters the orbit superior to the annulus of Zinn and runs below the orbital roof to innervate the superior oblique muscle joining the muscle within the posterior third.[33]

CN V: TRIGEMINAL NERVE

The trigeminal nerve (CN V) has the largest diameter of the CNs and serves sensation from the face with its three main segments (V.1 [ophthalmic], V.2 [maxillary], V.3 [mandibular]) (**Fig. 11**) as well as innervates the muscles of mastication through the V.3 segment. The nuclei and tracts of the trigeminal nerve are extensive, ranging from the midbrain through the upper cervical spinal cord.

CN V.c (Cisternal): Anatomy

The apparent origin of the trigeminal nerve is at the lateral aspect of the belly of the pons. The motor roots may arise separately from the main mass of the nerve and are typically seen as separate structures arising superiorly and medially. When seen separately, there may be between 1 and 3 motor roots.[41] The TZ of the sensory root of CN V.c is variously reported as extending, on average, approximately 3.6 mm from the apparent origin

(range 2.0–6.0 mm)[23] to 4.2 mm from the apparent origin (range 3.4–5 mm)[42] for the sensory root. For the motor roots, TZ is located, on average, 0.3 mm from the apparent origin (range 0–1.0 mm).[23]

CN V.c: Selected Pathologic Conditions

Facial pain caused by an abnormality of the trigeminal nerve, trigeminal neuralgia (TGN, also known as tic douloureux), is a particularly vexing clinical problem. When pain is associated with analgesia in the sensory distribution of the trigeminal nerve or one of its main 3 components, a mass is often suspected. In the absence of a mass, suspicion falls on the possibility of neurovascular compression (**Fig. 12**). The relationship of vascular structures within the cistern to CN V.c is often accurately depicted with CISS, although some investigators have not found predictions on high-resolution imaging to be entirely reliable.[43] Additionally, the finding of neurovascular compression is not uncommon in the asymptomatic population or on the asymptomatic side[44]; the surgical decision of microvascular decompression in patients with TGN should be made by the combination of clinical and radiological findings. The measurement of diameter and cross-sectional area on CISS has been reported to demonstrate decreased size of the CN V.c on the symptomatic side.[45] The combination of high-spatial-resolution imaging with DTI may allow for higher specificity for TGN[46] with substantially decreased FA associated with neurovascular compression.

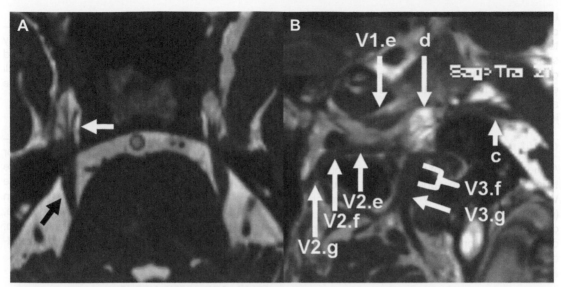

Fig. 11. (A) Axial noncontrast CISS demonstrates CN V.c emerging from the lateral pons (*black arrow*) extending through the porus trigeminus into the Meckel cave (*white arrow*) where fibers of CN V.d can be seen. (B) On sagittal oblique postcontrast CISS, CN V.c roots can be seen entering the Meckel cave (d) through the trigeminal porus with individual CN V.d fibers noted surrounded by CSF. CN V.1.e and CN V.2.e are seen extending anteriorly through the cavernous sinus. V.2.f continues through foramen rotundum into the pterygopalatine fossa as V.2.g. V.3.f extends caudally through foramen ovale with proximal branching of V.3.g visible in this image.

CN V.d: (Dural Cave) Anatomy

The dural cave of CN V is the most constant of all of the cranial nerves and is called Meckel cave (also known as the trigeminal cistern). The gasserian (also known as the semilunar or trigeminal) ganglion, which sits along the floor and anterior wall, is well visualized with contrast-enhanced

CISS.[47] Distal to the gasserian ganglion, the nerve divides into 3 divisions: V1 (ophthalmic), V2 (maxillary), and V3 (mandibular) (see **Fig. 11**B).

CN V.1.e (Interdural)

CN V.1.e, the interdural component of the ophthalmic division of the trigeminal nerve, enters

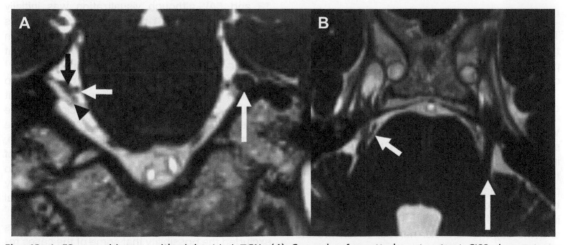

Fig. 12. A 52-year-old man with right-sided TGN. (A) Coronal reformatted postcontrast CISS demonstrates compression of the right CN V.c (*black arrow*) by a branch of the right superior cerebellar artery medially (*short white arrow*) and an enhancing venous structure (*black arrowhead*) coursing along its inferior and lateral aspect. The cross-sectional area of the right CN V.c is reduced when compared with the contralateral unaffected side (*long white arrow*). (B) On axial reformatted images, the right superior cerebellar artery (*short arrow*) can be seen traversing the superior margin of the right CN V.c. The left CN V.c (*long arrow*) is unimpinged.

the lower portion of the lateral wall of the cavernous sinus (see **Fig. 6C**) and extends anteriorly and superiorly (see **Fig. 11B**) toward the superior orbital fissure.[29] Dissections have demonstrated that the sympathetic fibers that extend from the adventitia of the internal carotid artery typically travel briefly with CN VI.e before joining CN V.1.e in this region.[48]

CN V.1.f (Foraminal)

At the anterior aspect of the cavernous sinus/posterior aspect of the superior orbital fissure, CN V.1.f is located laterally before final branching (see **Fig. 8B**). The frontal and lacrimal branches of V.1 pass anteriorly through the superior aspect of the superior orbital fissure, whereas the nasociliary branch of V.1 passes through the inferior aspect of the superior orbital fissure.[31]

CN V.1.g (Extraforaminal)

The frontal branch extends through the supraorbital foramen to supply sensation to the upper face. The lacrimal branch supplies sensation to the lacrimal gland. The nasociliary branch of V.1, through long and short ciliary branches, innervates the globe and is responsible for the afferent input for the corneal reflex with additional branches extending into the nasal cavity.

CN V.2.e (Interdural)

CN V.2.e, the interdural component of the maxillary division of the trigeminal nerve, enters the cavernous sinus just below CN V.1.e (see **Fig. 6C**).

CN V.2.f (Foraminal)

The V.2.f passes anteriorly through the foramen rotundum (see **Fig. 8B**) where it is surrounded by a perineural vascular plexus[49] and is well visualized on contrast-enhanced CISS.[47]

CN V.2.g (Extraforaminal)

V.2 emerges from the foraminal segment into the pterygopalatine fossa where CN V.2.g divides into 3 main branches: the infraorbital nerves, which travel anteriorly through the infraorbital foramen to provide sensation to the midportion of the face; the zygomatic nerve, which extends through the inferior orbital fissure to supply the lacrimal gland; and the superior alveolar nerves, which provide sensation to the maxillary teeth.[50]

CN V.3.e (Interdural)

The V.3.e segment is quite short because the nerve passes inferiorly from the Meckel cave.

CN V3.f (Foraminal)

The V.3 segment passes inferiorly and laterally through the foramen ovale where it is surrounded by a perineural vascular plexus[49] and is well visualized on contrast-enhanced CISS[47] (see **Fig. 12B**).

CN V.3.g (Extraforaminal)

CN V.3.g passes inferiorly into the masticator space. Multiple branch points of CN V.3.g are routinely visualized in the authors' experience (see **Fig. 12B**). Termination of distal branches in the muscles of mastication, which they innervate, is often visible. Sensory branches are also seen; the inferior alveolar nerve, for instance, can be followed to the mandibular foramen in most cases.

CN VI: ABDUCENS NERVE

The abducens nerve (also spelled *abducent*) has a single motor function: innervation of the lateral rectus muscle. The nucleus of the abducens nerve lies in the dorsal medial aspect of the caudal pons with fibers forming a tract and the fascicular segment extending anterolaterally toward the pontomedullary junction ventrally.

CN VI.c (Cisternal): Anatomy

The apparent origin of CN VI.c is typically found at the pontomedullary junction, although rootlets may arise from the caudal pons in approximately 18% of anatomic specimens.[51] The nerve extends superiorly within the prepontine cistern (see **Figs. 13** and **5A**); although visualization was initially limited to 79% with 1-mm sections,[52] CN VI.c is now well seen on CISS imaging, identifiable in nearly all cases.[53] Anatomic studies suggest that CN VI.c may arise as one or multiple rootlets[51] and, if the nerve arises as one root, may split into 2 roots within its cisternal course. Adjacent vascular structures may abut, encircle, or divide single roots or multiple rootlets.[51] A single nerve along the entirety of the course is most common, reported in approximately 87%[54] to 92%[55] of anatomic specimens. One study with 3D turbo spin echo reported 2 CN VI.c rootlets unilaterally in approximately 20% of individuals and bilateral double rootlets in approximately 5% of patients,[56] although it is not clear how the investigators excluded the possibility that some of the cases reflected vascular structures in the area studied, a factor that can lead to misidentification of cisternal segments of the cranial nerves in other contexts.[37] The TZ is located on average 0.3 mm from the apparent origin (range 0–1.0 mm).[23]

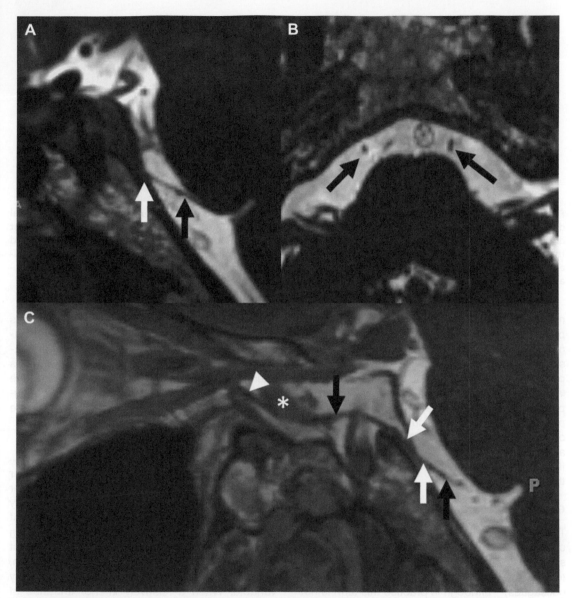

Fig. 13. (*A*) Sagittal oblique CISS without contrast demonstrates VI.c (*black arrow*) emerging from the pontomedullary junction and extending superiorly and anteriorly toward the dorsal clivus. CN VI.d is shallow in this case, without significant evagination of CSF (*white arrow*). (*B*) Axial CISS demonstrates both CN.c segments at the midcisternal component (*arrows*). (*C*) Postcontrast sagittal oblique CISS demonstrates CN VI.c (*black upward arrow*) extending to pierce the inner layer of dura without a significant CN VI.d segment (*white upward arrow*). CN VI.e extends through the petroclival (*white downward arrow*) into the cavernous segment (*black downward arrow*), passing adjacent to the cavernous internal carotid artery (*asterisk*) to enter the superior orbital fissure as CN VI.f (*arrowhead*).

CN VI.c: Selected Pathologic Conditions

The abducens nerve may be congenitally absent, a fact that is most easily verified in the cisternal segment.[57,58]

CN VI.d (Dural Cave): Anatomy

The dural cave segment of CN VI is defined on an imaging basis by visualization of CSF surrounding the nerve (**Fig. 14A**). The length of CN VI.c is variable, with corresponding variability on the position of CN VI.d. Additionally, the CN VI.d segment is variable in length and may be extremely short in some cases; however, imaging studies demonstrate that this segment measured 1 mm or greater in length approximately 57%[53] to 86% of the time.[59] Despite the apparently relatively diminutive length of this segment on imaging, the arachnoid

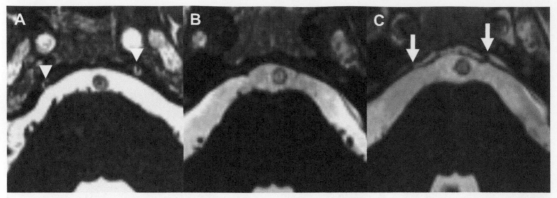

Fig. 14. (*A*) Axial precontrast CISS imaging through the level of the midpons in a patient with prominent bilateral dural caves. CN VI.d (*arrowheads*) is well visualized surrounded by CSF. (*B*) In other patients without a significant dural cave segment, CN VI.e is not well visualized at the same level before contrast administration, having passed through the junction of the CSF with the inner layer of dura. Note opacification of the petroclival venous confluence once intravenous contrast is administered (*C*) opacification of surrounding venous structures allows for visualization of the bilateral petroclival CN VI.e segments (*arrows*).

membrane may follow the nerve throughout the petroclival segment to the level of the petrosphenoidal ligament,[60] presumably creating a potential space. Anatomic studies suggest that when multiple CN VI.c roots are present, they pierce the inner layer of dura separately,[54] presumably with the potential for focal evagination of the CSF at each point of contact with the dura. For the purposes of imaging classification, CN VI.d is designated as the portion of the nerve surrounded by visible fluid within an evagination in communication with the subarachnoid space.

CN VI.e (Interdural): Anatomy

The segment of the abducens nerve is the longest of the cranial nerves and is itself divided into 2 subsegments. The proximal segment has been termed the *gulfar component* by Iaconetta and colleagues,[55] although in practice this term is not commonly used and the authors prefer the term *petroclival segment* as used by Yousry and colleagues,[53] Joo and colleagues,[61] and Umansky and colleagues.[62] CN VI.e extends superiorly through the inferior petrosal sinus (when individually defined and bilateral) or petroclival venous confluence[55] (when a venous plexus is present) into the Dorello canal typically coursing under the petrosphenoidal (Gruber) ligament before entering the cavernous segment. The usage of the term *Dorello canal* itself is somewhat confusing because it has sometimes been applied in the radiology literature[52] to the entirety of the petroclival segment, possibly in some instances including the dural cave segment.[52,53] Several investigators suggest that it should be properly reserved solely for the point at which the nerve passes under the

petrosphenoidal ligament.[60,62] For the purposes of this article, the authors use the term *Dorello canal* in the more narrow sense as that point of transition between the petroclival and cavernous interdural subsegments of CN VI.e, where the nerve passes under the Gruber ligament,[63] changing its course to extend anteriorly into the cavernous sinus.

CN VI.e: Petroclival Subsegment

The petroclival portion of CN VI.e courses over the dorsal aspect of the clivus between the inner and outer layers of dura surrounded by a variably robust network of venous channels, the confluent portion of which over the rostral clivus has been termed the *petroclival venous confluence*.[64] Just as the CN VI.d segment is variable in position, the CN VI.d/CN VI.e junction is correspondingly variable. When a relatively inferior entrance of the nerve into the interdural space is observed, CN VI.e may be seen as it extends superiorly surrounded by venous blood of the inferior petrosal sinus[61] coursing superiorly into the petroclival venous confluence. In some cases, particularly those with a more superior entrance to the dura, the proximal petroclival segment may begin surrounded by the petroclival venous confluence. Anatomic studies suggest that when 2 roots are present, one will depart the dorsal clival segment above and the other below the Gruber ligament.[54] On imaging, the distinction between CN VI.d and the petroclival CN VI.e is made by visualization of the presence of surrounding CSF; however, on anatomic studies, the arachnoid membrane[60] and an accompanying dural sleeve[61] actually follow the nerve as far

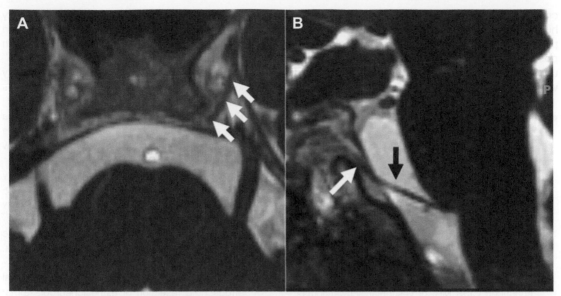

Fig. 15. Several-day history of abducens palsy on the right. Standard protocol MR imaging unremarkable. Post-contrast isotropic CISS. (*A*) Axial image. The left CN VI.e (*arrows*) is well visualized extending through Dorello canal into the cavernous sinus. The right abducens nerve is not visualized in the cavernous region because of pathologic enhancement. (*B*) In sagittal oblique reformatted views, CN VI.c (*black arrow*) and the proximal CN VI.e segment are seen with an abrupt transition to the region of pathologic enhancement (*white arrow*). Tolosa-Hunt syndrome was suggested. No significant CN VI.d segment was present in this individual, a feature of significant variation between patients.

superiorly as the Gruber ligament. Regardless, from an imaging perspective, the nerve is not typically visible in this region without the aid of contrast enhancement in the surrounding venous blood (see **Fig. 14**).

CN VI.e: Cavernous Subsegment

The cavernous segment of CN VI.e, alone among the CNs, traverses the main compartment of the cavernous sinus (rather than running in the fibrous lateral wall). The nerve can be found lateral to the cavernous carotid artery soon after it enters from the petroclival segment. Based on work with dissection, Harris and Rhoton[65] describe up to 5 roots of CN VI.e in this region, although in most cases only a single root was seen. In the authors' experience, CN VI.e may be obscured where it passes directly lateral to the cavernous internal carotid artery but is otherwise well seen in the cavernous interdural segment. The sympathetic nerves that ultimately innervate the orbit travel briefly with CN VI.e in this region before joining CN V.1.e.[48,66]

CN VI.e: Selected Pathologic Conditions

Fig. 15 demonstrates pathologic enhancement of CN VI.e, which was presumed to be caused

by inflammation, the so-called Tolosa-Hunt syndrome.

CN VI.f (Foraminal)

CN VI.f passes through the inferior aspect of the superior orbital fissure[31] within its central sector.[32]

CN VI.g (Extraforaminal)

The abducens nerve travels anteriorly along the medial aspect of the lateral rectus muscle to insert at the junction between the posterior one-third and anterior two-thirds of the muscle.[33]

SUMMARY

This article reviews the high-resolution anatomy and appearance of the cisternal through proximal extraforaminal segments of CN I to CN VI, following the classification scheme proposed in the accompanying article by Blitz, Choudhri, Chonka and colleagues on the segmental anatomy of the cranial nerves and imaging techniques. The cisternal and dural cave segments of the upper cranial nerves, with the possible exception of the fourth cranial nerve, are well evaluated with noncontrast CISS. The interdural and foraminal segments of the CNs are revealed after the administration of intravenous contrast. The proximal extraforaminal segments of the cranial nerves are also often well visualized on 3D high-resolution imaging with CISS. Evaluation for pathologic contrast enhancement is also now possible at a smaller scale and in regions of the upper cranial nerves which were previously not well seen.

REFERENCES

1. Casselman J, Kuhweide R, Deimling M, et al. Constructive interference in steady state-3DFT MR imaging of the inner ear and cerebellopontine angle. AJNR Am J Neuroradiol 1993;14(1):47–57.
2. Yagi A, Sato N, Taketomi A, et al. Normal cranial nerves in the cavernous sinuses: contrast-enhanced three-dimensional constructive interference in the steady state MR imaging. AJNR Am J Neuroradiol 2005;26(4):946–50.
3. Shigematsu Y, Korogi Y, Hirai T, et al. Contrast-enhanced CISS MRI of vestibular schwannomas: phantom and clinical studies. J Comput Assist Tomogr 1999;23(2):224.
4. Brazis PW, Masdeu JC, Biller J. Localization in Clinical Neurology. Philadelphia: Lippincott Williams & Wilkins; 2011.
5. Naidich TP, Duvernoy HM, Delman BN, et al. Duvernoy's Atlas of the Human Brain Stem and Cerebellum. Vienna (Austria): Springer-Verlag; 2009.
6. Nieuwenhuys R, Voogd J, Voogd J, et al. The Human Central Nervous System. New York: Springer Verlag; 2008.
7. Doucette R. PNS-CNS transitional zone of the first cranial nerve. J Comp Neurol 1991;312(3): 451–66.
8. Yousry I, Camelio S, Schmid U, et al. Visualization of cranial nerves I–XII: value of 3D CISS and T2-weighted FSE sequences. Eur Radiol 2000; 10(7):1061–7.
9. Borges A, Casselman J. Imaging the cranial nerves: part I: methodology, infectious and inflammatory, traumatic and congenital lesions. Eur Radiol 2007;17(8):2112–25.
10. Yousem DM, Geckle RJ, Bilker WB, et al. Olfactory bulb and tract and temporal lobe volumes: normative data across decades. Ann N Y Acad Sci 1998; 855(1):546–55.
11. Buschhüter D, Smitka M, Puschmann S, et al. Correlation between olfactory bulb volume and olfactory function. Neuroimage 2008;42(2):498–502.
12. Abolmaali N, Gudziol V, Hummel T. Pathology of the olfactory nerve. Neuroimaging Clin N Am 2008; 18(2):233–42.
13. Laitinen EM, Vaaralahti K, Tommiska J, et al. Incidence, phenotypic features and molecular genetics of Kallmann syndrome in Finland. Orphanet J Rare Dis 2011;6(1):41.
14. Rombaux P, Potier H, Markessis E, et al. Olfactory bulb volume and depth of olfactory sulcus in patients with idiopathic olfactory loss. Eur Arch Otorhinolaryngol 2010;267(10):1551–6.
15. Haehner A, Hummel T, Hummel C, et al. Olfactory loss may be a first sign of idiopathic Parkinson's disease. Mov Disord 2007;22(6):839–42.
16. Ponsen MM, Stoffers D, Twisk JW, et al. Hyposmia and executive dysfunction as predictors of future Parkinson's disease: a prospective study. Mov Disord 2009;24(7):1060–5.
17. Koss E, Weiffenbach JM, Haxby JV, et al. Olfactory detection and identification performance are dissociated in early Alzheimer's disease. Neurology 1988;38(8):1228–32.
18. Collet S, Grulois V, Bertrand B, et al. Post-traumatic olfactory dysfunction: a cohort study and update. B-ENT 2009;5(Suppl 13):97–107.
19. Gallia GL, Reh DD, Salmasi V, et al. Endonasal endoscopic resection of esthesioneuroblastoma: the Johns Hopkins Hospital experience and review of the literature. Neurosurg Rev 2011;34: 1–11.
20. Becker M, Masterson K, Delavelle J, et al. Imaging of the optic nerve. Eur J Radiol 2010;74(2): 299–313.
21. Watanabe K, Kakeda S, Yamamoto J, et al. Delineation of optic nerves and chiasm in close proximity to large suprasellar tumors with contrast-enhanced FIESTA MR Imaging. Radiology 2012; 264(3):852–8.
22. Killer H, Jaggi G, Flammer J, et al. Cerebrospinal fluid dynamics between the intracranial and the subarachnoid space of the optic nerve. Is it always bidirectional? Brain 2007;130(2):514–20.
23. Lang J. Clinical Anatomy of the Head. Berlin: Springer-Verlag; 1983.
24. Sun X, Liang C, Liu C, et al. Oculomotor paralysis: 3D-CISS MR imaging with MPR in the evaluation of neuralgic manifestation and the adjacent structures. Eur J Radiol 2010;73(2):221–3.
25. Mark AS, Casselman J, Brown D, et al. Ophthalmoplegic migraine: reversible enhancement and thickening of the cisternal segment of the oculomotor nerve on contrast-enhanced MR images. AJNR Am J Neuroradiol 1998;19(10):1887–91.
26. Gelfand AA, Gelfand JM, Prabakhar P, et al. Ophthalmoplegic "migraine" or recurrent ophthalmoplegic cranial neuropathy: new cases and a systematic review. J Child Neurol 2012;27(6): 759–66.
27. Martins C, Yasuda A, Campero A, et al. Microsurgical anatomy of the oculomotor cistern. Neurosurgery 2006;58(4):ONS-220–7.
28. Everton K, Rassner U, Osborn A, et al. The oculomotor cistern: anatomy and high-resolution imaging. AJNR Am J Neuroradiol 2008;29(7):1344–8.

29. Inoue T, Rhoton AL Jr, Theele D, et al. Surgical approaches to the cavernous sinus: a microsurgical study. Neurosurgery 1990;26(6):903.

30. Ettl A, Zwrtek K, Daxer A, et al. Anatomy of the orbital apex and cavernous sinus on high-resolution magnetic resonance images. Surv Ophthalmol 2000;44(4):303–23.

31. Morard M, Tcherekayev V, de Tribolet N. The superior orbital fissure: a microanatomical study. Neurosurgery 1994;35(6):1087–93.

32. Natori Y, Rhoton AL Jr. Microsurgical anatomy of the superior orbital fissure. Neurosurgery 1995; 36(4):762–75.

33. Lemke BN, Lucarelli MJ. Anatomy of the ocular adnexa, orbit, and related facial structures. In: Black EH, Nesi FA, Gladstone GJ, et al, editors. Smith and Nesi's Ophthalmic Plastic and Reconstructive Surgery. New York: Springer; 2012. p. 3–58.

34. Netter F. The Ciba Collection of Medical Illustrations, Volume 1: Nervous System; part 1: Anatomy and Physiology. West Caldwell: CIBA Limited; 1983.

35. Rhoton AL Jr. The posterior fossa cisterns. Neurosurgery 2000;47(3):S287–97.

36. Yousry I, Moriggl B, Dieterich M, et al. MR anatomy of the proximal cisternal segment of the trochlear nerve: neurovascular relationships and landmarks1. Radiology 2002;223(1):31–8.

37. Choi B, Kim J, Jung C, et al. High-resolution 3D MR imaging of the trochlear nerve. AJNR Am J Neuroradiol 2010;31(6):1076–9.

38. Tubbs RS, Oakes WJ. Relationships of the cisternal segment of the trochlear nerve. J Neurosurg 1998; 89(6):1015–9.

39. Bisaria K, Premsagar I, Lakhtakia P, et al. The superficial origin of the trochlear nerve with special reference to its vascular relations. J Anat 1990; 170:199.

40. Kim JH, Hwang JM. Absence of the trochlear nerve in patients with superior oblique hypoplasia. Ophthalmology 2010;117(11):2208–13.

41. Yousry I, Moriggl B, Holtmannspoetter M, et al. Detailed anatomy of the motor and sensory roots of the trigeminal nerve and their neurovascular relationships: a magnetic resonance imaging study. J Neurosurg 2004;101(3):427–34.

42. Guclu B, Sindou M, Meyronet D, et al. Cranial nerve vascular compression syndromes of the trigeminal, facial and vago-glossopharyngeal nerves: comparative anatomical study of the central myelin portion and transitional zone; correlations with incidences of corresponding hyperactive dysfunctional syndromes. Acta Neurochir 2011; 153(12):2365–75.

43. Yoshino N, Akimoto H, Yamada I, et al. Trigeminal neuralgia: evaluation of neuralgic manifestation and site of neurovascular compression with 3D CISS MR imaging and MR angiography1. Radiology 2003;228(2):539–45.

44. Lang E, Naraghi R, Tanrikulu L, et al. Neurovascular relationship at the trigeminal root entry zone in persistent idiopathic facial pain: findings from MRI 3D visualisation. J Neurol Neurosurg Psychiatr 2005;76(11):1506–9.

45. Erbay SH, Bhadelia RA, O'Callaghan M, et al. Nerve atrophy in severe trigeminal neuralgia: noninvasive confirmation at MR imaging— initial experience 1. Radiology 2006;238(2): 689–92.

46. Lutz J, Linn J, Mehrkens JH, et al. Trigeminal neuralgia due to neurovascular compression: high-spatial-resolution diffusion-tensor imaging reveals microstructural neural changes. Radiology 2011; 258(2):524–30.

47. Yousry I, Moriggl B, Schmid UD, et al. Trigeminal ganglion and its divisions: detailed anatomic MR imaging with contrast-enhanced 3D constructive interference in the steady state sequences. AJNR Am J Neuroradiol 2005;26(5):1128–35.

48. Mariniello G, Annecchiarico H, Sardo L, et al. Connections of sympathetic fibres inside the cavernous sinus: a microanatomical study. Clin Neurol Neurosurg 2000;102(1):1–5.

49. Williams LS, Schmalfuss IM, Sistrom CL, et al. MR imaging of the trigeminal ganglion, nerve, and the perineural vascular plexus: normal appearance and variants with correlation to cadaver specimens. AJNR Am J Neuroradiol 2003;24(7): 1317–23.

50. Lang J. Clinical Anatomy of the Masticatory Apparatus Peripharyngeal Spaces. New York: G. Thieme Verlag; 1995.

51. Marinkovic SV, Gibo H, Stimec B. The neurovascular relationships and the blood supply of the abducent nerve: surgical anatomy of its cisternal segment. Neurosurgery 1994;34(6): 1017–26.

52. Lemmerling M, De Praeter G, Mortele K, et al. Imaging of the normal pontine cisternal segment of the abducens nerve, using three-dimensional constructive interference in the steady state MRI. Neuroradiology 1999;41(5):384–6.

53. Yousry I, Camelio S, Wiesmann M, et al. Detailed magnetic resonance imaging anatomy of the cisternal segment of the abducent nerve: Dorello's canal and neurovascular relationships and landmarks. J Neurosurg 1999;91(2):276–83.

54. Nathan H, Ouaknine G, Kosary IZ. The abducens nerve. J Neurosurg 1974;41(5):561–6.

55. Iaconetta G, Fusco M, Cavallo LM, et al. The abducens nerve: microanatomic and endoscopic study. Neurosurgery 2007;61(3):7–14.

56. Alkan A, Sigirci A, Ozveren MF, et al. The cisternal segment of the abducens nerve in man:

three-dimensional MR imaging. Eur J Radiol 2004; 51(3):218–22.

57. Parsa CF, Ellen Grant P, Dillon WP, et al. Absence of the abducens nerve in Duane syndrome verified by magnetic resonance imaging. Am J Ophthalmol 1998;125(3):399–401.

58. Pilyugina SA, Fischbein NJ, Liao YJ, et al. Isolated sixth cranial nerve aplasia visualized with fast imaging employing steady-state acquisition (FIESTA) MRI. J Neuroophthalmol 2007;27(2): 127–8.

59. Ono K, Arai H, Endo T, et al. Detailed MR imaging anatomy of the abducent nerve: evagination of CSF into Dorello canal. AJNR Am J Neuroradiol 2004; 25(4):623–6.

60. Özveren MF, Erol FS, Alkan A, et al. Microanatomical architecture of Dorello's canal and its clinical implications. Neurosurgery 2007;60(2):1–8.

61. Joo W, Yoshioka F, Funaki T, et al. Microsurgical anatomy of the abducens nerve. Clin Anat 2012; 25(8):1030–42.

62. Umansky F, Valarezo A, Elidan J. The microsurgical anatomy of the abducens nerve in its intracranial course. Laryngoscope 1992;102(11):1285–92.

63. Umansky F, Elidan J, Valarezo A. Dorello's canal: a microanatomical study. J Neurosurg 1991;75(2): 294–8.

64. Destrieux C, Velut S, Kakou MK, et al. A new concept in Dorello's canal microanatomy: the petroclival venous confluence. J Neurosurg 1997; 87(1):67–72.

65. Harris FS, Rhoton AL Jr. Anatomy of the cavernous sinus. J Neurosurg 1976;45(2):169–80.

66. Parkinson D, Johnston J, Chaudhuri A. Sympathetic connections to the fifth and sixth cranial nerves. Anat Rec 1978;191(2):221–6.

Lower Cranial Nerves

Theodoros Soldatos, MD, PhD[a], Kiran Batra, MD[a],
Ari M. Blitz, MD[b], Avneesh Chhabra, MD[c],*

KEYWORDS

- Cranial nerves • Imaging assessment • Anatomy • Pathology • Magnetic resonance neurography
- Magnetic resonance imaging

KEY POINTS

- Enhancement of the intracanalicular and/or the labyrinthine portion of the facial nerve is always abnormal.
- Vestibulocochlear nerve schwannomas typically develop as intracanalicular–cisternal masses, whereas meningiomas develop as cisternal masses.
- Simultaneous glossopharyngeal, vagal, and spinal accessory neuropathy indicates a jugular foramen lesion. In the latter setting, paraganglioma constitutes the most common etiology.
- In isolated vagal neuropathy, detailed knowledge of the clinical findings is mandatory to tailor the examination and interpret the imaging findings.
- In hypoglossal neuropathy, the most important magnetic resonance imaging (MRI) feature is unilateral signal intensity denervation changes of the tongue musculature.
- Neurosarcoidosis, subarachnoid hemorrhage, basal meningitis, and viral neuritis may involve multiple lower cranial nerves and be demonstrated on MRI as nerve thickening and contrast enhancement.

INTRODUCTION

Imaging evaluation of cranial neuropathies (CNs) is a challenging task for radiologists, requiring thorough knowledge of the anatomic, physiologic, and pathologic features of the cranial nerves, as well as detailed clinical information, which is necessary for tailoring the examinations, locating the abnormalities, and interpreting the imaging findings. Although computed tomography (CT) provides excellent depiction of the skull base foramina, the nerves themselves can only be visualized in detail on magnetic resonance imaging (MRI).[1] This review provides clinical, anatomic, and radiological information on lower CNs (VII to XII), along with high-resolution magnetic resonance images as a guide for optimal imaging technique, so as to improve the diagnosis of cranial neuropathy.

ANATOMY
CN VII: Facial Nerve

The facial nerve is a complex mixed nerve, consisting of the facial nerve proper (the larger motor component) and the nervus intermedius (the smaller sensory component). The preganglionic fibers originate from the main motor nucleus, which is situated in the midpons. These join fibers from the superior salivatory nucleus, the nucleus solitarius, and the spinal tract of CN V. The facial nerve emerges at the ventrolateral aspect of the caudal pons, crosses the cerebellopontine angle (CPA) cistern, together with the vestibulocochlear nerve, and enters the temporal bone. The intratemporal course and central connections of the facial nerve can be roughly divided into the following segments:

[a] The Russell H. Morgan Department of Radiology and Radiological Science, The Johns Hopkins Hospital, 601 North Caroline Street, Baltimore, MD 21287, USA; [b] Division of Neuroradiology, The Russell H. Morgan Department of Radiology and Radiologic Science, The Johns Hopkins Hospital, Phipps B-100, 600 North Wolfe Street, Baltimore, MD 21287, USA; [c] University of Texas Southwestern, 5323 Harry Hines Blvd. Dallas, TX 75390-9178, USA
* Corresponding author.
E-mail address: avneesh.chhabra@utsouthwestern.edu

Neuroimag Clin N Am 24 (2014) 35–47
http://dx.doi.org/10.1016/j.nic.2013.03.022

The *meatal* segment runs within the internal acoustic canal (IAC), occupying the anterosuperior portion of the latter (**Fig. 1**).

Superior to the cochlea, the *labyrinthine segment* connects with the geniculate ganglion and provides the greater superficial petrosal nerve, which participates in the innervation of the lacrimal gland and mucous membranes of the nasal cavity and palate.[2]

The tympanic (horizontal) segment extends from the geniculate ganglion to the horizontal semicircular canal.

At the latter location, a second genu is formed, marking the beginning of the mastoid portion, which runs inferiorly within the mastoid bone and provides a) the nerve to the stapedius muscle b) the chorda tympani nerve, which provides secretomotor innervation to the submaxillary and sublingual glands, as well as sensory innervation to the anterior two thirds of the tongue c) the auricular branch of the vagus nerve, which participates in the sensory innervation of the posterior auditory canal.

The motor component of CN VII exits the skull through the stylomastoid foramen, and provides the posterior auricular nerve, which innervates the postauricular muscles, and two small branches, which innervate the posterior belly of the digastric muscle and the stylohyoid. Subsequently, the facial nerve penetrates the parotid gland, passes lateral to the retromandibular vein, and courses superficially into the muscles of facial expression.[3]

CN VIII: Vestibulocochlear Nerve

The vestibulocochlear nerve is a sensory nerve, consisting of a superior vestibular, an inferior vestibular, and a cochlear component. The fibers originate from vestibular nuclei located in the pons and medulla, and cochlear nuclei situated in the inferior cerebellar peduncles. The nerve emerges in the groove between the pons and the medulla oblongata, just posterior to the facial nerve, and courses together and parallel to the latter within the CPA cistern and the internal acoustic canal. The cochlear component runs in the anteroinferior aspect of the canal, whereas the superior and inferior vestibular components run in the posterosuperior and posteroinferior aspects, respectively (see **Fig. 1**).[4,5] The peripheral branches of the vestibular components are distributed in the utricle, saccule and semicircular ducts, whereas the respective branches of the cochlear component end at the organ of Corti.

CN IX: Glossopharyngeal Nerve

Among the six lower CNs, the glossopharyngeal is the smallest in terms of diameter, importance, and clinical significance.[6] The ninth nerve is a mixed nerve, which contains motor, somatosensory, visceral sensory, and parasympathetic fibers. The preganglionic fibers originate from the nucleus ambiguous, inferior salivatory nucleus, nucleus of tractus solitarius, and spinal trigeminal nucleus. The nerve exits the brain stem from the lateral aspect of the upper medulla along with cranial nerves X and XI, crosses the pontine cistern, and enters the pars nervosa of the jugular foramen (**Fig. 2**).[7] In passing through the latter, the nerve enters the superior and the petrous ganglia, from which final peripheral branches emanate. These include:

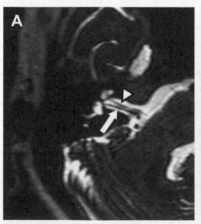 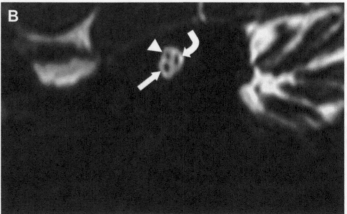

Fig. 1. Normal facial and vestibulocochlear nerves at the IAC fundus. Axial 3D DRIVE image (*A*) through the IAC demonstrates the facial nerve (*arrowhead*) and the vestibulocochlear nerve (*arrow*). The respective oblique sagittal image (*B*) shows the facial nerve anterosuperiorly (*arrowhead*), the cochlear branch of the vestibulocochlear nerve anteroinferiorly (*arrow*), and the superior and inferior vestibular branches posteriorly (*curved arrow*).

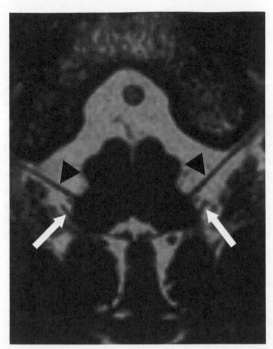

Fig. 2. Normal glossopharyngeal and vagus nerves. Axial CISS image through the brain stem demonstrates the origins of the glossopharyngeal nerves (*arrowheads*) and vagus nerves (*arrows*) from the sides of the upper medulla.

> The tympanic nerve (which forms the tympanic plexus that gives off the lesser superficial petrosal nerve, a branch to join the superficial petrosal nerve and branches to the tympanic cavity)
>
> Carotid branches (which connect with the vagus nerve and sympathetic branches)
>
> Pharyngeal branches (which supply the muscles and mucous membrane of the pharynx)
>
> Tonsilar branches (which supply the palatine tonsils)
>
> Lingual branches (which supply the posterior third of the tongue and communicate with the lingual nerve)
>
> A muscular branch (which is distributed to the stylopharyngeus)[8,9]

CN X: Vagus Nerve

The vagus nerve contains motor, sensory, and parasympathetic nerve fibers, and features the most extensive course and distribution among all CNs, coursing through the neck and traversing in the thorax and abdomen. The preganglionic fibers emanate from the nucleus ambiguous, dorsal motor nucleus, nucleus of tractus solitarius, and spinal trigeminal nucleus. The nerve emerges from the medulla oblongata, between the olive and the inferior cerebellar peduncle, just posterior to the glossopharyngeal nerve (see **Fig. 2**), entering the pars vascularis of the jugular foramen, where it forms the jugular and the nodose ganglia. Between the 2 latter ganglia, the vagus nerve gives off an auricular ramus, which innervates the skin of the concha of the external ear; a meningeal ramus, which runs to the dura matter of the posterior fossa; as well as a pharyngeal ramus, which forms the pharyngeal plexus with the glossopharyngeal nerve that supplies the muscles of the pharynx and soft palate (except the stylopharyngeus and tensor veli palatine muscles). Just distal to the nodose ganglion, the vagus nerve gives off the superior laryngeal nerve, which provides motor innervation to the cricothyroid muscle and sensory innervation to the larynx.[10] Subsequently, CN X descends in the neck within the carotid sheath, between the common carotid artery and the internal jugular vein. At the base of the neck, it provides the superior cardiac branches and the recurrent laryngeal nerves. The right recurrent laryngeal nerve bends upward and medially behind the subclavian artery, and ascends in the ipsilateral tracheoesophageal sulcus, whereas the left branch arises to the left of the aortic arch, loops beneath the ligamentum arteriosum, and ascends in the left tracheoesophageal sulcus. The recurrent laryngeal nerve innervates all the laryngeal muscles, except the cricothyroid, which is innervated by the superior laryngeal nerve. Subsequently, the vagus nerve enters the thorax, coursing over the subclavian artery on the right side, and between the common carotid and subclavian artery on the left side, and gives off branches to the pulmonary and esophageal plexuses. After crossing through the esophageal hiatus, the nerve terminates in multiple abdominal viscera.[11,12]

CN XI: (SPINAL) Accessory Nerve

The accessory nerve (often termed the spinal accessory nerve) is a motor nerve, composed of a small cranial part, which originates from the nucleus ambiguous and emerges from the side of the medulla oblongata, and a large spinal portion, which originates from the ventral horn of the spinal cord, between the C1 and C5 levels (**Fig. 3**). The 2 parts unite and enter the pars vascularis of the jugular foramen. The cranial part reaches the inferior vagal ganglion portion and is distributed to the striated muscles of the soft palate and larynx, whereas the spinal portion crosses the transverse process of C1 and provides innervation to the sternocleidomastoid and trapezius.[13,14]

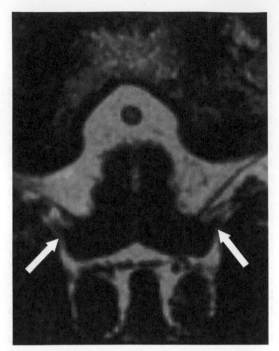

Fig. 3. Normal spinal accessory nerves. Axial CISS image at a slightly inferior level to Fig. 2 shows the origins of the bulbar spinal accessory nerves (*arrows*).

CN XII: Hypoglossal Nerve

The nucleus of the hypoglossal nerve is situated along the paramedian area of the anterior wall of the fourth ventricle in the medulla. The nerve emerges from the preolivary sulcus, runs through the hypoglossal canal, passes behind the inferior ganglion of the vagus nerve, and between the internal carotid artery and internal jugular vein (Fig. 4). After reaching the submandibular region, the hypoglossal nerve is distributed to the intrinsic muscles of the tongue (except the palatoglossus),

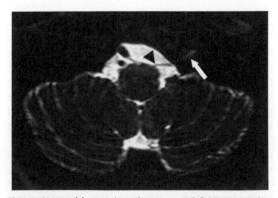

Fig. 4. Normal hypoglossal nerve. Axial 3D DRIVE image through the lower medulla demonstrates the left hypoglossal nerve (*arrowhead*) and entering the homonymous canal (*arrow*).

as well as the genioglossus, styloglossus, hyoglossus, and anterior strap muscles.[3]

IMAGING PROTOCOL

High-field imaging (3 T or newer 1.5 T scanners) is preferred to make use of the highest available signal-to-noise ratio and contrast-to-noise ratio, while keeping the imaging time in an acceptable range. A protocol that is commonly employed in most institutions and provides adequate high-resolution diagnostic evaluation is presented in Table 1. Thin-section imaging (1 mm) and low voxel size (0.6–1 mm for isotropic constructive interference in steady state [CISS] imaging) are essential to obtain the high-resolution evaluation of the posterior fossa CNs.

PATHOLOGIC CONDITIONS
CN VII: Facial Nerve

Facial palsy presents clinically with ipsilateral facial drop and difficulty in facial expression, pain around the jaw or behind the ear, increased sensitivity to sound, decreased ability to taste, headache, and changes in the amount of tears and saliva produced. It is crucial for clinicians to determine whether the forehead muscles are spared, which reflects pathology in the cerebral hemispheres (central facial palsy); or are affected, which implicates pathology in the facial nerve itself (peripheral facial palsy).[15]

After gadolinium administration, a thorough evaluation of all portions of the facial nerve is essential to detect areas of abnormal enhancement. Enhancement of the intracanalicular portion (which extends from the opening to the fundus of the IAC) and/or the labyrinthine portion (which extends from the fundus of the IAC to the facial hiatus) is always abnormal. The remaining portions of the nerve, as well as the geniculate ganglion, may normally enhance. In the case of abnormal facial nerve enhancement, the differential diagnosis includes Bell palsy, schwannoma, hemangioma, acute otitis media, lymphoma, sarcoidosis, viral neuritis, perineural tumor spread, Lyme disease, and Guillain-Barré and Ramsay-Hunt syndromes.[16]

In Bell palsy, there is enhancement of the intracanalicular and/or the labyrinthine portion of the ipsilateral facial nerve (Fig. 5), whereas some authors have also reported higher signal intensity ratio of the geniculate ganglion and tympanic segment on the affected side than on the normal side. The affected segment maintains linear morphology without any nodularity, and may be normal in size or slightly enlarged.[17–19] Although the diagnosis of Bell palsy is typically clinical,

Table 1
A commonly employed protocol for the MRI evaluation of the cranial nerves

Plane	Sequence	Technique	Comment
3-plane	Scout	GRE	
Sagittal	T1 W	TSE or 3D GRE	Thin (1 mm) slices
Axial	T2 W	TSE	Fat suppression
Axial	IR	FLAIR	
Axial	DWI		
Axial	T1 W	TSE	Thin (1 mm) slices
Axial	CISS	3D	Thin (0.6 mm) slices
Axial and coronal (+GD)	T1 W	TSE	Thin (1 mm) slices
Axial (+GD)	T1 W	TSE	Brain

For all sequences except the last one, the slice coverage is through the cavernous sinus and the brain stem.

Abbreviations: CISS, constructive interference in steady state; DWI, diffusion-weighted imaging; FLAIR, fluid-attenuated inversion recovery; GD, gadolinium administration; GRE, gradient echo; T1 W, T1 weighted; T2 W, T2 weighted; TSE, turbo spin echo.

MRI is reserved for patients in whom nerve decompression is planned, when there is suspected mass lesion in nonresolving neuropathy, or when there are indeterminate results of electromyography. Imaging can be used to confirm potential swelling of the nerve proximal to the meatal foramen and to detect any associated mass lesion.[20]

Schwannoma may develop in any portion of the facial nerve, although it has a predilection for the region of the geniculate ganglion. Typically, it presents as a well-demarcated space-occupying lesion, which is isointense to hypointense relative to gray matter on T1 weighted images and moderately hyperintense of T2 weighted images, and enhances homogeneously after gadolinium administration. Larger lesions undergo internal bleeding, presenting as hyperintense zones on T1 weighted images, or cystic degeneration or necrosis appearing as hyperintense areas on T2 weighted images.[21] CT demonstrates bony scalloping and remodeling rather than destruction.

Facial nerve venous vascular malformation (previously described as facial nerve hemangioma) also shows predilection for the geniculate ganglion. In the latter location, the lesion may be isointense to adjacent brain and only detectable on contrast-enhanced T1 weighted images, where it is expected to enhance intensely. Hemangiomas have similar signal characteristics compared with schwannomas, although in the former, the bony margins are indistinct, enabling differentiation from the latter, which feature well-defined remodeled margins. In addition, hemangiomas containing bone may feature foci of low signal intensity on MRI, and bone spicules or honeycomb morphology on CT. Associated widening of the facial nerve canal is sometimes present.[22–24] Meningiomas infrequently arise in the geniculate ganglion, are not readily differentiated from hemangiomas on imaging studies, and are included in the differential diagnosis solely based on the aforementioned location.[24]

In acute otitis media, there is obvious T2 hyperintensity and contrast enhancement of the tympanic segment of the facial nerve, although findings are difficult to assess because of the inflammation of the adjacent tissues. MRI is helpful in determining the degree of facial nerve involvement, as well as potential extension of the inflammation within the otic capsule and epidural and intradural spaces.[20]

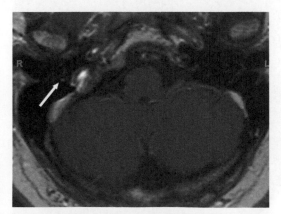

Fig. 5. Bels palsy. Contrast-enhanced axial T1 weighted image through the petrous bone demonstrates abnormal contrast enhancement of the labyrinthine portion of the right facial nerve (*arrow*).

Perineural spread of parotid malignancies and squamous cell carcinoma of the parotid or face may occur along the facial nerve. MRI demonstrates enlargement and enhancement of the involved nerve portion and commonly secondary enlargement of the stylomastoid foramen. The facial nerve may be involved by neurosarcoidosis and Lyme disease, and demonstrates nerve enhancement as well as diffuse or multifocal nodular enlargement, which tends to regress after therapy.[25,26] In Guillain-Barré syndrome, facial nerve involvement is acute, typically bilateral, and presents with enhancement.[27]

The facial nerve is susceptible to injury in cases of temporal bone fractures. In transverse fractures, the facial nerve is injured in up to 40% of cases, whereas in longitudinal fractures, it is injured in about 10% to 20% of cases. CT is the modality of choice for assessing the integrity of the facial canal, while the role of MRI is limited in these situations.[16]

CN VIII: Vestibulocochlear Nerve

Dysfunction of the vestibular branch of CN VIII presents clinically with dizziness, vertigo, disequilibrium, imbalance, ataxia, nausea, and/or vomiting. When the cochlear branch is affected, manifestations include tinnitus or ear ringing, poor hearing ability, or even deafness. Combinations of the aforementioned symptoms indicate simultaneous involvement of both nerve branches.

Schwannomas of the vestibulocochlear nerve (acoustic neuromas) usually develop as combined intracanalicular–cisternal masses, and less commonly as purely intracanalicular, extracanalicular, or intralabyrinthine lesions (**Figs. 6** and **7**). The lesions show the typical signal and enhancement characteristics of schwannomas, as previously described. In the IAC, intracanalicular lesions as well as segments of mixed intracanalicular–cisternal lesions demonstrate a funnel-shaped (ice cream cone) appearance with posterolateral epicenter on axial images and a short club-shaped configuration on coronal images.[28] In larger lesions, CT may demonstrate erosion of the temporal bone, which is limited to the boundaries of the IAC.[29]

Vestibulocochlear meningiomas are the most common intracranial extra-axial tumors in adults. They typically involve the cisternal portion of the nerve, assume a hemispherical configuration, and are eccentric to the IAC with anteromedial epicenter, although they may cross the latter or even extend into it. Typically, these neoplasms are isointense to gray matter on T1 weighted images, hyperintense on T2 weighted images, and enhance intensely after gadolinium administration. The margin of the tumor may elongate and flatten out along the bone, producing the dural tail sign.[30,31] On CT, associated calcifications and hyperostosis may be present.[32]

CN VIII, as well as CNs IX to XI, may be stretched or displaced by posterior fossa arachnoid cysts or lipomas. Whereas lipomas have signal characteristics of fat on all imaging sequences, arachnoid cysts show angled margins and have signal characteristics of cerebrospinal fluid, do not enhance, and can be differentiated

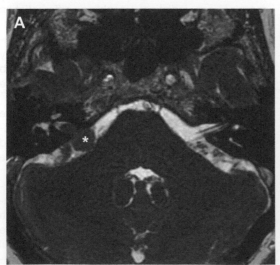
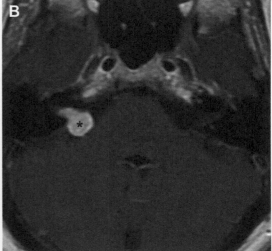

Fig. 6. Axial T2 weighted (*A*) and contrast-enhanced T1 weighted (*B*) images at the level of the cerebellopontine cisterns exhibit a round isointense, homogeneously enhancing space-occupying lesion (*asterisk*), extending in the right internal acoustic canal. On surgery, the lesion proved to be a vestibular schwannoma.

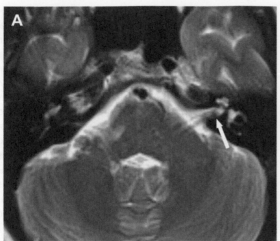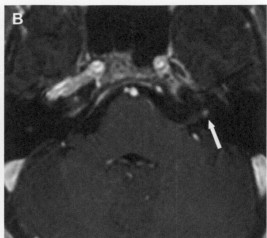

Fig. 7. Small acoustic schwannoma in a 52-year-old woman with gradual hearing loss in the left ear. Axial T2 weighted (A) and postcontrast T1 weighted (B) images at the level of the cerebellopontine cisterns demonstrate a tiny isointense enhancing lesion (arrow) within the left IAC.

from epidermoid cysts (lobulated margins) using diffusion-weighted imaging, on which the arachnoid cyst has low signal intensity, and the epidermoid cyst has high signal intensity.[30,33]

Although previously suspected to be associated with tinnitus, vascular loops of the anterior inferior cerebellar artery extending within the IAC are considered normal anatomic variations (Fig. 8). However, they should be reported if detected, because they could be symptomatic. Any vascular contacts with the vestibulocochlear nerves, especially with atrophic appearance of the ipsilateral

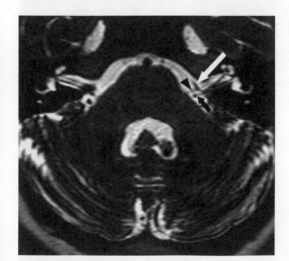

Fig. 8. Anterior inferior cerebellar artery looping within the IAC. Axial 3D DRIVE image through the IAC shows the left anterior inferior cerebellar artery (white arrow) in close anatomic relationship to the seventh (arrowhead) and eighth (black arrow), and entering the IAC.

nerves, should be reported.[34] Other vascular lesions that may compress the nerve include aneurysm of the anterior inferior cerebellar artery, tortuosity or dolichoectasia of the vertebrobasilar arteries, arteriovenous malformations, and dural fistulae. However, the aforementioned entities rarely cause neurogenic symptoms.[32]

Congenital pathologies of the vestibulocochlear nerve include

Aplasia, in which the nerve is absent, and the IAC is small containing only the facial nerve or no nerves at all

Hypoplasia, in which the cochlear branch is aplastic or hypoplastic

X-linked deafness, in which a wide neural aperture in the IAC fundus is associated with a broad communication between the cochlea and the IAC[30]

Within the CPA and/or the IAC, CNs VII and VIII may be affected due to meningitis, postmeningitic or postoperative fibrosis, and neoplastic dural or leptomeningeal disease. Nerve thickening and enhancement are apparent on MRI, although a definite differential diagnosis cannot be established, except from cases with multifocal cerebral involvement, which indicates a neoplastic process.[30] Similar to the facial nerve, the vestibulocochlear nerve may be involved by neurosarcoidosis, either in isolation or as part of multifocal disease.

CN IX, X, XI: Glossopharyngeal, Vagus, and Accessory Nerves

These nerves are reviewed in the same section, because of their close anatomic, and to some extent, functional relationship. The typical clinical scenario is complex neuropathy of CNs IX to XI, which indicates a lesion at the level of the medulla, CPA cistern, jugular foramen, or carotid space.[35] Intramedullary lesions, including demyelination, malignancy, motor neuron disease, syringobulbia, and infarction from occlusion of the posterior inferior cerebellar artery (PICA), can involve the nuclei of the aforementioned nerves, and present clinically as lateral medullary (Wallenberg) syndrome, which includes swallowing difficulty or dysphagia, slurred speech, ataxia, facial pain, vertigo, nystagmus, Horner syndrome, diplopia, and potentially palatal myoclonus.[36,37]

In the CPA cistern, the nerve roots of the glossopharyngeal and vagus nerves are subject to compression by the PICA, resulting in hyperactive rhizopathy, such as glossopharyngeal neuralgia or spasmodic torticollis (**Fig. 9**). However, this compressive relationship is not always possible to confirm on imaging, and the diagnosis is of exclusion and may be confirmed at the time of explorative surgery.[6]

Upon their entrance in the jugular foramen, CNs IX to XI are subject to simultaneous injury by various entities that develop locally. Combined neuropathy of the aforementioned nerves is known as jugular foramen (Vernet) syndrome. The most common entity is paraganglioma, arising from paraganglionic tissue situated in the adventitia of the jugular vein (glomus jugulare), or in and around

the vagus nerve (glomus vagale).[38] Paragangliomas are generally benign and locally aggressive, but may undergo malignant degeneration in approximately 3% to 4% of cases.[39] On imaging, these tumors are centered at the jugular foramen or the nasopharyngeal carotid space, respectively, demonstrate ovoid or lobulated margins, and may extend in the posterior fossa or inferiorly, toward the carotid bifurcation. Unlike carotid body tumor (glomus caroticus), which splays the internal and external carotid arteries, glomus vagale displaces both vessels anteromedially.[40,41] On MRI, paragangliomas are identified as isointense lesions that enhance avidly after gadolinium administration. Larger lesions may show a characteristic salt-and-pepper appearance on MRI, with T1 hyperintense foci representing areas of subacute hemorrhage, and T2 hypointense foci reflecting high-velocity flow voids (**Fig. 10**).[42] High-resolution, thin-section CT images using bone windows exhibit moth-eaten permeative destructive bone changes around the jugular foramen (**Fig. 11**).[16,35,43] The jugular foramen may also be involved by metastatic tumors (usually from prostate, breast or lung). In such cases, the contour of the foramen appears irregular on CT.[42] Other neoplasms that may arise at the jugular foramen and cause bone destruction include meningioma, fibrous dysplasia, Paget disease, histiocytosis X, multiple myeloma, and primitive ectodermal tumor. The latter is an irregular destructive mass,

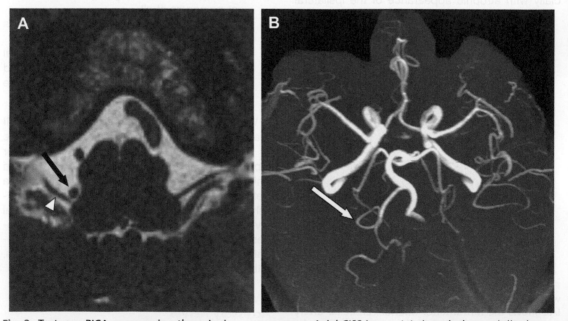

Fig. 9. Tortuous PICA compressing the spinal accessory nerve. Axial CISS image (*A*) though the medulla demonstrates a vessel (*arrow*) indenting the right glossopharyngeal nerve (*arrowhead*). Magnetic resonance angiography image (*B*) from the same case indicates the corresponding vessel is a tortuous right PICA (*arrow*).

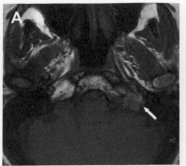
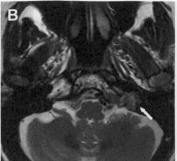
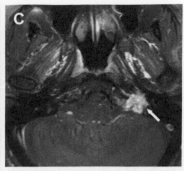

Fig. 10. Paraganglioma of the left jugular foramen. Axial T1 weighted (*A*), T2 weighted (*B*), and fat-suppressed contrast-enhanced T1 weighted (*C*) images display an enhancing space-occupying lesion (*arrow*) centered in the left jugular foramen, exhibiting a salt-and-pepper configuration.

which is isointense and slightly hyperintense to muscle on T1 and T2 weighted images, respectively. Additionally, it enhances homogeneously after contrast administration, demonstrates no tumor blush on angiography, and is surrounded by eroded bone on CT. Skull base fractures extending to the jugular foramen may also injure CNs IX to XI. Finally, the foramen may be infiltrated by extrinsic processes, which commonly originate from the temporal bone or the clivus, including cholesteatoma, epidermoid tumor, cholesterol granuloma, petrositis, abscess, mucocele, meningioma, chordoma, chondrosarcoma, chondroblastoma, osteoclastoma, fibrosarcoma, endolymphatic sac tumor, rhabdomyosarcoma, and osteomyelitis (**Fig. 12**).[42] Distal to the jugular foramen, the nerves may be involved by lymphoma or extension of nasopharyngeal carcinoma.

Isolated glossopharyngeal palsy is a rare entity, which, apart from PICA compression over the nerve root zone, may be caused by intramedullary lesions, entrapment by an elongated styloid process, or an ossified stylohyoid ligament (Eagle syndrome), as well as by lesions of the

retropharyngeal or retroparotid space, such as nasopharyngeal carcinoma, adenopathy, aneurysm, abscess, trauma (eg, birth injury), and surgical procedures (eg, carotid endarterectomy).[10] The disease presents as paroxysms of unilateral and severe lancinating pain in the oropharyngeal or otitic region, which is either spontaneous or elicited by actions that stimulate the region supplied by the nerve (eg, yawning, coughing, swallowing, and talking).[44]

Isolated vagal neuropathy may be of peripheral or central type, corresponding to isolated impairment of the recurrent laryngeal nerve or complete vagal dysfunction, respectively. In the former case, there is injury of the recurrent laryngeal branch in the infrahyoid neck or upper thorax, with common causes including iatrogenic trauma (thyroidectomy, cervical spine, skull base, carotid or thoracic surgery, intubation), trauma (eg, motor vehicle accident), and extralaryngeal neoplasm (particularly esophageal or lung cancer). Due to its relatively medial location, the right recurrent laryngeal nerve is more susceptible to injury during thyroid or esophageal surgery. However, in up to one-third

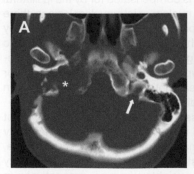
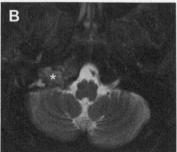
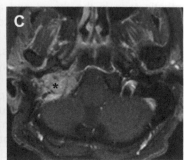

Fig. 11. Glomus tumor. CT image (*A*) at the level of the skull base demonstrates erosion of the right jugular foramen (*asterisk*), with a moth-eaten pattern. Note the normal left jugular foramen (*arrow*). Corresponding axial T2 weighted (*B*) and contrast-enhanced (*C*) images exhibit an isointense, avidly enhancing, mass centered within the jugular foramen (*asterisk*).

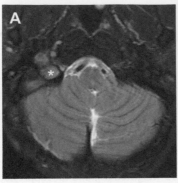 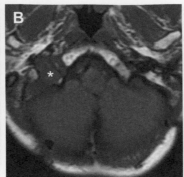 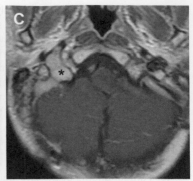

Fig. 12. Jugular foramen meningioma. Axial T2 weighted image (*A*) through the jugular foramina demonstrates absence of the normal flow void on the right (*asterisk*). Axial T1 weighted image (*B*) shows intermediate signal in this region (*asterisk*). Following contrast administration (*C*), an enhancing mass (*asterisk*) is evident extending inferiorly into the right carotid space.

of cases, no cause is identified, and the entity is considered idiopathic.[10,45] The disease presents clinically with hoarseness, resulting from paralysis of all ipsilateral laryngeal muscles (except the cricothyroid). In the case of bilateral nerve damage, there is breathing difficulty and aphonia. Cross-sectional imaging, either CT or MRI, should cover the area between the skull base and the carina, and thorough evaluation of the carotid space, tracheoesophageal groove, and aortopulmonary window is mandatory to detect the causative lesion.[46] On the ipsilateral side, imaging findings suggestive of vocal cord paralysis include paramedian vocal cord position (100%), pyriform sinus and laryngeal ventricle dilatation (100%), thickening and medial deviation of the aryepiglottic fold (>75%), anteromedial deviation of the arytenoid cartilage (>45%), true vocal cord fullness (>45%), subglottic fullness, vallecula dilatation, subglottic arch flattening, posterior cricoarytenoid atrophy, and thyroarytenoid muscle atrophy.[47]

In central type vagal neuropathy, the aforementioned clinical picture and imaging findings are supplemented by alterations of the parasympathetic tone in the thorax and abdomen. The injury of the vagus nerve distal to the origin of the recurrent laryngeal nerve may be caused by thoracic or abdominal neoplasms, compression by aortic aneurysm, cardiomegaly, or tuberculous sequelae.[48]

Isolated spinal accessory nerve palsy may be a complication of surgery. Other causes includeinternal jugular vein cannulation in the posterior triangle of the neck, following carotid endarterectomy, coronary bypass surgery, and radiation therapy, as well as with shoulder blunt trauma or dislocation.[49] On MRI, signal intensity denervation changes of sternocleidomastoid and trapezius muscles are apparent. In chronic cases, compensatory hypertrophy of the ipsilateral levator scapulae is a common finding, and should not erroneously be interpreted as a tumor.[35]

As with all CNs, the glossopharyngeal, vagus, and spinal accessory nerves may be involved by nerve sheath tumors, and viral neuritis due to varicella zoster virus infection. In the latter case, MRI demonstrates thickening and contrast enhancement of the affected nerve(s), reflecting breakdown of the blood–brain barrier. As the clinical picture improves, nerve swelling regresses, but contrast enhancement may persist for a long period.[50]

CN XII: Hypoglossal Nerve

Palsy of the hypoglossal nerve is relatively uncommon, produces distinctive clinical findings, and may be caused by injury at any point throughout its course from the medulla oblongata to the tongue.[51] In supranuclear lesions, there is weakening or paralysis of the contralateral side of the tongue, although no dysfunction is usually apparent, since it is compensated for by the ipsilateral normal side. In nuclear or intranuclear lesions, there is ipsilateral tongue deviation, supplemented by muscle atrophy and fasciculation in chronic stages.[52] After gadolinium administration, enhancement of the hypoglossal canal with minor anterior extension beneath into the nasopharyngeal region is a normal finding.[53]

In hypoglossal nerve dysfunction, the most important MRI feature is unilateral signal intensity denervation changes of the tongue musculature, which manifest as low and high signal intensity on T1 and T2 weighted images, respectively, in the subacute phase, signifying edema, and as high signal intensity on both sequences and loss of volume in the chronic cases, representing fatty infiltration and atrophy, respectively.[54] Once detected, the aforementioned finding should prompt for a comprehensive evaluation of skull base along the course of the nerve. Lipomas and dermoids of the tongue musculature may contain abundant amounts of fat, and caution is warranted not to misInterpret them as fatty infiltration.[52]

The medullary portion of the 12th nerve may be affected by cerebral infarcts, gliomas and metastatic neoplasms, and less commonly, by encephalitis, multiple sclerosis and pseudobulbar palsy, amyotrophic lateral sclerosis, or poliomyelitis.[51,55]

Skull base primary (eg, chordoma, meningioma) and secondary tumors involve the cisternal and skull base portions of the nerve. Nerve sheath tumors (schwannomas, neurofibromas) are uncommon and show typical MRI findings, whereas when located in the hypoglossal canal, they may cause expansion and bone remodeling, but no cortical rupture.[52,56] In addition, the cisternal portion may be involved by sarcoidosis or undergo compression by aneurysm or dolichoectasia of the vertebral artery or the PICA, although, similar to the vestibulocochlear nerve, the clinical significance of this finding remains questionable. Traumatic injury to the skull base segment may be caused by occipital condyle fracture and odontoid process subluxations, and is rarely bilateral.[51,57,58] The cisternal and skull base portions may also be damaged by subarachnoid hemorrhage or infections of the skull base (eg, osteomyelitis or basal meningitis).[52]

The extracranial segment of CN XII may be invaded by malignancies of the nasopharynx, oropharynx, and sublingual spaces. Hypoglossal nerve palsy may also be caused by carotid artery aneurysm, ectasia or dissection, venous thrombosis, deep neck infections, odontogenic abscesses, and neck surgery (carotid endarterectomy, vascular puncture, or operations on the upper cervical spine or submandibular gland).[51,57,58] Finally, hypoglossal nerve palsy has been reported after skull base radiation therapy.[59]

SUMMARY

In the vast majority of lower CN pathologies, MRI enables accurate detection and characterization of the causative entity. Thorough knowledge of the anatomy, pathology, and radiologic appearance, as well as appropriate imaging technique and correlation with the clinical findings are mandatory for a precise diagnosis, which will help avoid surgical pitfalls and optimize management planning.

REFERENCES

1. Casselman J, Mermuys K, Delanote J, et al. MRI of the cranial nerves—more than meets the eye: technical considerations and advanced anatomy. Neuroimaging Clin N Am 2008;18(2):197–231.
2. Ginsberg LE, De Monte F, Gillenwater AM. Greater superficial petrosal nerve: anatomy and MR findings in perineural tumor spread. AJNR Am J Neuroradiol 1996;17(2):389–93.
3. Yousem DM, Grossman RI. Cranial anatomy. In: Yousem DM, Grossman RI, editors. Neuroradiology: the requisites. 3rd edition. Philadelphia: Mosby; 2010. p. 46.
4. Rubinstein D, Sandberg EJ, Cajade-Law AG. Anatomy of the facial and vestibulocochlear nerves in the internal auditory canal. AJNR Am J Neuroradiol 1996;17(6):1099–105.
5. Tian GY, Xu DC, Huang DL, et al. The topographical relationships and anastomosis of the nerves in the human internal auditory canal. Surg Radiol Anat 2008;30(3):243–7.
6. Soh KB. The glossopharyngeal nerve, glossopharyngeal neuralgia and the Eagle's syndrome—current concepts and management. Singapore Med J 1999;40(10):659–65.
7. Rubinstein D, Burton BS, Walker AL. The anatomy of the inferior petrosal sinus, glossopharyngeal nerve, vagus nerve, and accessory nerve in the jugular foramen. AJNR Am J Neuroradiol 1995;16(1):185–94.
8. Zhao H, Li X, Lv Q, et al. A large dumbbell glossopharyngeal schwannoma involving the vagus nerve: a case report and review of the literature. J Med Case Rep 2008;2:334.
9. Suzuki F, Handa J, Todo G. Intracranial glossopharyngeal neurinomas. Report of two cases with special emphasis on computed tomography and magnetic resonance imaging findings. Surg Neurol 1989;31(5):390–4.
10. Brazis PW, Masdeu JC, Biller J. Cranial nerves IX and X (the glossopharyngeal and vagus nerves). Localization in clinical neurology. 6th edition. Philadelphia: Lippincott Williams & Wilkins; 2011. p. 361–368.
11. Dionigi G, Chiang FY, Rausei S, et al. Surgical anatomy and neurophysiology of the vagus nerve (VN) for standardised intraoperative neuromonitoring (IONM) of the inferior laryngeal nerve (ILN) during thyroidectomy. Langenbecks Arch Surg 2010; 395(7):893–9.
12. Binder D, Sonne DC, Fischbein N. Vagus nerve. Cranial nerves: anatomy, pathology, imaging. New York: Thieme Medical Publishers; 2010. p. 158–171.
13. Lloyd S. Accessory nerve: anatomy and surgical identification. J Laryngol Otol 2007;121(12):1118–25.

14. Cappiello J, Piazza C, Nicolai P. The spinal accessory nerve in head and neck surgery. Curr Opin Otolaryngol Head Neck Surg 2007;15(2):107–11.

15. Hazin R, Azizzadeh B, Bhatti MT. Medical and surgical management of facial nerve palsy. Curr Opin Ophthalmol 2009;20(6):440–50.

16. Yousem DM, Grossman RI. Temporal bone. neuroradiology: the requisites. 3rd edition. Philadelphia: Mosby, Inc; 2010. p. 385–418.

17. Kohsyu H, Aoyagi M, Tojima H, et al. Facial nerve enhancement in Gd-MRI in patients with Bell's palsy. Acta Otolaryngol Suppl 1994;511:165–9.

18. Murphy TP, Teller DC. Magnetic resonance imaging of the facial nerve during Bell's palsy. Otolaryngol Head Neck Surg 1991;105(5):667–74.

19. Al-Noury K, Lotfy A. Normal and pathological findings for the facial nerve on magnetic resonance imaging. Clin Radiol 2011;66(8):701–7.

20. Kumar A, Mafee MF, Mason T. Value of imaging in disorders of the facial nerve. Top Magn Reson Imaging 2000;11(1):38–51.

21. Wiggins RH 3rd, Harnsberger HR, Salzman KL, et al. The many faces of facial nerve schwannoma. AJNR Am J Neuroradiol 2006;27(3):694–9.

22. Friedman O, Neff BA, Willcox TO, et al. Temporal bone hemangiomas involving the facial nerve. Otol Neurotol 2002;23(5):760–6.

23. Phillips CD, Hashikaki G, Veilon F, et al. Anatomy and development of the facial nerve. In: Swartz JD, Loevner LA, editors. Imaging of the temporal bone. New York: Thieme Medical Publishers; 2009. p. 444–79.

24. Larson TL, Talbot JM, Wong ML. Geniculate ganglion meningiomas: CT and MR appearances. AJNR Am J Neuroradiol 1995;16(5):1144–6.

25. Oki M, Takizawa S, Ohnuki Y, et al. MRI findings of VIIth cranial nerve involvement in sarcoidosis. Br J Radiol 1997;70(836):859–61.

26. Saremi F, Helmy M, Farzin S, et al. MRI of cranial nerve enhancement. AJR Am J Roentgenol 2005; 185(6):1487–97.

27. Ramsey KL, Kaseff LG. Role of magnetic resonance imaging in the diagnosis of bilateral facial paralysis. Am J Otol 1993;14(6):605–9.

28. Jeng CM, Huang JS, Lee WY, et al. Magnetic resonance imaging of acoustic schwannomas. J Formos Med Assoc 1995;94(8):487–93.

29. Feghali JG, Kantrowitz AB. Atypical invasion of the temporal bone in vestibular schwannoma. Skull Base Surg 1995;5(1):33–6.

30. De Foer B, Kenis C, Van Melkebeke D, et al. Pathology of the vestibulocochlear nerve. Eur J Radiol 2010;74(2):349–58.

31. Pickett BP, Kelly JP. Neoplasms of the ear and lateral skull base. In: Bailey BJ, Johnson JT, editors. Head and neck surgery—otolaryngology,

vol. 6. Philadelphia: Lippincott Williams & Wilkins; 2006. p. 2003–26.

32. Enterline DS. The eighth cranial nerve. Top Magn Reson Imaging 1996;8(3):164–79.

33. Aribandi M, Wilson NJ. CT and MR imaging features of intracerebral epidermoid—a rare lesion. Br J Radiol 2008;81(963):e97–9.

34. Swartz JD. Pathology of the vestibulocochlear nerve. Neuroimaging Clin N Am 2008;18(2): 321–46.

35. Ong CK, Chong VF. The glossopharyngeal, vagus and spinal accessory nerves. Eur J Radiol 2010; 74(2):359–67.

36. Sacco RL, Freddo L, Bello JA, et al. Wallenberg's lateral medullary syndrome. Clinical–magnetic resonance imaging correlations. Arch Neurol 1993; 50(6):609–14.

37. Kim JS, Lee JH, Suh DC, et al. Spectrum of lateral medullary syndrome. Correlation between clinical findings and magnetic resonance imaging in 33 subjects. Stroke 1994;25(7):1405–10.

38. Ramina R, Maniglia JJ, Fernandes YB, et al. Jugular foramen tumors: diagnosis and treatment. Neurosurg Focus 2004;17(2):E5.

39. Caldemeyer KS, Mathews VP, Azzarelli B, et al. The jugular foramen: a review of anatomy, masses, and imaging characteristics. Radiographics 1997; 17(5):1123–39.

40. Weissman JL. Case 21: glomus vagale tumor. Radiology 2000;215(1):237–42.

41. Lee KY, Oh YW, Noh HJ, et al. Extraadrenal paragangliomas of the body: imaging features. AJR Am J Roentgenol 2006;187(2):492–504.

42. Vogl TJ, Bisdas S. Differential diagnosis of jugular foramen lesions. Skull Base 2009;19(1):3–16.

43. Rao AB, Koeller KK, Adair CF. From the archives of the AFIP. Paragangliomas of the head and neck: radiologic-pathologic correlation. Armed Forces Institute of Pathology. Radiographics 1999;19(6): 1605–32.

44. Pearce JM. Glossopharyngeal neuralgia. Eur Neurol 2006;55(1):49–52.

45. Blau JN, Kapadia R. Idiopathic palsy of the recurrent laryngeal nerve: a transient cranial mononeuropathy. Br Med J 1972;4(5835):259–61.

46. Chin SC, Edelstein S, Chen CY, et al. Using CT to localize side and level of vocal cord paralysis. AJR Am J Roentgenol 2003;180(4):1165–70.

47. Escott EJ, Bakaya S, Bleicher AG, et al. Vocal cord lesions and paralysis. In: Lin EC, Escott EJ, Garg KD, et al, editors. Practical differential diagnosis for CT and MRI. New York: Thieme Medical Publishers; 2008. p. 109–10.

48. Hartl DM, Travagli JP, Leboulleux S, et al. Clinical review: current concepts in the management of unilateral recurrent laryngeal nerve paralysis after

thyroid surgery. J Clin Endocrinol Metab 2005; 90(5):3084–8.

49. Brazis PW, Masdeu JC, Biller J. Cranial nerve XI (the spinal accessory nerve). Localization in clinical neurology. 6th edition. Philadelphia: Lippincott Williams & Wilkins; 2011. p. 369–76.

50. Sniezek JC, Netterville JL, Sabri AN. Vagal paragangliomas. Otolaryngol Clin North Am 2001; 34(5):925–39.

51. Thompson EO, Smoker WR. Hypoglossal nerve palsy: a segmental approach. Radiographics 1994;14(5):939–58.

52. Alves P. Imaging the hypoglossal nerve. Eur J Radiol 2010;74(2):368–77.

53. Voyvodic F, Whyte A, Slavotinek J. The hypoglossal canal: normal MR enhancement pattern. AJNR Am J Neuroradiol 1995;16(8):1707–10.

54. Russo CP, Smoker WR, Weissman JL. MR appearance of trigeminal and hypoglossal motor denervation. AJNR Am J Neuroradiol 1997;18(7):1375–83.

55. Laine FJ, Underhill T. Imaging of the lower cranial nerves. Neuroimaging Clin N Am 2004; 14(4):595–609.

56. Biswas D, Marnane CN, Mal R, et al. Extracranial head and neck schwannomas—a 10-year review. Auris Nasus Larynx 2007;34(3):353–9.

57. Delamont RS, Boyle RS. Traumatic hypoglossal nerve palsy. Clin Exp Neurol 1989;26:239–41.

58. Freixinet J, Lorenzo F, Hernandez Gallego J, et al. Bilateral traumatic hypoglossal nerve paralysis. Br J Oral Maxillofac Surg 1996;34(4):309–10.

59. Billan S, Stein M, Rawashdeh F, et al. Radiation-induced hypoglossal nerve palsy. Isr Med Assoc J 2007;9(2):134.

Peripheral Neuropathy
Clinical and Electrophysiological Considerations

Tae Chung, MD[a], Kalpana Prasad, MBBS[a],
Thomas E. Lloyd, MD, PhD[a,b],*

KEYWORDS

- Neuroimaging • Peripheral neuropathy • Electromyography • Nerve conduction study
- Entrapment neuropathy • Hereditary neuropathy

KEY POINTS

- Distal symmetric sensorimotor polyneuropathy due to "dying-back" axonal degeneration is the most common form of polyneuropathy and is typically caused by a toxic/metabolic condition, such as diabetes.
- Electromyography and nerve conduction study (EMG/NCS) is an extremely useful test in determining the localization (anatomic and nerve fiber type), pathophysiology (axonal or demyelinating), acuity, and severity of neuropathies.
- Axonal neuropathies typically demonstrate decreased amplitude action potentials on NCS and neurogenic motor units on EMG.
- Demyelinating neuropathies show decreased conduction velocity, temporal dispersion, and prolonged distal and F-wave latencies.
- MR neurography plays an important role in the evaluation of proximal, focal nerve lesions that are difficult to evaluate by EMG/NCS.

INTRODUCTION

Although neuroimaging has been used routinely to help diagnose focal nerve lesions such as trauma and tumors for years, the utility of high-resolution MR neurography in the evaluation of multifocal and systemic polyneuropathies is just now being investigated.[1] For the neurologist, the anatomic distribution, temporal progression, and electrophysiological properties of neuropathies guide the differential diagnosis, workup, and management of most forms of peripheral neuropathy; at present, MR neurography is not part of the standard workup for patients with peripheral neuropathy. For example, both Charcot-Marie-Tooth disease and amyloid neuropathy may show diffuse nerve enlargements that may not be readily distinguishable from one another on MR neurography,[2] whereas a nerve conduction study (NCS) will reveal dramatic reduction of conduction velocity in Charcot-Marie-Tooth type 1A, but normal velocity in amyloid neuropathy. As neuroimaging technology improves, novel MR imaging techniques such as molecular imaging may make MR neurography more useful in the evaluation of patients with neuropathy.

In the first part of this article, the way in which neurologists approach peripheral nerve lesions is reviewed, based on the anatomic, pathophysiological, and electrophysiological properties of peripheral nerves. Later in this article, the characteristics of various peripheral nerve lesions are summarized.

[a] Department of Neurology, The Johns Hopkins Hospital, 600 N. Wolfe Street, Baltimore, MD 21287, USA;
[b] Department of Neuroscience, The Johns Hopkins Hospital, 600 N. Wolfe Street, Baltimore, MD 21287, USA
* Corresponding author. Department of Neuroscience, The Johns Hopkins Hospital, 600 N. Wolfe Street, Baltimore, MD 21287.
E-mail address: tlloyd4@jhmi.edu

Neuroimag Clin N Am 24 (2014) 49–65
http://dx.doi.org/10.1016/j.nic.2013.03.023
1052-5149/14/$ – see front matter © 2014 Elsevier Inc. All rights reserved.

BASIC STRUCTURE OF PERIPHERAL NERVOUS SYSTEM

The peripheral nervous system refers to the part of the nervous system outside of the brain and spinal cord. Functionally, peripheral nerves are categorized into motor, sensory, and autonomic nerves. The cell bodies (soma) of motor neurons reside in the ventral gray matter of the spinal cord and are called anterior horn cells. Motor fibers often have very long axons that extend all the way to the neuromuscular junction. A motor unit consists of an anterior horn cell, its motor axon, and all the muscle fibers it innervates, forming a synapse at the neuromuscular junction. Sensory neurons are bipolar with an afferent axon receiving sensory input from the periphery and an efferent axon entering the central nervous system via the dorsal root. The cell body of the sensory neuron resides in the dorsal root ganglion or one of the sensory ganglia of sensory cranial nerves. The autonomic nervous system is classified into sympathetic and parasympathetic nerves. The neurons of sympathetic nerves are located in the lateral horn of the spinal cord from T1 to L2, whereas the neurons of parasympathetic nerves are located in the brain stem and sacral spinal cord (S2, S3, and S4).

Peripheral nerves have multiple layers of connective tissue surrounding axons; epineurium contains blood vessels and other connective tissues that surround multiple fascicles of nerves (Fig. 1A). Each fascicle is encased in perineurial connective tissue. Inside of each fascicle, individual myelinated and/or unmyelinated axons are surrounded by endoneurial connective tissue. Blood vessels (vasa vasorum) and nerves (nervi nervorum) are also contained within the nerve.

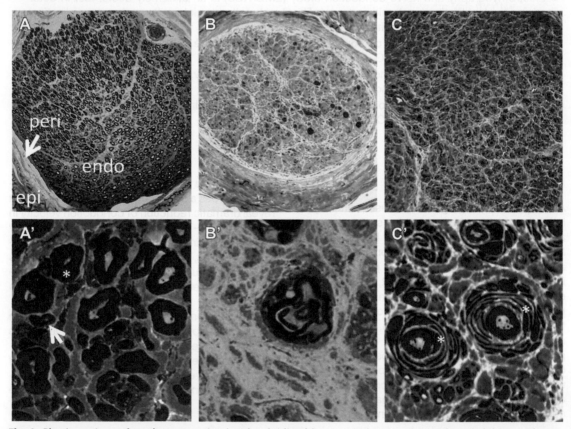

Fig. 1. Plastic sections of sural nerves stained with toluidine blue at ×10 (A–C) and ×100 (A'–C'). (A) Normal nerve showing normal density of myelinated nerve fibers. Endo, endoneurium; peri, (arrow) perineurium surrounding fascicles; epi, epineurium. At high magnification (A'), large, thickly myelinated fibers (asterisk) can be distinguished from smaller, thinly myelinated fibers (arrow). (B) Sural nerve from a patient with axonal neuropathy showing a fascicle with markedly reduced nerve fiber density. (B') shows a fiber with a "myelin ovoid," which can be seen in Wallerian degeneration. (C) Sural nerve from a patient with Charcot-Marie-Tooth disease type 1A. The nerve is diffusely enlarged (C), and at high magnification (C'), shows nerve fibers undergoing cycles of demyelination and remyelination, resulting in the typical "onion-bulb" appearance (asterisk).

PATHOPHYSIOLOGY OF PERIPHERAL NERVE INJURY

Regardless of its cause and nature of injury, peripheral nerve reaction to injury is limited to certain types of physiologic changes, depending on the extent of injury (Table 1). Minor, local insult to a peripheral nerve will result in a transient, focal conduction block, whereas intermediate insult may cause focal demyelination that requires a longer period of time for recovery. If the extent of nerve injury is severe enough to disrupt its axonal contents, a series of physiologic changes known as Wallerian degeneration follow to ensure removal and reformation of the nerve's damaged portion. The distal, degenerating portion of the axon undergoes stereotyped morphologic changes and is subsequently digested by Schwann cells to pave the way for regenerating axons from the proximal portion.

Immediately after nerve transection, there are microstructural changes in the distal portion of the axon without any gross light microscopic abnormalities until 48 hours. During this period, a nerve conduction study of the distal portion will show only a mild decrease in amplitude and nearly normal conduction velocity.[3,4] At about 48 to 72 hours, the axons begin to fragment and form spiral or hooklike segments; in a cross-section of a nerve biopsy, this fragmentation will appear as "myelin ovoids" (see Fig. 1B'). At 7 days, there is a complete absence of axon organelles. By this time, there is significant reduction or absence of motor/sensory responses in nerve conduction studies. Considering the length of the entire axon, how these reactions occur in a concerted way within a relatively short period of time remains unknown. In the case of toxic or metabolic neuropathy where the entire nerve fiber, from cell body to neuromuscular junction, is affected, retrograde degeneration appears to take place, possibly due to an insufficient supply of energy or other resource from the soma. This phenomenon is also called "dying-back" neuropathy and typically affects the longest nerves first, thus causing symptoms initially in the feet.

Peripheral nerve injury is often classified into 3 basic categories based on its cause, histologic features, and clinical manifestations: neuropraxia, axonotmesis, and neurotmesis (Table 2).[5] Prognosis following trauma is poor if there is loss of continuity of the endoneurial tube.

Following nerve transection, the regeneration process begins at the distal end of the proximal stump. By 3 to 8 days after injury, small clublike branches will appear at the terminal axon. This distal extension is called a "growth cone." By 48 hours, only a few of these collaterals reach the zone of injury. In optimal situations, it may take 8 to 15 days for growing axons to reach the distal portion. However, the closer to the cell body the site of injury is, the faster the rate of growth. The ability of nerves to regenerate depends on maintenance of the endoneurial tube, which practically speaking, depends on the severity of nerve injury and length that the axon needs to regenerate. After approximately 9 to 20 days, the regenerating axon remyelinates; however, it should be noted that the myelination of the regenerating axon is often incomplete and has shorter internodal distances compared with the preinjured axon, delaying the propagation of action potentials.

ELECTROPHYSIOLOGY IN PERIPHERAL NEUROPATHY

Nerve Conduction Study

Peripheral neuropathy can be divided into those that primarily affect axons and those that primarily affect the myelin sheath. Primary axon loss may be seen after trauma to the nerve or as a result of toxic, ischemic, metabolic, or genetic conditions. Demyelination may be seen in compressive neuropathies, hereditary neuropathies, and acquired immune-mediated neuropathies like Guillain-Barré syndrome (GBS) and chronic inflammatory demyelinating polyneuropathy (CIDP). Nerve conduction studies provide information to differentiate primary axon loss lesion from a primary demyelinating lesion.

Table 1
Peripheral nerve reaction to injury

Insult	Physiologic Status	Etiology	Electrophysiology
Minimal	Conduction block, rapidly reversible	Focal ischemia, mild compression	Focal conduction block
Intermediate	Conduction block, prolonged	Focal demyelination	Focal conduction block and slowing
Severe	Wallerian degeneration	Loss of axon and myelin sheath	Absent response

Table 2
Classification of nerve injury

Classification	Physiology	Histology	Prognosis
Neuropraxia	Focal conduction block	Local myelin injury; no axonal injury	Recovery in weeks to months
Axonotmesis	Loss of nerve conduction at injury site and distally	Loss of continuity of axon, but endoneurial tube, perineurium, and epineurium are intact	Good
		Loss of continuity of axon and endoneurial tube, but perineurium and epineurium are intact	Poor
Neurotmesis	Loss of nerve conduction at injury site and distally	Severance of entire nerve	Regeneration only possible if distal stump reconnected

Axon Loss

Amplitude of compound muscle action potential (CMAP) correlates with the number of motor nerve axons, and similarly, the amplitude of the sensory nerve action potential (SNAP) reflects the number of sensory nerve axons. Lesions causing axon loss generally result in reduced CMAP and SNAP amplitudes. It is important to keep in mind, however, that secondary axonal loss often occurs in severe or chronic demyelinating lesions. Furthermore, in axonal neuropathies, mild slowing of conduction velocity and prolongation of the distal latency (measure of distal conduction velocity) may occur if the fastest and largest axons are lost.

Demyelination

Loss of myelin is associated with slowing of conduction velocity (slower than 75% of the lower limit of normal), marked prolongation of distal latency (longer than 130% of the upper limit of normal), or both. Amplitude changes can also occur with demyelination because of secondary axonal loss. Reduced motor amplitude may also occur in demyelination if there is conduction block. In conduction block, the amplitude will be low when the nerve is stimulated proximal to the site of demyelination, but will be normal when stimulated below the block (**Fig. 2**). Any drop in CMAP amplitude or area of more than 20% implies conduction block and any increase in the CMAP duration of more than

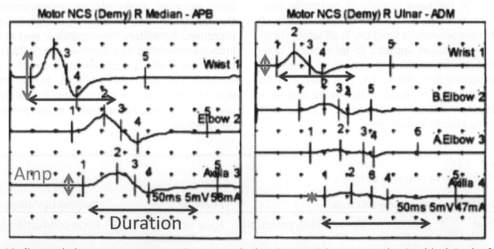

Fig. 2. Median and ulnar motor nerve conduction study showing partial motor conduction block in the forearm segment in a patient with acquired demyelinating polyneuropathy. Note that with stimulation above the elbow, the amplitiude (*Amp, vertical blue lines*) of the motor response is diminished (due to conduction block) when compared with the response at the wrist. Also, the duration of the response (*horizontal red lines*) is prolonged with stimulation above the elbow due to temporal dispersion, a common feature of demyelination.

15% signifies temporal dispersion; both are hallmarks of demyelination. In patients with demyelinating polyneuropathies, conduction block at nonentrapment sites helps to differentiate acquired (GBS and CIDP) from inherited neuropathies (Charcot-Marie-Tooth disease [CMT]).

Another useful measurement obtained in nerve conduction studies is the "F-wave" response, which is derived by antidromic travel of the action potential up the nerve to the anterior horn cell, which then backfires in a small proportion of anterior horn cells, leading to orthodromic travel back down the nerve, past the stimulation site, to the muscle. The F response measures conduction along the entire length of a nerve and is typically markedly prolonged in demyelinating lesions.

In patients with entrapment neuropathy, the exact entrapment site can be obtained by finding evidence of focal demyelination, either by slowing or by conduction block across the lesion site. Recovery from entrapment may occur quickly over several weeks if the compression is reversible and causes only focal demyelination. In contrast, entrapment causing significant axonal loss, evidenced by marked decrease in motor and sensory amplitudes, will have a longer and less complete recovery.

Electromyography

EMG is the recording of muscle electrical activity at rest (spontaneous) and with exertion (voluntary motor units) with an insertional electrode. The presence of abnormal spontaneous activity (positive sharp waves and fibrillation potentials) suggests active denervation. Analysis of motor unit potentials on needle EMG helps determine the acuity and severity of nerve injury. Long duration, large amplitude, and polyphasic motor unit potentials are seen in chronic axonal neuropathies, because of uninjured motor axons innervating denervated muscle fibers. During muscle contraction, there are 2 ways to increase muscle force: either motor units can increase their firing rate or additional motor units can start firing. Recruitment refers to the ability to add motor units as the firing rate increases. In neuropathic diseases, recruitment is reduced and may be the earliest physiologic sign of nerve injury. Thus, several weeks following a focal traumatic nerve injury, EMG will show abnormal spontaneous activity and reduced recruitment of normal-appearing motor units, whereas several months later, the spontaneous activity will be normal, recruitment will remain reduced, and now the motor units will have prolonged duration and enlarged amplitude. In this way, EMG cannot only help localize nerve lesions, but also can determine the chronicity of the neuropathic process.

CLINICAL ASSESSMENT OF PERIPHERAL NERVE INJURY

When evaluating patients with neuropathy or nerve injury, it is very important to assess the physiologic status of peripheral nerves with nerve conduction studies to correlate their physiology with their clinical symptoms. Once the physiologic status of the nerve injury is assessed, its temporal progression, severity, and anatomic distribution should be carefully determined to reach an accurate diagnosis.

Anatomic Distribution

Localization of nerve lesions is the most important aspect of the neurologic examination. A careful history and examination in conjunction with a thorough understanding of the anatomy of the peripheral nervous system should allow one to localize the lesion. In addition, EMG/NCS can further localize the lesion and aid in understanding the pathophysiology. Table 3 summarizes common types of neuropathies that should be considered according to their characteristic patterns of neurologic findings.

Nerve Fiber Type

Motor, sensory, and/or autonomic; large and/or small fibers. Careful attention to patients' symptomatology and clinical examination often reveals the type of fibers that are involved in disease. Typically, the involvement of motor fibers can cause weakness, fasciculations, or muscle atrophy, whereas sensory involvement causes numbness, tingling, and/or altered perception of pain. Also, the damage of large fibers causes imbalance and reduced vibratory and proprioceptive sensation, whereas small-fiber dysfunction causes decreased pinprick and temperature sensations. Autonomic involvement can result in altered sweating, orthostasis, constipation, urinary retention, or palpitations. Nerve conduction studies can only evaluate large motor and sensory nerve fibers, whereas, if there is selective damage to small fibers, other tests, such as a skin biopsy, are required to evaluate these small unmyelinated nerve fibers.

Pathophysiology: Demyelinating or Axonal

A nerve conduction study is necessary to determine whether a nerve injury is primarily demyelinating, axonal, or both, and is essential in the assessment of peripheral nerve injury. Demyelinating neuropathy characteristically shows a reduction in conduction velocity and prolongation of distal and F-wave latencies, whereas axonal neuropathy shows a reduction in amplitude. In some situations, a nerve biopsy may be

Table 3
Pattern of neurologic symptoms

Pattern	Neuropathies that Should be Considered
Symmetric, length-dependent distal weakness with sensory loss (most common type)	Metabolic neuropathies (eg, diabetes), toxic neuropathies, Charcot-Marie-Tooth disease
Symmetric proximal and distal weakness with sensory loss and areflexia	Inflammatory demyelinating polyneuropathies (CIDP and GBS)
Multiple mononeuropathies	Vasculitic neuropathy, hereditary neuropathy with liability to pressure palsies
Asymmetric weakness with intact sensory examination and SNAPs	Motor neuron disease, multifocal motor neuropathy
Asymmetric weakness with pain in a dermatomal distribution	Radiculopathy
Sensory ataxia with or without weakness	Sensory neuronopathies from paraneoplastic syndrome, Sjogren syndrome
Significant autonomic involvement	Amyloidosis, diabetic neuropathy

considered to evaluate the cause of neuropathy and is most useful in diagnosing vasculitic or amyloid neuropathy and infiltrative neuropathies due to tumor. When possible, the sural or superficial radial sensory nerves are typically resected for pathologic analysis so as to leave minimal neurologic deficit. When other nerves are considered for biopsy, MR neurography is often helpful in determining the optimal biopsy site. Although diagnosis of demyelinating neuropathies (eg, CIDP or CMT) can be aided by biopsy, nerve biopsy is rarely needed for diagnosis.

Severity

In addition to the examination, EMG/NCS is extremely helpful in determining severity of nerve injury. The amplitude of motor and sensory responses is a good measure of the degree of axonal loss and correlates with disability. EMG can assess whether muscles are denervated, and if so, can also determine the acuity and severity of denervation. There are different quantitative methods for measuring severity of nerve injury, often using simple tools such as the Rydel-Seiffer tuning fork, Von Frey monofilaments, and hand-held dynamometer. Various measurement formulas have also been suggested, using a combination of the above quantitative testing results. Among them, total neuropathy score (TNS) is widely used for many systemic neuropathies; its interreliability and intrareliability are well established[6,7] and are particularly useful in assessing therapeutic responses.

Clinical Course

Careful evaluation of the temporal progression of the patients' symptoms, when correlated with the examination and physiology, can provide crucial information about the disease process. For example, a toxic or nutritional neuropathy might present with a monophasic course when adequately treated, whereas chronic inflammatory neuropathy can present with a relapsing and remitting course.

ENTRAPMENT MONONEUROPATHIES

Carpal tunnel syndrome is the most common mononeuropathy and is caused by entrapment of the median nerve as it runs in the carpal tunnel at the wrist. Other common entrapment neuropathies include ulnar neuropathy at the elbow (cubital tunnel syndrome), radial neuropathy at the spiral groove, and peroneal neuropathy at the fibular head. Conditions that predispose to carpal tunnel and cubital tunnel syndrome include occupations that undergo repetitive flexion/contraction of the wrists and elbows, diabetes, obesity, hypothyroidism, arthritis, and underlying peripheral neuropathies leading to nerve hypertrophy. Examination shows sensory with or without motor deficits in the distribution of the peripheral nerve and may show a "positive Tinel's sign" in which percussion over the site of nerve injury reproduces the patient's sensory symptoms. Diagnosis is typically made with EMG/NCS, but imaging modalities such as ultrasound and MR neurography are increasingly being used to help surgeons determine cause, severity, prognosis, and treatment of entrapment mononeuropathies.

NEUROPATHIES ASSOCIATED WITH METABOLIC DISEASE

Neuropathies associated with metabolic disease typically present with a slowly progressive, distal (length-dependent) symmetric sensorimotor polyneuropathy (DSPN) with physiologic features of axonal loss.

Diabetes Mellitus

Diabetes mellitus is the most common cause of peripheral neuropathy in the United States and Europe. The risk of developing peripheral neuropathy correlates with the duration of diabetes mellitus, glycemic control, and presence of retinopathy and nephropathy.[8] DSPN is by far the most common form of diabetic neuropathy; however, multiple forms of neuropathy are associated with diabetes (**Box 1**). Nerve conduction studies typically show length-dependent, mixed demyelinating, and axonal polyneuropathy, and this correlates with the nerve biopsy findings of axonal degeneration, regenerative clusters, and segmental demyelination. Autonomic and sensory nerve fibers are prominently involved in diabetic DSPN. Some diabetic patients develop "diabetic amyotrophy," also known as "diabetic lumbosacral radiculoplexopathy," which presents with relatively abrupt-onset, severe, asymmetric pain in the proximal thighs, often lasting months. Muscle weakness and atrophy in proximal thigh muscles often develop, although the course of diabetic amyotrophy is monophasic, and patients will usually improve without treatment. Some pathologic studies revealed infiltration of inflammatory cells in various locations in roots and peripheral nerves in patients with diabetic amyotrophy, suggesting an autoimmune cause.[9,10] However, efficacy of immunotherapy with intravenous immunoglobulin or prednisone is questionable because of its favorable outcome even without any treatment.

Hypothyroidism

Hypothyroidism most commonly predisposes patients to entrapment neuropathies, such as carpal tunnel syndrome, but rarely can cause generalized

---

Box 1
Neuropathy associated with diabetes

Distal symmetric sensory motor polyneuropathy

Autonomic neuropathy

Diabetic polyradiculoneuropathy

- Asymmetric, painful lumbosacral radiculoplexopathy (diabetic amyotrophy)
- Symmetric, painless, polyradiculopathy
- Cervical or thoracic radiculopathy

Focal mononeuropathies

- Cranial neuropathy
- Entrapment mononeuropathy

Diabetic small-fiber neuropathy

---

sensory neuropathy, characterized by painful paresthesias and numbness in distal limbs.[11]

Vitamin B12 (Cobalamin)

Vitamin B12 (Cobalamin) deficiency causes peripheral neuropathy in addition to the classic presentation of "subacute combined degeneration," referring to a loss of dorsal columns and corticospinal tracts within the spinal cord, leading to loss of proprioception and vibratory sensation in addition to hyperreflexia. Vitamin B12 deficiency–related neuropathy can be seen in patients who undergo bariatric surgery in addition to strict vegetarians.

Other Vitamin Deficiencies

Other vitamin deficiencies, especially vitamin B1 (thiamine) and vitamin E deficiency, are rare causes of peripheral neuropathy. Thiamine deficiency can occur in patients with chronic alcoholic consumption. Both deficiency and overdose of vitamin B6 (pyridoxine) can cause peripheral neuropathy.

Uremic Neuropathy

Uremic neuropathy refers to neuropathy associated with renal failure. Approximately 60% of patients with chronic renal failure (usually when glomerular filtration rate is less than 12 mL/min) develop DSPN.[12] Mononeuropathies, especially carpal tunnel syndrome, are common and thought to be related to the accumulation of β2-microglobulin during hemodialysis.

Chronic Liver Disease

Chronic liver disease is another cause of neuropathy. In one study, DSPN was found in 71% of patients and autonomic neuropathy was found in 48% of patients.[13]

INFLAMMATORY AND IMMUNE-MEDIATED NEUROPATHY

The immune-mediated neuropathies are a heterogeneous group of disorders wherein the immunologic process may be directed to either peripheral nerves or the supporting blood vessels. Peripheral nerve myelin is the usual target in demyelinating neuropathy. In vasculitic neuropathy, the pathologic process originates in the blood vessels and leads to nerve ischemia, resulting in a neuropathy characterized by multifocal sensory and motor axonal loss.

Guillain-Barré Syndrome

GBS is the most frequent cause of acute flaccid paralysis worldwide.[14] GBS is not a single disorder, but rather encompasses several types of acute immune-mediated polyneuropathies (Box 2).

Antecedent illness

About two-thirds of patients with GBS have an illness during the preceding few weeks, usually a respiratory or gastrointestinal infection. Cytomegalovirus is the most commonly associated viral infection. *Campylobacter jejuni*, which causes gastroenteritis, is the most frequently associated bacterial infection. Vaccination may increase GBS risk.

AIDP clinical features

AIDP clinical features include the following: GBS usually initially presents with numbness and tingling in the feet and hands. Even at an early stage, the muscle stretch reflexes are usually lost or diminished. Progressive weakness accompanies the sensory disturbance, classically in an ascending pattern. However, in some patients, weakness from the onset involves proximal or axial muscles, and facial weakness is often apparent in at least half of the patients during the course of the illness. Ophthalmoparesis and bulbar paralysis may develop in some patients, and the most concerning feature is respiratory insufficiency due to diaphragm weakness.

Axonal GBS

Axonal GBS is uncommon in the United States and Europe, but is common in Asia.[15] AMAN has exclusively motor findings with weakness typically beginning in the legs. Tendon reflexes are preserved until weakness is severe. Respiratory insufficiency may occur. AMSAN is clinically and physiologically similar, but with detectable sensory involvement.

MFS

MFS is characterized by ataxia, areflexia, and ophthalmoplegia. There is a spectrum between MFS and Bickerstaff encephalitis that is characterized by ataxia, ophthalmoplegia, abnormalities in consciousness, and pyramidal tract dysfunction associated with brain MR imaging showing gadolinium-enhancing brainstem lesions. These syndromes typically are preceded by *C jejuni* or Mycoplasma infection and are associated with anti-GQ1b antibodies.[16]

Electrophysiology

NCS in AIDP shows typical features of demyelination including prolonged distal latencies, slow conduction velocities, temporal dispersion, conduction block, and prolonged F-wave latencies. In axonal GBS, NCS reveals low-amplitude or unobtainable CMAPS and/or SNAPs, and EMG shows acute and chronic denervation. In MFS, NCS reveals reduced amplitudes of SNAPs out of proportion to any prolongation of the distal latencies or slowing of sensory conduction velocities. CMAPs in the upper and lower limbs are usually normal.

Investigations

Cerebrospinal fluid shows albuminocytologic dissociation (elevated cerebrospinal fluid protein levels accompanied by few mononuclear cells) in greater than 80% of GBS patients after 2 weeks. Enhancement of nerve roots may be seen on spine MR imaging in AIDP. Antiganglioside antibodies, particularly GM1 immunoglobulin G (IgG) antibodies, are found in some patients with AIDP and correlate with recent *C jejuni* infection. Serologic evidence of recent *C jejuni* infection with GM1 or GD1a antibodies are demonstrated in most patients with AMAN; GM1 antibodies are found in most patients with AMSAN[17] and GQ1b antibodies are evident in many patients with MFS.[16] Molecular mimicry between gangliosides expressed on nerve fibers and glycolipids present on *C jejuni* may account for their association and may play a role in the pathogenesis of the disorder.

Prognosis

The rate of progression in GBS is variable; in greater than 90% of patients, the nadir is reached within 1 month. The severity of involvement varies from minimal weakness to complete quadriplegia and need for mechanical ventilation. Autonomic dysfunction can occur in many patients. The progression phase is followed by a plateau phase followed by recovery. Poor prognostic predictors include advanced age, fast rate of progression, axonal loss on NCS, and severe weakness at the nadir. Immunotherapy is believed to hasten recovery, but does not alter ultimate prognosis.[18–20] Recovery may take many months and may be incomplete. Approximately 15% of GBS patients have functionally significant residual deficits.[21]

Box 2
The Guillain-Barré syndromes

Acute inflammatory demyelinating polyneuropathy (AIDP)

Miller Fisher syndrome (MFS): ataxia, areflexia, and ophthalmoplegia

Axonal forms

Acute motor axonal neuropathy (AMAN)

Acute motor-sensory axonal neuropathy (AMSAN)

Chronic Inflammatory Demyelinating Polyneuropathy

CIDP is an acquired immune-mediated peripheral neuropathy that presents as either a chronic progressive or a relapsing-remitting disorder.[22]

Clinical features

In typical CIDP, motor and sensory deficits develop insidiously over months (minimum of 8 weeks), often leading to significant disability. Most patients manifest with progressive, symmetric, proximal, and distal weakness of the upper and lower limbs with numbness and paresthesias in extremities. As in AIDP, reflexes are usually absent or markedly attenuated, and examination reveals a loss of large-fiber sensory modalities (vibration and proprioception). Involvement of cranial nerves (ophthalmoparesis, facial, or bulbar weakness) may be observed in approximately 15% of cases. Patients with long-standing CIDP can have symptoms typical of lumbar stenosis and cauda equina dysfunction. In some cases, hypertrophy of nerve roots may cause crowding and entrapment of the roots in the lumbar thecal sac and lumbar spinal canal, including the neural foramina.[23]

Investigations

As in AIDP, diagnosis of CIDP is supported by findings of cytoalbuminergic dissociation and electrodiagnostic evidence of demyelination in multiple motor nerves. Nerve biopsy is performed in unusual cases, such as those patients with asymmetrical presentations and pain, in whom there is concern about other pathologies such as a vasculitis. Biopsies typically show inflammation and demyelination in addition to mild axonal degeneration. Laboratory testing should include a quantitative assessment of serum immunoglobulins and screening for monoclonal gammopathies in serum and urine with immunoelectrophoresis and immunofixation. If κ or λ light-chains are detected, follow-up with hematology consultation and bone marrow biopsy is often necessary to rule out a lymphoproliferative disorder or malignant plasma cell dyscrasia. A radiologic skeletal survey should be performed to search for either osteosclerotic or osteolytic myeloma.

Prognosis

The course of CIDP may be continuous or stepwise progressive or relapsing. Most patients respond to immunotherapy (steroids, plasmapheresis, or intravenous gammaglobulin), and clinical response may aid in diagnosis. In patients who do not respond well to immunotherapy, variants of CIDP should be considered (**Box 3**).

Box 3
CIDP with concurrent disease

HIV infection

Lymphoma

Osteosclerotic myeloma, POEMS (polyneuropathy, organomegaly, endocrinopathy, monoclonal protein, and skin changes)

Monoclonal gammopathy

Chronic active hepatitis, hepatitis C

Inflammatory bowel disease

Connective tissue disease

Bone marrow and organ transplants

Central nervous system demyelination

Nephrotic syndrome

Diabetes mellitus

Hereditary neuropathy

Thyrotoxicosis

Multifocal Motor Neuropathy

Multifocal motor neuropathy (MMN) is an acquired, immune-mediated asymmetrical motor neuropathy with focal motor conduction block on electrophysiologic testing.

Clinical features

Generally, MMN has onset between the ages of 20 and 50, and men are affected 3 times more frequently than women. As its name suggests, MMN is an asymmetric motor neuropathy that has a predilection for the upper limbs, particularly the nerves innervating the forearm and the intrinsic hand muscles leading to wrist drop. Sensory involvement is minimal. Fasciculations and cramps may be seen, often raising a concern for a diagnosis of motor neuron disease. Most of the cases follow a slow progressive course.

Electrophysiology

Focal conduction block of motor fibers outside common entrapment sites is the hallmark of MMN. Sensory conduction studies obtained across the same sites of motor block are normal. Conduction block is defined as a significant reduction of the evoked CMAP amplitude, or area between distal and proximal sites of stimulation along a focal nerve segment, in the absence of abnormal temporal dispersion.

Investigations

IgM anti-GM1 antibodies are present in ~50% of cases.[24]

Paraproteinemic Neuropathy

Monoclonal gammopathy (or paraprotein) identified on serum or urine electrophoresis is often found in patients with neuropathy.[25] IgG is the most common paraprotein, followed by IgM and IgA. Monoclonal gammopathy can be associated with hematological disorders like multiple myeloma, lymphoma, plasmacytoma, Waldenstrom globulinemia, amyloidosis, cryoglobulinemia, and chronic lymphocytic leukemia. If a detailed hematologic evaluation is normal, the term monoclonal gammopathy of undetermined significance is used. Even if the initial evaluation is normal, these patients should be followed periodically. The association between paraprotein and neuropathy is strongest with IgM. Some paraproteinemic neuropathies may be caused by immunoreactivity of the paraprotein, whereas in patients with known hematological disease, pathogenic mechanisms, such as nerve infiltration, cryoglobulinemia, amyloidosis, or hyperviscosity, may play a role. In others, the paraprotein may not be the cause of neuropathy.

IgM gammopathy

Most neuropathies seen in association with IgM gammopathy are demyelinating. About 50% of patients with peripheral neuropathy and IgM gammopathy have IgM antibodies that bind to myelin-associated glycoprotein. These patients present with slowly progressive distal limb paresthesias, sensory loss, gait ataxia, and tremor, with mild or no weakness. This condition has also been called distal acquired demyelinating symmetric neuropathy. Nerve conduction study often shows markedly prolonged distal latency with only mildly reduced conduction velocities.

POEMS syndrome

POEMS syndrome (Polyneuropathy, organomegaly, endocrinopathy, monoclonal gammopathy, and skin changes) is a rare paraneoplastic disorder that usually occurs in patients with osteosclerotic myeloma, but may occur in association with Waldenstrom macroglobulinemia or plasmacytoma. The most common paraprotein is IgG or IgA lambda chain. The clinical and electrophysiological features of neuropathy are similar to CIDP, but are usually refractory to immunosuppressive treatment. Serum vascular endothelial growth factor levels are often markedly elevated.

VASCULITIC NEUROPATHY

Vasculitic neuropathy is an immune-mediated disorder directed against blood vessels, resulting in ischemia and infarction to the peripheral nervous system.[26] Vasculitic involvement of the peripheral nerves typically causes multiple, focal areas of ischemic injury. The clinical presentation is typically initially one of multiple mononeuropathies (also called mononeuritis multiplex), but over time, may develop into a distal symmetric polyneuropathy. Patients typically present with an acute onset of pain and progressive sensory and motor deficits in the distribution of specific nerves. The clinical course may be stepwise or progressive (Box 4).

Diagnosis

Electrodiagnostic testing often shows a mononeuritis multiplex pattern. Laboratory evaluations are performed to evaluate for systemic forms of vasculitis (see Box 4), including complete blood count, erythrocyte sedimentation rate, C-reactive protein, renal and liver functions, electrolytes, urinalysis, glycated hemoglobin, serum immunofixation electrophoresis, complement levels, cryoglobulins, hepatitis B surface antigen, hepatitis C antibody, human immunodeficiency virus (HIV)

Box 4
Vasculitis associated with neuropathy

Primary systemic vasculitis

    Large vessels

        Giant cell arteritis

    Medium vessels

        Polyarteritis nodosa

    Small vessels

        Microscopic polyangiitis

        Churg-Strauss syndrome

        Wegener's granulomatosis

Secondary systemic vasculitis

    Connective tissue diseases

        Rheumatoid arthritis

        Systemic lupus erythematosus

        Sjogren syndrome

        Dermatomyositis

    Inflammatory bowel disease

    Behcet disease

    Sarcoidosis

    Infection

        Hepatitis B and C, HIV

    Malignancy

Nonsystemic vasculitis

antibody, antinuclear antibodies, rheumatoid factor, SSA and SSB antibodies, and antineutrophil cytoplasmic antibodies. The definitive diagnosis of vasculitic neuropathy is made with biopsy of a clinically or electrophysiologically involved nerve, preferably the sural or superficial radial sensory nerve. The pathologic features of vasculitic neuropathy include vessel wall changes of transmural inflammation, fibrinoid necrosis, endothelial damage and hemorrhage, thrombosis, endothelial hyperplasia, fibrosis of vessel wall, fragmentation of the elastic membrane, narrowing or occlusion of the lumen, recanalization, wedge-shaped axon loss, centrafascicular degeneration, subperineural edema, and fascicle-to-fascicle variability (see **Fig. 3**). A combined nerve and muscle biopsy increase the diagnostic sensitivity.

HEREDITARY NEUROPATHY

Also known as Charcot-Marie-Tooth disease, the hereditary motor and sensory neuropathies encompass the largest group of inherited neuropathies. These diseases are commonly classified based on clinical presentation (age of onset and inheritance pattern) and pathologic abnormality/electrophysiology (axonal: CMT2 vs demyelinating: CMT1).[27,28]

Clinical Features

Most patients with CMT develop slowly progressive weakness and atrophy in their feet beginning in childhood or early adulthood. Pain or sensory loss is variable, but is usually not a chief complaint. Foot deformities (pes cavus, or high arches, and

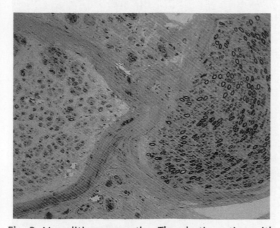

Fig. 3. Vasculitic neuropathy: The plastic section with toluidine blue staining shows a striking fascicle-to-fascicle variation of fiber density in the 2 adjacent fascicles. Mild subperineurial edema can also be appreciated in this section.

hammertoes) are common and may lead to disability. Because of the insidious nature of this disease, most patients do not complain of motor or sensory symptoms until late in the course of the disease, and most patients remain ambulatory. On examination, patients typically have distal weakness and atrophy in the feet, areflexia, and length-dependent sensory loss of both large-fiber and small-fiber sensory modalities. More severely affected patients will develop sensory ataxia or tremor (Roussey-Levey syndrome), palpably enlarged nerves (CMT1), and weakness, atrophy, and sensory loss of the hands. Patients without evidence of sensory involvement on examination or electrodiagnostic testing are classified as having hereditary motor neuropathy, whereas patients without evidence of motor involvement are classified as hereditary sensory or hereditary sensory and autonomic neuropathy.

Electrophysiology

When CMT is clinically suspected, the most useful test is nerve conduction study. Nerve conduction studies usually can classify the disease as primarily axonal or demyelinating. For example, the most common form of CMT, CMT1A, typically shows marked and uniform reduction of motor and sensory conduction velocities (typically 10–30 m/s). Hereditary neuropathy with liability for pressure palsies shows milder slowing of conduction velocities, but frequently shows focal slowing or conduction block at common sites of entrapment. Classification of the disease as axonal or demyelinating can frequently limit the genetic testing required, as the common mutations causing CMT1 (demyelinating) are in general different than those causing CMT2 (axonal).

Diagnosis

CMT is usually suspected when there is a family history of peripheral neuropathy, as most forms of CMT are autosomal-dominant. Less commonly, CMT can be X-linked, autosomal-recessive, or sporadic. Approximately two-thirds of CMT is type 1, and approximately two-thirds of CMT1 is CMT1A, caused by duplication of the peripheral myelin protein 22 gene. The most common cause of axonal CMT (CMT2A) is caused by mutations in the mitofusin2 gene; as its name implies, mitofusion regulates fusion of mitochondria, a process thought to be important in the maintenance of axonal health. Although treatments are not yet available for specific forms of CMT, genetic testing can potentially give a definitive diagnosis not available by any other means and can obviate invasive testing (eg, nerve biopsy) and unnecessary treatment (eg, intravenous gammaglobulin). Genetic testing also has important implications for other family members and family planning and should be performed along with genetic counseling. When nerve biopsy is performed in CMT1 patients, they typically show the classic appearance of "onion bulbs" (see **Fig.** 1C′), caused by severe, chronic demyelination and remyelination.

NEUROPATHIES ASSOCIATED WITH AMYLOID PROTEIN

Amyloids are insoluble aggregates of various proteins that share common 3-dimensional structure of β-pleated sheets and are resistant to proteolytic decomposition. Amyloidosis refers to a variety of conditions whereby amyloid protein accumulates in any organ, including peripheral nerves, leading to dysfunction. Amyloid deposits have characteristic apple-green birefringence when stained with Congo red and seen under a polarizing microscope and may be detected on nerve biopsy (**Fig. 4**). Amyloidosis can be either acquired or hereditary. Acquired amyloidosis can be due to abnormal protein accumulation in the setting of

multiple myeloma, Waldenstrom macroglobulinemia, lymphoma, or lymphoproliferative disorders. Polyneuropathy develops in about 30% of patients with acquired primary amyloidosis, which can be a presenting symptom.[29] There is a predilection for small-fiber neuropathy causing a painful burning sensation in the distal limbs. Nerve conduction study typically shows a symmetric, length-dependent sensorimotor polyneuropathy; however, some patients present with asymmetric, multiple mononeuropathies. In the case of primary amyloidosis, carpal tunnel syndrome is also very common. Familial amyloidosis is most commonly caused by mutations in the transthyretin gene, but rarely can be caused by mutations in apolipoprotein A1 or gelsolin.

TOXIC NEUROPATHY

From a practical perspective, it is often difficult to prove causality when a toxic neuropathy is suspected.[30] However, finding the cause should not be neglected, as toxic neuropathy is one of those conditions whereby treatments are available, if diagnosed timely. Although many clinicians regard

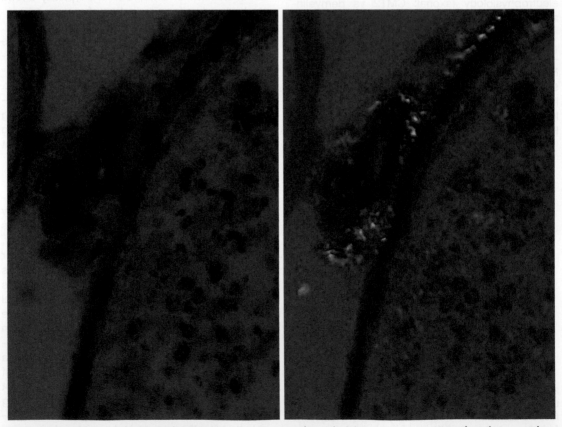

Fig. 4. Congo red stain shows apple-green birefringence under polarizing microscope. Note that the amorphous birefringent material invades into the vessel wall.

toxic neuropathy as a diagnosis of exclusion, it was found to be very helpful to use quantitative measurement tools, such as the TNS to appreciate the temporal relation of disease's severity and a suspected toxin better. In some chemotherapy-induced neuropathies, TNS is shown to correlate with the dose of chemotherapeutic agents, validating its use to establish causality.[7]

Most toxic neuropathies cause distal, length-dependent peripheral neuropathy, regardless of toxin. As briefly mentioned in the previous section, neurotoxins affect entire length of nerve, from its cell body to terminal axon, affecting more severely in the distal portion. This "dying-back" neuropathy is very common in most forms of neuropathy, making toxic neuropathy difficult to diagnose. Hence, other systemic features can be a clue to diagnose certain toxic neuropathies. For example, toxic neuropathy due to arsenic poisoning can show not only typical length-dependent neuropathy, but also systemic symptoms, such as gastrointestinal symptoms, psychosis, and/or Mee's line in fingernails. Toxins that can cause neuropathy and its pathophysiologic characteristics are summarized in **Table 4**.

NEUROPATHIES ASSOCIATED WITH AUTOIMMUNE DISEASE
Sjogren Syndrome

Peripheral neuropathy is present in 10% to 22% of all patients with Sjogren syndrome.[31,32] Common forms of neuropathy include length-dependent axonal sensorimotor neuropathy, small-fiber neuropathy, and sensory neuronopathy.

Rheumatoid Arthritis

About 50% of patients with rheumatoid arthritis are reported to have neuropathy, most frequently due to entrapment.[33] Vasculitic neuropathy can also develop in patients with rheumatoid arthritis, making it the third most common cause of vasculitic neuropathy in one case series,[34] after polyarteritis nodosa and isolated peripheral nervous system vasculitis. It is also important to rule out toxic neuropathy related to disease-modifying anti-rheumatic drugs.

Systemic Sclerosis

Although sensory complaints are common and reported in up to 50% of scleroderma patients, the prevalence of polyneuropathy is thought to be low.[35,36] Multiple mononeuropathies have been described in patients with CREST (calcinosis, Raynaud phenomenon, esophageal dysmotility, sclerodactyly, and telangiectasia) syndrome.

Systemic Lupus Erythematosus

Systemic lupus erythematosus (SLE) is a relatively common multisystem disease, often affecting the nervous system. Although SLE more frequently affects the central nervous system, about a quarter of patients with SLE are reported to have peripheral neuropathy.[37] Patients typically complain of

Table 4		
Common toxins that can cause neuropathy		
Toxins	**Clinical Features**	**Pathophysiology**
Vinca alkaloids	Symmetric, sensorimotor, large-fiber and small-fiber polyneuropathy	Mixed axonal degeneration and demyelination
Cisplatin	Predominantly large-fiber sensory neuronopathy	Sensory neuronopathy
Taxanes	Symmetric, predominantly sensory polyneuropathy	Axonal degeneration
Amiodarone	Severe proximal and distal weakness, affecting legs more than arms	Demyelinating
Colchicine	Proximal weakness from concomitant myopathy and loss of touch/vibratory sensation	Axonal degeneration
Lead	Insidious-onset, progressive weakness in upper extremities, with minimal sensory involvement; gastrointestinal symptoms, bluish-black line coloration of gums ("lead line")	Axonal degeneration
Alcohol	Slowly progressive parasthesia, numbness, and burning pain, more severe in legs; autonomic dysfunction is common	Generalized sensorimotor, primarily axonal polyneuropathy

slowly progressive distal sensory loss. Multiple mononeuropathies are reported, but seem to be less common.

Mixed Connective Tissue Disease

A mild distal axonal sensorimotor polyneuropathy reportedly occurs in about 10% of patients.[38]

Sarcoidosis

The central and peripheral nervous system can be affected in sarcoidosis. Characteristically, cranial nerves are frequently involved, mostly commonly the facial nerve. In one study, clinical features of 57 patients with sarcoid neuropathy were analyzed; the most common pattern was mono-phasic, asymmetric, and non-length-dependent.[39]

Celiac Disease

About 10% of patients with celiac disease have neurologic complications, with ataxia and periph-eral neuropathy being most common. The periph-eral neuropathy associated with celiac disease manifests as distal sensory.[40] Generalized senso-rimotor polyneuropathy, motor neuropathy, multi-ple mononeuropathies, autonomic neuropathy, and neuromyotonia are also reported.

Inflammatory Bowel Disease

Ulcerative colitis and Crohn disease are inflamma-tory disorders of the bowel associated with various neurologic complications, including peripheral neuropathy. AIDP, CIDP, sensory neuropathy, sen-sorimotor neuropathy, small-fiber neuropathy, bra-chial plexopathy, multiple mononeuropathies, and cranial neuropathy have been reported.[41]

Primary Biliary Sclerosis

Peripheral neuropathy associated with primary biliary sclerosis is characterized by distal numb-ness and tingling. Large-fiber sensory modalities are predominantly affected by primary biliary sclerosis.[42]

Hypereosinophilic Syndrome

A generalized peripheral neuropathy of multiple mononeuropathies occurs in 6% to 14% of pa-tients with hypereosinophiic syndrome.[43]

NEUROPATHIES ASSOCIATED WITH INFECTION
Leprosy

Leprosy is caused by the acid-fast bacteria *Myco-bacterium leprae* and is the most common cause of peripheral neuropathy in the developing world, including Southeast Asia, Africa, and South Amer-ica. A slowly progressive sensorimotor polyneurop-athy gradually develops because of widespread invasion of the bacilli into the nerve fibers.[44]

Lyme Disease

Lyme disease is caused by infection with *Borrelia burgdorferi*, which is transmitted by ticks. There are 3 stages of Lyme disease: the first stage be-ing early infection with erythema migrans; the second stage being disseminated infection; and the third stage being late infection. Neurologic complications may develop during the second and third stages of infection. Various neuropa-thies can occur with Lyme disease, facial neurop-athy being most common. Mononeuropathies, polyradiculopathy, and plexopathy are also asso-ciated with Lyme disease.[45] The presentation of polyradiculopathy may resemble GBS. It is also important to note that false-positive results of Lyme serology tests are common, and therefore, Western blot must be performed to confirm the results.

Diphtheritic Neuropathy

Diphtheritic neuropathy is caused by a toxin re-leased by the bacteria, *Corynebacterium diphther-iae*. Cranial nerves can be affected 3 to 4 weeks after the infection. Generalized polyneuropathy may develop 2 to 3 months following the initial symptom presentation.

Human Immunodeficiency Virus

HIV infection can cause various neurologic com-plications, including peripheral neuropathy. About 20% of patients with HIV infection develop neurop-athy as a result of virus infection itself, opportunistic infections, such as cytomegalovirus infection, or neurotoxicity from antiviral medications. The most common forms of HIV-related peripheral neuropa-thies include distal symmetric polyneuropathy, in-flammatory demyelinating polyneuropathy (either acute or chronic), multiple mononeuropathies, pol-yradiculopathy, autonomic neuropathy, and sen-sory ganglinitis.[46] Among them, distal symmetric polyneuropathy is the most common form and is usually seen in patients with AIDS. Acute inflamma-tory demyelinating polyneuropathy can occur at the time of seroconversion.

Human T-lymphocyte Type 1 Virus

Human T-lymphocyte type 1 virus is associated with an axonal, length-dependent, sensorimotor polyneuropathy, which can be seen in the absence of myelopathy.[47]

Cytomegalovirus

Cytomegalovirus can cause acute lumbosacral polyradiculopathy and multiple mononeuropathies in immunocompromised patients.

Epstein-Barr Virus

Epstein-Barr virus is associated with acute inflammatory demyelinating neuropathy, cranial neuropathy, multiple mononeuropathies, brachial plexopathy, lumbosacral radiculoplexopathy, and sensory neuronopathies.

Varicella-zoster Virus

Varicella-zoster virus can cause neuropathy because of reactivation of latent virus or a primary infection. Primary infection causes "chicken pox" and reactivation of the virus later in life results in dermal zoster. Most adult patients develop severe pain and parasethesias in a dermatomal region with a vesicular rash. Some patients also develop muscle weakness in the same myotomal area. Rarely, patients with varicella-zoster virus develop acute inflammatory demyelinating neuropathy.

Hepatitis B and C Viruses

Hepatitis B and C viruses can cause vasculitic neuropathy, often associated with cryoglobulinemia.

NEUROPATHIES ASSOCIATED WITH MALIGNANCY
Paraneoplastic Neuropathy

Paraneoplastic neuropathy is relatively rare and most commonly associated with lung cancer. In particular, paraneoplastic sensory neuronopathy/ganglinopathy most commonly occurs with small cell lung cancer (often associated with anti-Hu antibody) and can precede the diagnosis of cancer by 4 to 12 months.[48–50] The causes of sensory neuronopathy are limited, and on recognition, should prompt a thorough evaluation for malignancy. In addition, symmetric, sensorimotor polyneuropathy and paraneoplastic autonomic neuropathy can develop in patients with underlying cancer.

Neuropathy Secondary to Tumor Infiltration

Direct infiltration of tumor cells into leptomeninges, cranial nerves, and nerve roots can cause peripheral nervous system dysfunction, which is particularly common with leukemia and lymphoma, resulting in mononeuropathy, multiple mononeuropathies, polyradiculopathy, plexopathy, and generalized symmetric distal or proximal polyneuropathy. Polyradiculopathies are especially common, and MR imaging may show compression of multiple nerve roots by the tumor.

Peripheral Neuropathies Associated with Lymphoproliferative Disorders

There is an increased incidence of peripheral neuropathy in patients with monoclonal gammopathies, and there is a well-established causal relationship between IgM monoclonal gammopathy and demyelinating sensorimotor polyneuropathy.[51] Antibodies against myelin-associated glycoprotein are found in patients with lymphoproliferative disorders or plasmacytomas, whereas IgA and IgG monoclonal gammopathies are much less common. Multiple myeloma is commonly related to distal axonal, sensorimotor polyneuropathy. Osteosclerotic myeloma is rare, but commonly associated with polyneuropathy, sometimes simultaneously presenting with hepatosplenomegaly, cutaneous pigmentation, hypertrichosis, edema, pericardial and pleural effusions, so-called POEMS syndrome. POEMS syndrome is also known to be associated with Castleman disease (angiofollicular lymph node hyperplasia).

Graft-versus-host Disease

Graft-versus-host disease can cause various immune-mediated disorders, including the one against the peripheral nervous system. GBS, multiple mononeuropathies, and cranial neuropathy have been reported in patients with graft-versus-host disease.[52]

SUMMARY

Peripheral nerves are affected by a broad spectrum of disorders. With technical advances that permit high-resolution MR, peripheral neuroimaging is gaining utility in evaluation of peripheral nerve disorders. MR neurography is especially useful in evaluating proximal nerve lesions that are not easily assessable with nerve conduction study; for example, MR neurography will not only provide better diagnosis of a tumor compressing the brachial plexus than an electrophysiological study but also aid neurosurgeons in their plan for treatment. However, it is important for radiologists to have an understanding of the various peripheral nervous disorders and communicate the findings to the referring physicians including neurologists and neurosurgeons for optimal patient management.

REFERENCES

1. Chhabra A, Andreisek G, Soldatos T, et al. MR neurography: past, present, and future. AJR Am J Roentgenol 2011;197:583–91.

2. Thawait SK, Chaudhry V, Thawait GK, et al. High-resolution MR neurography of diffuse peripheral nerve lesions. AJNR Am J Neuroradiol 2011;32: 1365–72.

3. Williams IR, Gilliatt RW. Regeneration distal to a prolonged conduction block. J Neurol Sci 1977; 33:267–73.

4. Gutmann E, Holubar J. The degeneration of peripheral nerve fibers. J Neurol Neurosurg Psychiatry 1950;13:89–105.

5. Seddon HJ, Medawar PB, Smith H. Rate of regeneration of peripheral nerves in man. J Physiol 1943; 102:191–215.

6. Cornblath DR, Chaudhry V, Carter K, et al. Total neuropathy score: validation and reliability study. Neurology 1999;53:1660–4.

7. Cavaletti G, Frigeni B, Lanzani F, et al. The Total Neuropathy Score as an assessment tool for grading the course of chemotherapy-induced peripheral neurotoxicity: comparison with the National Cancer Institute-Common Toxicity Scale. J Peripher Nerv Syst 2007;12:210–5.

8. Dyck PJ, Kratz KM, Karnes JL, et al. The prevalence by staged severity of various types of diabetic neuropathy, retinopathy, and nephropathy in a population-based cohort: the Rochester Diabetic Neuropathy Study. Neurology 1993;43: 817–24.

9. Dyck PJ, Norell JE. Microvasculitis and ischemia in diabetic lumbosacral radiculoplexus neuropathy. Neurology 1999;53:2113–21.

10. Said G, Elgrably F, Lacroix C, et al. Painful proximal diabetic neuropathy: inflammatory nerve lesions and spontaneous favorable outcome. Ann Neurol 1997;41:762–70.

11. Nemni R, Bottacchi E, Fazio R, et al. Polyneuropathy in hypothyroidism: clinical, electrophysiological and morphological findings in four cases. J Neurol Neurosurg Psychiatry 1987;50: 1454–60.

12. Ogura T, Makinodan A, Kubo T, et al. Electrophysiological course of uraemic neuropathy in haemodialysis patients. Postgrad Med J 2001; 77:451–4.

13. Chaudhry V, Corse AM, O'Brien R, et al. Autonomic and peripheral (sensorimotor) neuropathy in chronic liver disease: a clinical and electrophysiologic study. Hepatology 1999;29:1698–703.

14. Yuki N, Hartung HP. Guillain-Barre syndrome. N Engl J Med 2012;366:2294–304.

15. Griffin JW, Li CY, Ho TW, et al. Guillain-Barre syndrome in northern China. The spectrum of neuropathological changes in clinically defined cases. Brain 1995;118(Pt 3):577–95.

16. Paparounas K. Anti-GQ1b ganglioside antibody in peripheral nervous system disorders:

pathophysiologic role and clinical relevance. Arch Neurol 2004;61:1013–6.

17. Ogawara K, Kuwabara S, Mori M, et al. Axonal Guillain-Barre syndrome: relation to anti-ganglioside antibodies and Campylobacter jejuni infection in Japan. Ann Neurol 2000;48:624–31.

18. Lawn ND, Fletcher DD, Henderson RD, et al. Anticipating mechanical ventilation in Guillain-Barre syndrome. Arch Neurol 2001;58:893–8.

19. Cornblath DR, Mellits ED, Griffin JW, et al. Motor conduction studies in Guillain-Barre syndrome: description and prognostic value. Ann Neurol 1988;23:354–9.

20. McKhann GM, Griffin JW, Cornblath DR, et al. Plasmapheresis and Guillain-Barre syndrome: analysis of prognostic factors and the effect of plasmapheresis. Ann Neurol 1988;23:347–53.

21. Fletcher DD, Lawn ND, Wolter TD, et al. Long-term outcome in patients with Guillain-Barre syndrome requiring mechanical ventilation. Neurology 2000; 54:2311–5.

22. Koller H, Kieseier BC, Jander S, et al. Chronic inflammatory demyelinating polyneuropathy. N Engl J Med 2005;352:1343–56.

23. Ginsberg L, Platts AD, Thomas PK. Chronic inflammatory demyelinating polyneuropathy mimicking a lumbar spinal stenosis syndrome. J Neurol Neurosurg Psychiatry 1995;59:189–91.

24. Adams D, Kuntzer T, Burger D, et al. Predictive value of anti-GM1 ganglioside antibodies in neuromuscular diseases: a study of 180 sera. J Neuroimmunol 1991;32:223–30.

25. Latov N. Pathogenesis and therapy of neuropathies associated with monoclonal gammopathies. Ann Neurol 1995;37(Suppl 1):S32–42.

26. Burns TM, Schaublin GA, Dyck PJ. Vasculitic neuropathies. Neurol Clin 2007;25:89–113.

27. Lloyd TE, Chaudhry V. Treatment and management of hereditary neuropathies. In: Bertorini T, editor. Neuromuscular disorders: treatment and management. Philadelphia: Elsevier; 2011. p. 191–213.

28. Patzko A, Shy ME. Charcot-Marie-Tooth disease and related genetic neuropathies. Continuum (Minneap Minn) 2012;18:39–59.

29. Kelly JJ Jr, Kyle RA, O'Brien PC, et al. The natural history of peripheral neuropathy in primary systemic amyloidosis. Ann Neurol 1979;6:1–7.

30. Morrison B, Chaudhry V. Medication, toxic, and vitamin-related neuropathies. Continuum (Minneap Minn) 2012;18:139–60.

31. Gemignani F, Marbini A, Pavesi G, et al. Peripheral neuropathy associated with primary Sjogren's syndrome. J Neurol Neurosurg Psychiatry 1994;57: 983–6.

32. Lopate G, Pestronk A, Al-Lozi M, et al. Peripheral neuropathy in an outpatient cohort of patients

with Sjogren's syndrome. Muscle Nerve 2006;33: 672–6.

33. Chamberlain MA, Bruckner FE. Rheumatoid neuropathy. Clinical and electrophysiological features. Ann Rheum Dis 1970;29:609–16.

34. Scott DG, Bacon PA, Tribe CR. Systemic rheumatoid vasculitis: a clinical and laboratory study of 50 cases. Medicine (Baltimore) 1981;60: 288–97.

35. Averbuch-Heller L, Steiner I, Abramsky O. Neurologic manifestations of progressive systemic sclerosis. Arch Neurol 1992;49:1292–5.

36. Poncelet AN, Connolly MK. Peripheral neuropathy in scleroderma. Muscle Nerve 2003;28:330–5.

37. Sivri A, Hascelik Z, Celiker R, et al. Early detection of neurological involvement in systemic lupus erythematosus patients. Electromyogr Clin Neurophysiol 1995;35:195–9.

38. Rosenbaum R. Neuromuscular complications of connective tissue diseases. Muscle Nerve 2001; 24:154–69.

39. Burns TM, Dyck PJ, Aksamit AJ. The natural history and long-term outcome of 57 limb sarcoidosis neuropathy cases. J Neurol Sci 2006;244:77–87.

40. Chin RL, Sander HW, Brannagan TH, et al. Celiac neuropathy. Neurology 2003;60:1581–5.

41. Gondim FA, Brannagan TH 3rd, Sander HW, et al. Peripheral neuropathy in patients with inflammatory bowel disease. Brain 2005;128:867–79.

42. Charron L, Peyronnard JM, Marchand L. Sensory neuropathy associated with primary biliary cirrhosis. Histologic and morphometric studies. Arch Neurol 1980;37:84–7.

43. Dorfman LJ, Ransom BR, Forno LS, et al. Neuropathy in the hypereosinophilic syndrome. Muscle Nerve 1983;6:291–8.

44. Ooi WW, Srinivasan J. Leprosy and the peripheral nervous system: basic and clinical aspects. Muscle Nerve 2004;30:393–409.

45. Halperin J, Luft BJ, Volkman DJ, et al. Lyme neuroborreliosis. Peripheral nervous system manifestations. Brain 1990;113(Pt 4):1207–21.

46. Barohn RJ, Gronseth GS, LeForce BR, et al. Peripheral nervous system involvement in a large cohort of human immunodeficiency virus-infected individuals. Arch Neurol 1993;50:167–71.

47. Kiwaki T, Umehara F, Arimura Y, et al. The clinical and pathological features of peripheral neuropathy accompanied with HTLV-I associated myelopathy. J Neurol Sci 2003;206:17–21.

48. Amato AA, Collins MP. Neuropathies associated with malignancy. Semin Neurol 1998;18:125–44.

49. Denny-Brown D. Primary sensory neuropathy with muscular changes associated with carcinoma. J Neurol Neurosurg Psychiatry 1948;11:73–87.

50. Dalmau J, Graus F, Rosenblum MK, et al. Anti-Hu–associated paraneoplastic encephalomyelitis/sensory neuronopathy. A clinical study of 71 patients. Medicine (Baltimore) 1992;71:59–72.

51. Latov N, Sherman WH, Nemni R, et al. Plasma-cell dyscrasia and peripheral neuropathy with a monoclonal antibody to peripheral-nerve myelin. N Engl J Med 1980;303:618–21.

52. Amato AA, Barohn RJ, Sahenk Z, et al. Polyneuropathy complicating bone marrow and solid organ transplantation. Neurology 1993;43:1513–8.

Magnetic Resonance Neurography
Technical Considerations

Avneesh Chhabra, MD[a],*, Aaron Flammang, MBA[b],
Abraham Padua Jr, RT[c], John A. Carrino, MD, MPH[d],
Gustav Andreisek, MD[e]

KEYWORDS

- MR neurography • MRN • Technique • 3 T • 1.5 T

KEY POINTS

- Magnetic resonance (MR) neurography (MRN) is a technically demanding examination requiring the knowledge of appropriate clinical questions, regional nerves, and perineural anatomy as well as the various available MR imaging pulse sequences.
- A good MRN examination should involve the referring clinician, protocoling radiologist, performing technologist, as well as the patient and interpreting radiologist as a team, and should follow the guidelines presented in this article.

INTRODUCTION

Magnetic resonance (MR) neurography (MRN) is a technique to enhance peripheral nerve visualization with a variety of available high-resolution and high-contrast nerve-nonselective and nerve-selective imaging pulse sequences. MRN has been performed for more than 2 decades with great emphasis being on two-dimensional (2D) imaging.[1,2] Although 2D imaging remains the standard for the primary examination interpretation, high-quality three-dimensional (3D) imaging is essential for display and problem solving when current clinical and imaging evaluations show unclear or ambiguous results. A good MRN technique should enhance the visualization of peripheral nerves in various planes to provide assistance to the referring physician in understanding the disease process and its localization.[3] This article discusses the technical considerations of MRN, various imaging pulse sequences available on current clinical scanners, as well as their relative advantages and disadvantages. In addition, a guide to the optimal use of high-resolution and high-contrast imaging technique is provided, which will aid clinicians in attaining a good-quality examination.

ESSENTIALS OF MRN TECHNIQUE

A good MRN examination should involve the referring clinician, protocoling radiologist, performing technologist, as well as the patient and interpreting

Disclosures: A.C. acknowledges research grant support from GE-AUR, Siemens, Integra Life Sciences. A.C. also serves as MSK CAD development consultant with Siemens. G.A. is coapplicant for US patent (USPTO Number 12/947,256); has received grants from SNSF, Holcim, and Siemens; is PI, Co-PI or sub-PI in several third-party–funded clinical trials (Millennium Pharmaceuticals, Eli Lilly, GlaxoSmithKline, Cytheris SA, Roche, BioChemics, Novartis, Bristol-Meyers Squibb, TopoTarget, and Merck Sharp & Dohme); and his department receives grants from Bayer, GE, Phillips, Cordis, and Guerbet.

[a] The University of Texas Southwestern, 5323 Harry Hines Blvd, Dallas, TX 75390, USA; [b] Siemens AG, Health-care sector - MRI, Erlangen, Germany; [c] Siemens Healthcare, Malvern, Pennsylvania, USA; [d] The Russell H. Morgan Department of Radiology and Radiological Science, The Johns Hopkins Hospital, Baltimore, Maryland; [e] Department of Radiology, University Hospital Zurich, Ramistrasse 100, Zurich, CH 8091, Switzerland
* Corresponding author.
E-mail address: avneesh.chhabra@utsouthwestern.edu

Neuroimag Clin N Am 24 (2014) 67–78
http://dx.doi.org/10.1016/j.nic.2013.03.032
1052-5149/14/$ – see front matter © 2014 Elsevier Inc. All rights reserved.

radiologist as a team and should follow the guidelines presented in this article.

Referring Clinician

Close interaction between the referring clinician and radiologists is important for good interpretation of image findings. Clinicians should be informed about the technical limitation of MR imaging including the maximum size of field of view (FOV) as well as that the greater the anatomy to be covered, the longer the examination usually takes. Especially in older patients with peripheral neuropathies (eg, with tremor), reduced image quality must be expected. The use of gadolinium-based contrast agents should be discussed with regard to the various indications. In addition, preferred reconstructions should be discussed because some clinicians like maximum-intensity projections (MIPs) or 3D reconstructions. Although the latter may or may not useful for the radiologist's interpretation, they might be an important preoperative guide for surgeons.

Patient Coaching

The technologist plays an important role in patient coaching for successful performance of the examination. The patient should fill out a form with most relevant acute/chronic complaints, any relevant electrodiagnostic information, history of diabetes mellitus/family history of neuropathy, and any prior regional nerve surgery, and so forth. A marker should ideally be placed at the most symptomatic site, and the patient should be asked to remain still during the image acquisition, as well as to breathe normally. The extremity should be well padded and coil(s) tightly wrapped around it to restrict motion during the examination. The urinary bladder should be voided in pelvic or lumbosacral (LS) plexus imaging because it interferes with the MIP images.

Scanner

The imaging is ideally performed on a 3-T scanner to make use of the higher signal/noise ratio (SNR) available on these scanners. Higher SNR translates into higher contrast and potentially faster imaging, and the slice thickness is kept to a minimum (Fig. 1). Minimal slice thickness results in excellent through-plane resolution for 2D sequences and thinner isotropic resolution for 3D imaging. If 3 T scanners are not available, 1.5 T can be used, with some drawbacks such as limits with respect to 3D imaging capability and prolonged examination times. Nevertheless, the authors encourage the use of MRN techniques for 1.5 T as well, because they show better performance than standard MR imaging techniques. Use of 1.5 T might even be advantageous, such as in patients with metal in the imaging FOV, for whom 3 T is expected to produce artifacts.[4]

Coil Selection

Dedicated multichannel joint coils should be used in extremities for tunnel imaging (carpal, cubital, and tarsal tunnel) and proper use of parallel imaging should be used with acceleration factors of 2 to 3. For additional contiguous area imaging, multichannel flex (surface or body matrix) coils can be tightly wrapped around the larger extremity portion, such as upper arm, forearm, or thigh and can be combined with joint-specific coils, if needed. Clinicians should not try to wrap the joint and extremity together and image them both in the same FOV, because this produces low-quality images with a lot of blank (air) space around the region of interest. For pelvic, LS, or brachial plexus imaging, the spine array coils can be combined with body array coils on the front of the patient; in some systems, dedicated array designs may be used.

FOV

FOV should be determined based on the physician request and should be kept as small as possible, both in longitudinal and transverse planes, to obtain high-resolution imaging. Therefore, clinicians should describe the location of the lesion as precisely as possible (discussed earlier). However, lesion localization is often difficult clinically and, this is frequently the main indication for the imaging. Blank space around the extremity should be no more than approximately 20% of the diameter of the extremity for optimal assessment of small nerves. However, this method may result in wraparound artifacts, especially in off-center imaging. Phase oversampling or fold-over suppression techniques may be used to avoid such artifacts (Fig. 2). In the case of nonspecific or nonlocalizing symptoms, the radiologist should make use of all available clinical and electrodiagnostic test information to best tailor the high-resolution examination across the known injury or entrapment sites of the extremity and perform the remaining examination as well-spaced images (axial and coronal thickness 5–6 mm) to keep the imaging time of the study short and within acceptable limits (less than 45–60 minutes).

2D Imaging

High-quality 2D imaging with both non–fat-suppressed T1-weighted (W) and fat-suppressed fluid-sensitive T2-W images is essential. These

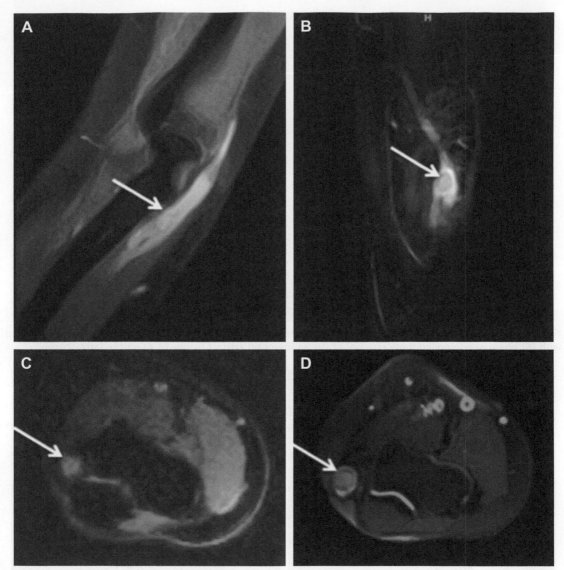

Fig. 1. 1.5 T versus 3 T: oblique coronal (*A*) and axial (*C*) fat-suppressed T2–weighted (W) images on 1.5-T scanner and similar plane 3D SPAIR (spectral adiabatic inversion recovery) SPACE (sampling perfection with application optimized contrasts using different flip angle evolution) (*B*) and axial T2 SPAIR (*D*) images on 3-T scanner show higher resolution and better delineation of the target sign (*arrows*) on the latter images in a known case of ulnar nerve schwannomatosis.

images should be sequential and ideally be obtained at similar table positions to allow the reader to evaluate the images with different tissue contrasts in tandem for various intraneural and perineural nerve anatomic and pathologic imaging characteristics.[5,6] In case of patient motion, the imaging should be repeated and patient coaching may be required. The coronal and sagittal planes should be obtained in long axes, parallel and perpendicular to the extremity and not the body. For smaller nerves in the hindfoot, nerve-perpendicular, oblique axial images across the

axis of calcaneus are useful for optimal evaluation of medial plantar, lateral plantar, and calcaneal nerves (**Fig. 3**).[7] It is usually helpful for the radiologist to control the correct image planes during the MR examination and to adjust or add planes and sequences, respectively.

2D Imaging Parameters

Axial images should have in-plane resolution of 0.3 to 0.4 mm and should not have slice thicknesses of more than 2 to 3 mm in distal extremities, and no

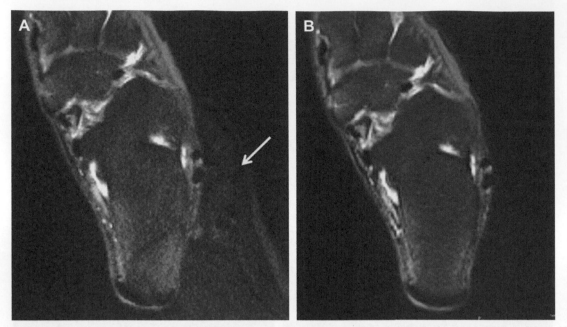

Fig. 2. Wraparound artifacts: axial T2 SPAIR images through lower aspect of the tarsal tunnel without (*A*) and with (*B*) phase oversampling show removal of the wraparound artifact (*arrow* in *A*) on the latter image.

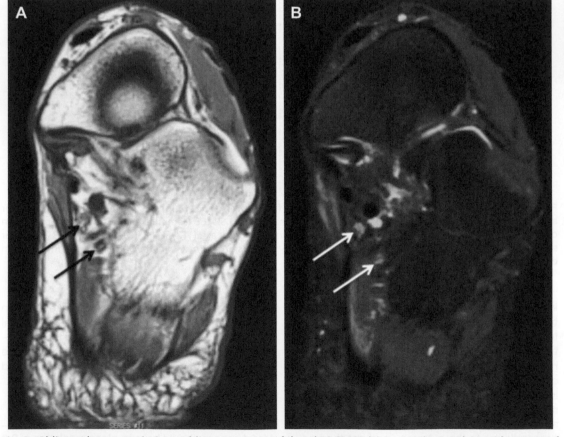

Fig. 3. Oblique plane prescriptions: oblique axial T1-W (*A*) and T2 SPAIR (*B*) images in a patient with suspected tarsal tunnel syndrome show abnormally hyperintense medial and lateral plantar nerves (*arrows*) in their respective canals, separated by the fibrous septum.

more than 4 to 5 mm in proximal extremities with minimal or no interslice gap. For fluid-sensitive T2-W images, the fat suppression should be homogeneous and the effective echo time (TE) should be 60 to 70 milliseconds to minimize magic angle artifacts. Axial short tau inversion recovery (STIR) imaging is not routinely used in our practice, but if used in cases of failed fat suppression, should have a lower TE (30–50 milliseconds) to maintain good SNR. Dixon-type fat suppression is a good alternative in regions with inhomogeneous fat suppression using standard techniques (discussed later). The echo train length can vary from 3 to 8 for T1-W, 8 to 22 for T2-W, and 44 to 68 for 3D imaging. Parallel imaging with an acceleration factor of 2 to 3 is frequently used.

3D Imaging

3D imaging is essential for good multiplanar nerve display and is currently available as high-contrast spin-echo type multislab acquisition on most vendor types. 3D imaging can be obtained with or without fat suppression. For non–fat-suppressed 3D T2-W imaging, the effective TE should be more than 90 milliseconds (ideally 100–105 milliseconds), and for 3-D fat-saturated (fs) T2 W imaging, effective TE can be lowered to 60 to 80 milliseconds. It can be obtained in acceptable imaging times of 5 to 6 minutes with isotropic resolution of 1 to 1.5 mm. MIP with or without curved planar reconstructions from 3D fsT2 W imaging allows excellent nerve visualization, and the abnormal nerve and the related lesion is easier to depict because the nerve gets brighter with

abnormality (Fig. 4).[8,9] Gradient echo–type 3D imaging should be avoided because it is more prone to susceptibility artifacts and produces poorer contrast. However, it is frequently used with contrast imaging to obtain isotropic multiplanar depiction of contrast-enhancing lesions (Fig. 5). With the addition of diffusion weighting, nerve-selective and functional images can be obtained with effective vascular signal suppression, as discussed later. Shimming is essential for any diffusion imaging to obtain the maximum field homogeneity and good fat suppression.

Semiautomatic Multiplanar Image Reconstructions

Technologist-generated after-scan semiautomatic multiplanar image reconstructions are useful in decreasing the image interpretation times of radiologists. Thick-slab (12–20 mm) predefined curved planar and multiplanar reconstructions (Fig. 6) are useful to show the nerve along its long axis for excellent depiction of course alterations, discontinuity, and lesions along its long axis.[9,10] These images can be obtained from nerve-nonselective as well as nerve-selective images, and it is advantageous to know that the more the nerve is abnormal; the easier it is to show the abnormality on these images.

RELATIVE MERITS OF AVAILABLE PULSE SEQUENCES
Axial T1-W Sequence

This is an essential pulse sequence and can be obtained as spin-echo or fluid-attenuated inversion

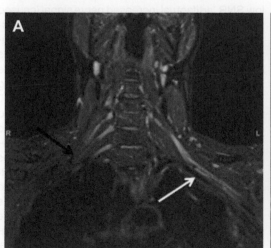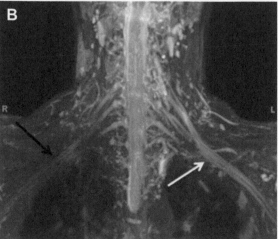

Fig. 4. 3D isotropic imaging in left brachial plexopathy. Coronal 3D STIR SPACE (original acquisition, *A*) and MIP reconstruction (*B*) show asymmetric hyperintensity and enlargement of the left C6 nerve, upper trunk, and distal segments of the left brachial plexus (*white arrows*) in this patient with radiation neuropathy. Compare with normal brachial plexus on the right (*black arrows*).

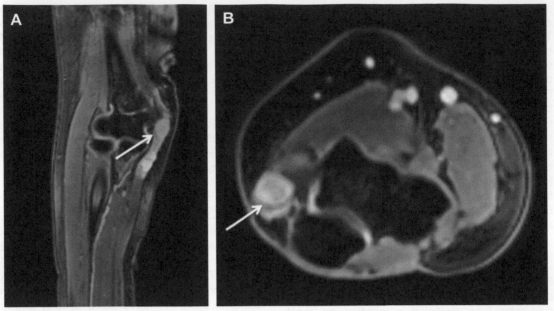

Fig. 5. 3D postcontrast isotropic imaging. Same subject as in Fig. 1. Multiplanar depiction of the enhancing lesion (*arrows*) on postcontrast isotropic fat-suppressed T1 3D gradient echo (coronal, *A*) and (axial, *B*) images.

recovery image. It should have in-plane resolution of 0.3 to 0.4 mm. It is the best image to depict intraneural fat, perineurial and epineurial thickening, and effacement of perineural fat plane by mass lesion/focal fibrosis.[11] Regional muscle fatty infiltration and atrophy is also best depicted on these images.

Axial fs Fluid-sensitive Sequence

This is the best image to show the lesions as well as their relationship to normal or abnormal fascicles within the nerve. Options include fat-suppressed

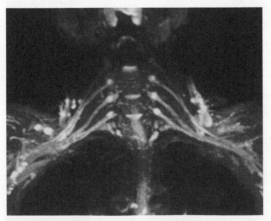

Fig. 6. Semiautomated, technologist-generated, thick-slab (18 mm) MIP image from 3D STIR SPACE along an angled coronal plane oriented in the cervical spine axis. Note the symmetric normal appearance of the bilateral brachial plexuses.

fast spin-echo T2-W sequence with inherent advantages of high contrast, minimal to no pulsation artifacts, and less susceptibility artifact. Frequency-selective fat suppression should be avoided with metal in the imaging FOV. The major disadvantage of the fsT2 W sequence is poor fat suppression in off-center areas or inhomogeneous fat suppression, especially along the extremity curvatures. STIR sequence has the advantages of excellent and uniform fat suppression; however, it is often marred by several disadvantages during routine use, such as frequent pulsation artifacts, low SNR, artifactual increased nerve signal (caused by better dynamic range of contrast and accentuated signal from endoneurial fluid), and long imaging times. It is heavily used for fat suppression as a fallback sequence if fat saturation fails for some reason, or if there is known metal in the FOV, using various modifications, such as lower TE (30–40 milliseconds) and higher echo train length and bandwidth (400–500 Hz/Px). T2 spectral adiabatic inversion recovery (SPAIR) is an excellent sequence for MRN examinations because it provides similar fat suppression as STIR in both well-centered and off-center areas with almost no pulsation artifacts and higher SNR (Fig. 7). It is also more responsive to specific absorption rate than STIR and produces an isointense nerve signal similar to the skeletal muscle signal in normal nerves. It comes in both weak and strong contrast types for user preferences. Although weak SPAIR fat saturation provides more homogeneity throughout the transverse imaging FOV, the strong

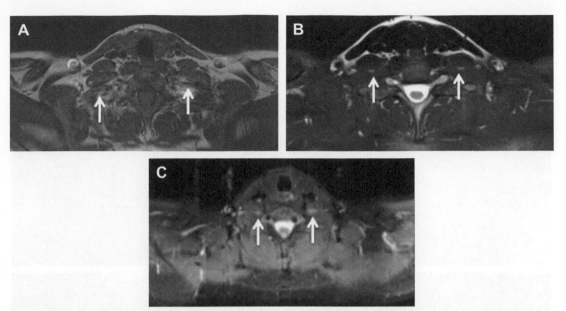

Fig. 7. 2D image comparison. Axial T1-W (*A*), T2 SPAIR (*B*), and STIR (*C*) images through the lower neck show high-resolution brachial plexus imaging at the level of the roots (*arrows*). Note the decreased SNR and pulsation artifacts on STIR imaging (*C*) and suboptimal fat suppression anteriorly on SPAIR imaging (*B*).

SPAIR pulse group produces more isointense signal to the nerve. It should be obtained with high resolution.[12] The main disadvantage is that it is sometimes partially degraded by poor fat suppression in the first couple of images at the extremes of FOV, especially in off-center areas. However, it is less sensitive than fsT2 W to susceptibility artifacts in the presence of metal; STIR is still preferred in these circumstances. Another disadvantage is that it is not available with all vendors. Water-selective fat suppression also produces good fluid-sensitive images and is currently used for 3D diffusion-weighted (DW) reversed steady-state free precession (PSIF) sequences, as discussed later. Similarly, Dixon type fat suppression produces excellent fat suppression for T2 W imaging with multiple images possible using the 2-point Dixon technique; however, is currently limited to only 2D imaging because of its long acquisition time (**Fig. 8**), and again fat suppression may be affected in the off-center areas.

Long-axis 2D Imaging

In addition to axial T1-W and fsT2-W imaging, 1 or more images of the long axis should be obtained (4–5 mm thick: coronal T1, eg, in pelvis; proton density [PD], eg, around extremity joints; or STIR, eg, in brachial and LS plexus) for global evaluation of the region of interest and exclusion of regional lesions as a potential cause of neurogenic symptoms.

3D Nonselective Nerve Imaging

3D isotropic imaging is available in a variety of contrasts and can be obtained in nerve-selective or nonselective fashion. The commonly used imaging pulse sequence is a nerve-nonselective type that involves turbo spin-echo–type acquisition. It was introduced only in the past few years by different vendors. Acronyms for these MR sequences are SPACE (sampling perfection with application optimized contrasts using different flip angle evolution, Siemens Health care, Erlangen, Germany), CUBE (GE Health care, Waukesha, WI), and VISTA (volumetric isotropic T2-weighted acquisition, Philips, Best, The Netherlands). Because thin slice 2D imaging is often affected by magnetization transfer–related cross talk among slices on high-field scanners, the 3D isotropic technique better allows thinner slices and multiplanar reconstructions from isotropic voxels. In addition, these can be obtained in a variety of contrasts (eg, PD, T1, T2), and can be used with fat-suppression techniques such as SPAIR and STIR. As an example, non–fat-suppressed T2 SPACE is often used for spine imaging as part of plexus evaluation because it allows isotropic spine reformats in multiple planes as well as showing the spinal cord and preganglionic intradural rootlets. It is also a good sequence to show anatomic variants of peripheral nerves, such as split sciatic nerves. However, the sequence is not recommended for the detection of nerve signal changes, which are in general better seen with fat-suppressed 3D

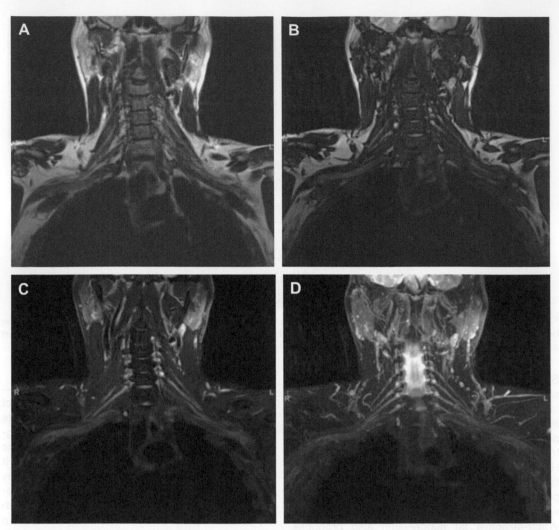

Fig. 8. Dixon imaging. Coronal brachial plexus imaging using 2-point Dixon method. Note the good 2D depiction of nerves on in-phase (*A*), opposed phase (*B*), water-only (*C*), and MIP water-only (*D*) images. Also note the flow artifact from subclavian veins bilaterally overlapping the plexuses.

imaging. In clinical routine, the authors heavily use 3D STIR SPACE for plexus imaging (because of better fat suppression) and 3D SPAIR SPACE for extremities (because of higher SNR).[3,8–10,13] These sequences allow curved and/or multiplanar reconstructions as well as creation of MIP images of the nerves for excellent display of normal and abnormal nerves along their long axes (see **Figs. 1**B, **4** and **6**). The main disadvantage of these sequences is frequent contamination with vessel signal caused by similar signal hyperintensity and, if not properly performed, the images may turn out to be grainy and noisy. For ideal performance, the coil selection as described earlier is important. In the author's experience, careful shimming helps, and the effective TE (whether kept as variable or constant evolution) should be in the range of 60 to 80 milliseconds, whereas recovery time (TR) is kept between 1500 and 2000 milliseconds. Although 3D STIR SPACE and SPAIR SPACE sequences are most widely used and are time tested, other sequences must be considered as works in progress, such as 3D PD SPACE with variable echo times, which has shown good image quality in the author's preliminary work (**Fig. 9**). It remains to be seen whether other MR techniques, such as Dixon in combination with SPACE, will be available in the future, and whether such sequences can be obtained in reasonable scan durations while providing the necessary isotropic spatial resolution as well good tissue contrast resolution.

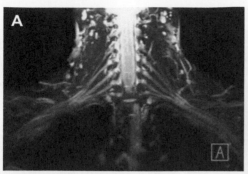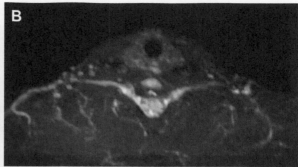

Fig. 9. PD variable SPACE. Coronal (*A*) and reconstructed axial (*B*) isotropic 3D STIR SPACE with PD variable contrast show the brachial plexus with good fat suppression and maintained SNR.

3D Selective Anatomic Nerve Imaging

Because saturation bands do not work well for obliquely coursing neurovascular bundles in extremities, any selective nerve imaging includes some sort of diffusion weighting (with a diffusion moment $\sim$80–200 s/mm^2) to suppress the flowing vascular signal and to enhance the relative nerve signal within the neurovascular bundle. As diffusion gradient is added to the 3D imaging, the SNR is reduced and the image quality can be degraded. The anatomic sequences include 3D DW PSIF, DW STIR SPACE, and simple monopolar or bipolar gradient DW imaging (DWI) with background tissue suppression.[14–16] 3D DW PSIF creates nice vessel-suppressed nerve-selective images in a 3D isotropic fashion (**Fig. 10**). Disadvantages include susceptibility to local inhomogeneities, sensitivity to motion artifacts, and being prone to poor fat suppression. Water-selective fat suppression currently works well with 3D DW PSIF with b values of $\sim$80 s/mm^2. DW SPACE allows a larger diffusion moment ($\sim$200 s/mm^2), but is currently only available for research purposes (**Fig. 11**). MIP images from DW PSIF and DW SPACE remove the added image noise from the diffusion gradients, and provide excellent nerve-selective depiction in both anatomic and pathologic states. With further pulse sequence development, Dixon-type fat suppression might be added to DW PSIF instead of water-selective fat suppression, or improvements might be made to DW SPACE sequences so that they can be obtained in acceptable time periods while keeping the advantages of nerve selectivity. Simple DWI imaging also produces good nerve-selective images with diffusion gradients applied perpendicular to the nerve axis, but, because of surrounding tissue suppression and low SNR, the relationship to the regional anatomy is usually not well seen and therefore these are not practical. In addition, not much functional information is attainable from these images.

3D Selective Functional Nerve Imaging

Functional imaging of the peripheral nerves primarily includes diffusion tensor imaging (DTI). Single-shot echo-planar imaging (EPI) is the most widely used technique. Multishot techniques are currently not feasible but might be tested in future. At least 6 directions of interrogation are needed for DTI, although most investigators have used 12 to 20 directions to obtain better imaging information and reproducible data.[17,18] We routinely use 3 diffusion moments (0, 800, and 1000 s/mm^2) and 12 directions of interrogation. These images can frequently be degraded by

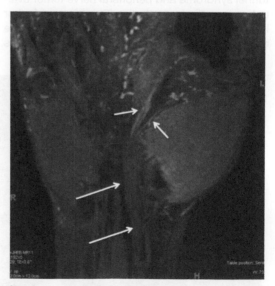

Fig. 10. 3D DW PSIF. Coronal MIP reconstruction from 3D DW PSIF sequence shows normal median nerve in the carpal tunnel with isointense signal (*large arrows*) and injured hyperintense radial sided branches (*small arrows*) distally in the palm. Note the excellent fat and vascular signal suppression with selective nerve depiction and thenar muscle edema in this case of recurrent carpal tunnel syndrome.

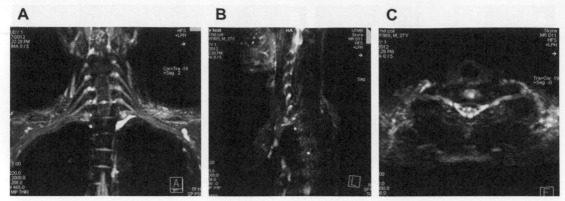

Fig. 11. DW STIR SPACE. Coronal (*A*), sagittal (*B*), and axial (*C*) 3D isotropic STIR SPACE images of the brachial plexus following application of diffusion moment of 200 s/mm². Note the selective depiction of the brachial plexus with effective suppression of vascular signal but decreased SNR compared with the traditional STIR SPACE.

motion and ghosting artifacts, therefore tight echo spacing, frequency-selective fat suppression, high-quality shim before image acquisition, and patient coaching to prevent motion degradation are essential to obtain good and reproducible DTI data.[19] Axial images obtained with 2–5 mm slice thickness with 0-mm gap can be reconstructed in multiple planes without artifacts. These images then allow reliable tensor calculation, fractional anisotropy, and apparent diffusion coefficient (ADC) measurements as well as tractography. DTI has been shown to be useful in carpal tunnel syndrome and peripheral nerve tumor evaluation in preliminary studies (**Fig. 12**), and further investigations are underway to evaluate the role of DTI in other types of neuropathy. DTI is

currently the only quantitative MR imaging method that produces reliable and reproducible quantitative data that provide (in contrast with visual assessments) the basis for the detection of neuropathies based on threshold values, and allow objective longitudinal observation, such as in preoperative-postoperative comparisons or for monitoring nonoperative therapies.

GUIDE TO OPTIMAL MRN IMAGING TECHNIQUE

With knowledge of techniques described earlier, the examination can be tailored to the extremities or plexuses with prudent use of various 2D and 3D pulse sequences.

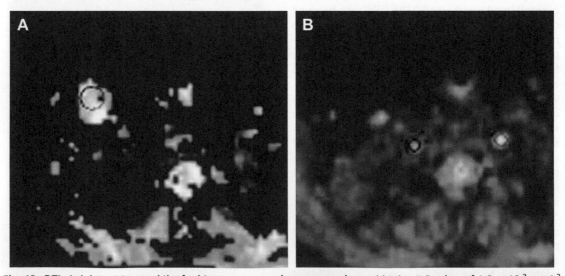

Fig. 12. DTI. Axial ADC image (*A*) of a biopsy-proven schwannoma showed high ADC value of 1.8 × 10⁻³ mm/s² (benign range) obtained with a circular region of interest (ROI) (*red*) and tensor image (*B*) at the level of the neural foramina showed asymmetrically lower fractional anisotropy (0.2) (*red*) of the involved right nerve root compared with normal left nerve root (0.4) (*green*).

Table 1
The imaging protocol used in the MRN examination for the LS plexus

MR Sequence	Slice Thickness (mm)	TR/TE (ms)	TF	Base Resolution (Pixels)
Axial T1	4	800/12	6	832
Coronal T1	4	960/12	5	384
Axial T2 SPAIR	4	4890/70	22	384
Sagittal T2 3D SPACE	1	1000/97	81	256
Sagittal STIR (optional)	4	3700/18	22	256
Coronal STIR 3D SPACE	1.5	1500/78	48	256

Abbreviation: TF, turbo factor.

Extremities

A good combination of sequences includes axial T1 W (anatomy), axial T2 SPAIR or T2 Dixon (pathology), coronal or sagittal PD (regional abnormalities), 3D SPAIR SPACE (nerve-nonselective longitudinal depiction), 3D DW PSIF (nerve-selective depiction), and axial DTI (for clinical and research applications). An optional sequence is STIR (failed fat suppression/regional metal).

Brachial Plexus

A good combination of sequences includes axial or coronal T1 W (anatomy), sagittal STIR (pathology), T2 SPACE (spine evaluation), 3D STIR SPACE (nerve-nonselective longitudinal depiction), and axial DTI (for clinical and research applications). Axial SPAIR/T2 Dixon may be added for suspected tumors/concomitant chest wall evaluation (**Table 1**).

LS Plexus

A good combination of sequences includes coronal T1 W (regional anatomy, obturator and sciatic nerves), axial T1 (anatomy), axial T2 SPAIR/T2 Dixon (pathology), T2 SPACE (spine evaluation), 3D STIR SPACE (nerve-nonselective longitudinal depiction), and axial DTI (for clinical and research applications). An optional sequence is STIR (failed fat suppression/regional metal).

MRN plus Contrast

Normal nerves do not enhance as because of the blood-nerve barrier created by perineurium. Contrast imaging (gadolinium-based agent) does not add much in trauma or entrapment neuropathy cases because these cases mostly present in subacute stages. In those cases, only denervated muscles enhance, the demonstration of which is already apparent on T1-W and fat-suppressed fluid-sensitive images. Contrast administration is recommended in other cases, such as suspected neural and perineural mass lesions (nerve sheath tumors, perineurioma), polyneuropathy conditions including lymphoma, amyloidosis, demyelinating neuropathies, and hereditary neuropathies, and so forth.[20] Before and after T1-W 3D gradient echo (VIBE-volume–interpolated breath-hold examination) imaging with subtraction is useful to show the enhancing lesion in multiple planes.

SUMMARY

MRN is a technically demanding examination requiring knowledge of appropriate clinical questions, regional nerves, and perineural anatomy as well as the various available MR imaging pulse sequences. Its proper performance is essential to the generation and accurate interpretation of optimal images.

REFERENCES

1. Aagaard BD, Maravilla KR, Kliot M. MR neurography. MR imaging of peripheral nerves. Magn Reson Imaging Clin North Am 1998;6:179–94.
2. Filler AG, Kliot M, Howe FA, et al. Application of magnetic resonance neurography in the evaluation of patients with peripheral nerve pathology. J Neurosurg 1996;85:299–309.
3. Chhabra A, Lee PP, Bizzell C. 3 Tesla MR neurography - technique, interpretation, and pitfalls. Skeletal Radiol 2011;40(10):1249–60.
4. Chhabra A, Flammang A, Andreisek G. Magnetic resonance neurography technique. Chapter 3. 1st edition. New Delhi, India: Jaypee Brothers Medical Publishers; 2012. p. 10–22.
5. Maravilla K, Bowen B. Imaging of the peripheral nervous system: evaluation of peripheral neuropathy and plexopathy. AJNR Am J Neuroradiol 1998;19: 1011–23.
6. Grant GA, Britz GW, Goodkin R, et al. The utility of magnetic resonance imaging in evaluating peripheral nerve disorders. Muscle Nerve 2002;25:314–31.

7. Chhabra A, Subhawong TK, Williams EH, et al. High-resolution MR neurography: evaluation before repeat tarsal tunnel surgery. AJR Am J Roentgenol 2011;197(1):175–83.

8. Vargas MI, Viallon M, Nguyen D, et al. New approaches in imaging of the brachial plexus. Eur J Radiol 2010;74(2):403–10.

9. Chhabra A, Thawait GK, Soldatos T, et al. High-resolution 3T MR neurography of the brachial plexus and its branches, with emphasis on 3D imaging. AJNR Am J Neuroradiol 2012;34(3):486–97.

10. Mallouhi A, Marik W, Prayer D, et al. 3T MR tomography of the brachial plexus: structural and microstructural evaluation. Eur J Radiol 2011;81(9): 2231–45.

11. Thakkar RS, Del Grande F, Thawait GK, et al. Spectrum of high-resolution MRI findings in diabetic neuropathy. AJR Am J Roentgenol 2012;199(2):407–12.

12. Thawait SK, Wang K, Subhawong TK, et al. Peripheral nerve surgery: the role of high-resolution MR neurography. AJNR Am J Neuroradiol 2012;33(2):203–10.

13. Chhabra A, Andreisek G, Soldatos T, et al. MR neurography: past, present, and future. AJR Am J Roentgenol 2011;197(3):583–91.

14. Chhabra A, Subhawong TK, Bizzell C, et al. 3T MR neurography using three-dimensional diffusion-weighted PSIF: technical issues and advantages. Skeletal Radiol 2011;40(10):1355–60.

15. Zhang Z, Song L, Meng Q, et al. Morphological analysis in patients with sciatica: a magnetic resonance imaging study using three-dimensional high-resolution diffusion-weighted magnetic resonance neurography techniques. Spine (Phila Pa 1976) 2009;34: E245–50.

16. Takahara T, Hendrikse J, Yamashita T, et al. Diffusion-weighted MR neurography of the brachial plexus: feasibility study. Radiology 2008;249(2): 653–60.

17. Andreisek G, White LM, Kassner A, et al. Evaluation of diffusion tensor imaging and fiber tractography of the median nerve: preliminary results on intrasubject variability and precision of measurements. AJR Am J Roentgenol 2010;194:W65–72.

18. Tagliafico A, Calabrese M, Puntoni M, et al. Brachial plexus MR imaging: accuracy and reproducibility of DTI-derived measurements and fiber tractography at 3.0-T. Eur Radiol 2011;21(8):1764–71.

19. Chhabra A, Thakkar RS, Chalian M, et al. Anatomic MR imaging and functional diffusion tensor imaging of peripheral nerve tumor and tumor like conditions. AJNR Am J Neuroradiol 2013;34(4):802–7.

20. Thawait SK, Chaudhry V, Thawait GK, et al. High-resolution MR neurography of diffuse peripheral nerve lesions. AJNR Am J Neuroradiol 2011;32(8): 1365–72.

Peripheral MR Neurography
Approach to Interpretation

Avneesh Chhabra, MD

KEYWORDS

- Magnetic resonance neurography • Interpretation • Peripheral neuropathy
- Peripheral nerve imaging

KEY POINTS

- Normal peripheral nerves demonstrate a size similar to the adjacent arteries, and the size and signal intensity are nearly symmetrical bilaterally.
- Systemic and polyneuropathy conditions may be incidentally discovered on magnetic resonance neurography; however, their diagnosis is primarily based on clinical and electrodiagnostic findings.
- In entrapment neuropathy, the signal, fascicular, and size abnormality of the peripheral nerve are maximum at and just proximal to the site of entrapment with distal gradual return to normalcy.
- In nerve injury, it is important to differentiate stretch injury from neuroma in continuity and nerve discontinuity because of the different treatment implications.
- The triple-B sign is a sign of severe peripheral neuropathy, which will require surgery, in many cases.
- Muscle denervation change usually shows diffuse involvement with a lack of associated perimuscular edema, hemorrhage, or nearby fascial involvement as opposed to myopathy/myositis cases, which usually involve multiple muscle compartments and are frequently associated with above findings.
- Two-dimensional imaging is most useful for the depiction of detailed nerve architecture and regional pathology.
- Three-dimensional imaging is useful to produce a longitudinal display of the nerves for discussing cases with referring physicians, depicting course deviations/focal changes in nerve caliber, and demonstrating the relationship to the adjacent space-occupying lesions for presurgical planning.

INTRODUCTION

Magnetic resonance neurography (MRN) is an exquisite technique for the visualization of peripheral nerve anatomy and lesions. Proper performance of MRN requires an understanding of nerve anatomy; a high-strength MR machine; good-quality gradient coils; and high-resolution as well as high-contrast, 2-dimensional (2D) and 3D, predominantly spin echo–type imaging techniques.[1–3] For accurate MRN interpretation, it requires a detailed understanding of nerve anatomy and pathophysiology, normal and abnormal imaging appearances of the peripheral nerves on various imaging techniques, and a systematic approach to evaluate the spectrum of nerve lesions.[4–6] This article outlines the MRN technical considerations, normal and abnormal peripheral nerve imaging appearances, current indications of MRN, and a systematic approach to diagnose these lesions.

NERVE ANATOMY

Peripheral nerves form a part of the neurovascular bundle, and their caliber is usually similar to an

Research grants for patient scans: GE-AUR/Siemens Medical solutions/Integra Life Sciences.
Consultant: Siemens: MSK CAD system development unrelated to this research.
The University of Texas Southwestern, 5323 Harry Hines Blvd, Dallas, TX-75390-9178, USA
E-mail address: avneesh.chhabra@utsouthwestern.edu

Neuroimag Clin N Am 24 (2014) 79–89
http://dx.doi.org/10.1016/j.nic.2013.03.033

neuroimaging.theclinics.com

adjacent artery. The nerve size gradually decreases along its distal course with minimal variations near the ramifications and joints. Peripheral nerves encompass a unique organizational structure.[5,7] The smallest unit is an axon enveloped by a layer of Schwann cells and connective tissue stroma and is referred to as the *endoneurium*. The axons are bathed by endoneurial fluid, which shows antegrade and, possibly, retrograde axoplasmic flow. The axons are bundled together to form a fascicle, which in turn is covered by another connective tissue layer called the *perineurium*. The fascicular bundles may range from 2 to 10 on imaging in commonly visualized peripheral nerves and may contain motor, sensory, or sympathetic fibers in various combinations. The final connective tissue layer, named the *epineurium*, covers all of the fascicles within the nerve.[7] There are internal and external epineurium layers surrounding and enveloping the fascicles, respectively. The epineurium and perineurium are uniformly thin structures. On current high-resolution MRN techniques, the normal peripheral nerves (more than 2–3 mm) are easily distinguished from the surrounding vessels because of their unique fascicular appearance, nonbranching, relatively straight course in most parts, and lack of flow voids.[1,3] The normal nerves are expected to show isointense signal intensity on T1-weighted (W) and T2-W MR images (**Fig. 1**).[5] Minimal T2 hyperintense signal alteration is commonly observed on the inversion recovery images because of the increased sensitivity to endoneurial fluid, better fat suppression, and increased dynamic range of contrast. The hyperintensity is particularly prominent on 3D inversion recovery images; however, it should be symmetric from side to side. Using good surface coils, the fascicles are consistently depicted in normal nerves that are 3 mm or larger.[3] The pencil-thin epineurial layer can also be seen forming the outer covering of the nerve in larger nerves. The perineurial and epineurial layers are relatively imperceptible, unless abnormally thickened (**Fig. 2**). Normal and abnormal nerve MRN imaging appearances are outlined in **Table 1**.

NERVE PATHOPHYSIOLOGY

Peripheral nerves may be involved in a variety of pathologies, which are broadly divided as systemic and local conditions. The systemic pathologies include vasculitis; toxic and metabolic diseases, such as diabetes mellitus (DM), amyloidosis, and hyperlipidemia; hereditary conditions, such as Charcot-Marie-Tooth (CMT) disease; idiopathic conditions, such as multifocal motor neuropathy (MMN); acute or chronic demyelinating conditions, such as chronic demyelinating polyneuropathy (CIDP); and neurocutaneous syndromes, such as neurofibromatosis (NF) and schwannomatosis (SW). The local conditions include compressive or adhesive neuropathies, such as tunnel syndromes; nerve injury; infection; peripheral nerve sheath tumor (PNST) and perineural tumor; or functional or traction neuropathy from activities, such as repeated typing, bad footwear, ankle instability, and functional compartment syndromes.[8,9]

In systematic conditions, the spinal cord, dorsal nerve root ganglion, axons, or the surrounding

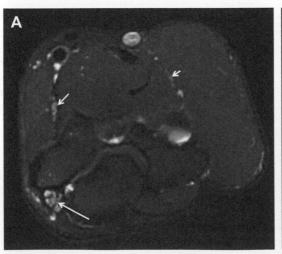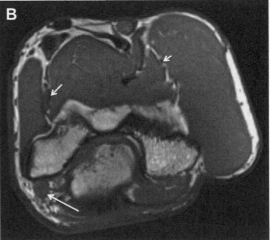

Fig. 1. Normal and abnormal nerve appearances: axial T2 spectral adiabatic inversion recovery (*A*) and T1-W (*B*) images show normal radial nerve (*small arrows*), mildly hyperintense median nerve (*medium arrows*), and moderate-severely hyperintense ulnar nerve (*large arrows*) with abnormal enlargement in this case of mild median and moderate-severe ulnar neuropathy.

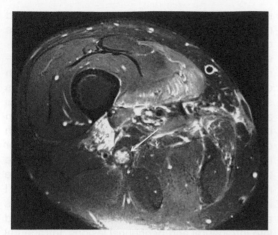

Fig. 2. Thickened epineurium. Axial T2 spectral adiabatic inversion recovery image through the midthigh shows enlarged and severely hyperintense sciatic nerve with prominent fascicles and thickened epineurium (*arrow*) from prior penetrating injury.

myelin sheath are affected in various combinations. The diagnosis is generally clinical and biochemical with frequently multi-compartment or multifocal nerve abnormality observed in the aforementioned pathologies. Electrodiagnostic studies, such as electromyography and nerve conduction study, are currently the diagnostic technique of choice to evaluate these lesions. MRN is uncommonly used to evaluate these subjects and might be used in cases when there are worsening focal/regional symptoms to exclude a superimposed entrapment or a mass lesion. Sometimes, the neuropathy related to the systemic conditions may be incidentally observed in studies performed for suspected nerve entrapment or injury, especially diabetic neuropathy, which is not uncommonly encountered during joint/extremity imaging. Therefore, the reader should be aware of neuropathy findings related to such conditions. Although hereditary neuropathy leads to symmetric disease with marked nerve thickening and hyperintensity, especially in CMT type IA (demyelinating type) (**Fig. 3**), acquired conditions commonly lead to asymmetrical nerve thickening or hyperintensity. Diabetic neuropathy is seen as abnormal T2 hyperintensity with or without prominent fascicles, symmetric and multi-nerve involvement, nerve enlargement, and internal fat proliferation with chronicity.

Table 1
MR interpretation criteria: normal versus abnormal nerve

Nerve	Normal	Abnormal
Size	Similar to adjacent artery Gradually decreases distally	Focal or diffuse enlargement Larger than the adjacent artery
Signal intensity	T1W & T2W: isointense to skeletal muscle STIR/fat suppressed T2W: isointense to minimally hyperintense 3D TSE (turbo spin echo): uniform and symmetric hyperintensity	T2 hyperintensity (becoming similar to adjacent veins) Asymmetric hyperintensity on 3D TSE
Fascicular pattern	T1W & T2W: present and uniform	Single or multiple fascicles enlargement/disruption Loss of fascicular pattern
Course	Smooth without focal deviations	Focal or diffuse deviations Discontinuity
Enhancement	Absent (except in areas of deficient blood-nerve barrier, such as dorsal nerve root ganglion)	In tumors & infections (disruption of the blood-nerve barrier)
Perineural fat	Clean fat planes	Perineural strand like T1 & T2 hypointensities/nerve encasement
Diffusion tensor imaging, tracts	Normal tracts	Abnormal tracts, disrupted or displaced
Diffusion tensor imaging, quantitative	Normal fractional anisotropy values (>0.4–0.5)	Abnormal fractional anisotropy values (<0.4–0.5)
Diffusion tensor imaging, qualitative	Symmetric brightness of nerves on tensor images	Asymmetrical hyperintensity of the neuropathic nerve

Abbreviations: SPACE, sampling perfection with application optimized contrasts using varying flip angle evolutions; STIR, short tau inversion recovery.

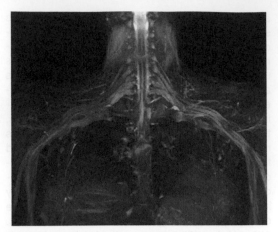

Fig. 3. Symmetric polyneuropathy. CMT type 1A. Coronal, maximum intensity projection, 3D, short tau inversion recovery, sampling perfection with application optimized contrasts using varying flip angle evolutions (SPACE, Siemens, Erlangen, Germany) image shows symmetric bilateral nerve thickenings in this genetically proven case of CMT type 1A.

Most commonly imaged local conditions can be subdivided into nerve entrapment or nerve injury.[10] Nerve entrapment caused by increased pressure within a tunnel (confined space through which the nerve traverses) or from a space-occupying lesion leads to the blockade of axoplasmic flow, venous congestion, hyperemia, epineurial edema at and proximal to the site of entrapment, as well as wallerian degeneration distally. The larger myelinated axons situated in the outer portions of the nerve are the earliest and most affected, supporting the theory that the primary mechanism of injury is a shear force, which is followed by ischemia. These pathologic abnormalities lead to hyperintense nerve signal change on T2-W MR images, with signal intensity approaching approximately 90%, similar to adjacent vessels confirming neuropathy. The signal abnormality is also maximum at and just proximal to the site of entrapment with distal fading/resolution to normal signal intensity. Associated nerve enlargement and fascicular abnormality becomes apparent with increasing severity of neuropathy (see Fig. 1).[4,5,7] Both proximal and distal nerve enlargement may be seen with entrapment on MRN. The proximal enlargement is much more common and pronounced than the distal enlargement, and the latter is usually observed in more severe cases of entrapment. This finding also supports the theory of bidirectional axoplasmic flow. With chronic entrapment, the epineurial edema incites fibrotic changes causing further nerve entrapment, axonal degeneration, and myelin loss. Thus, mild entrapment neuropathy is identified as mild-moderate hyperintensity or mild nerve flattening. Moderate entrapment shows one or a combination of imaging findings of moderate to severe hyperintensity, fascicular abnormality, and proximal nerve enlargement with distal flattening; whereas severe neuropathy is seen as the aforementioned findings as well as abrupt changes in the nerve signal intensity from bright-black-bright (triple-B sign) along the length of the nerve. Signal intensity on diffusion tensor imaging (DTI) also increases nearly proportionate to the degree of neuropathy; however, more research is needed to establish the value of DTI in nerve imaging (Fig. 4). Space-occupying lesions affecting the nerves can be broadly characterized into intraneural and perineurial lesions. Intraneural lesions lead to nerve enlargement and/or fascicular involvement (Fig. 5), whereas perineurial lesions cause nerve encasement or displacement.

Nerve injuries have been traditionally classified by the Seddon and Sunderland grading systems based on injury to various layers of the nerve.[5] However, for practical management planning and while interpreting MRN examinations, nerve injuries can be conveniently divided into the following: (1) stretch injury (which could be mild- observed as abnormally hyperintense nerve, otherwise in continuity and with nearly similar size to the adjacent vessels or contralateral nerves; or Moderate-observed as moderate diffuse nerve enlargement more than the size of the adjacent vessels or contralateral nerves because of axonal degeneration and the expansion of fluid space within the

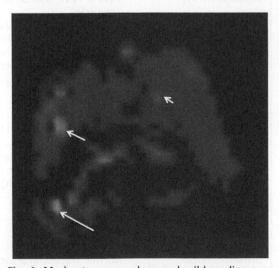

Fig. 4. Moderate-severe ulnar and mild median neuropathy on DTI. Same case as Fig. 1. Notice the hyperintensities of the nerves at the level of the elbow joint on the tensor image, ulnar (large arrow) is greater than the median (medium arrow), which is greater than the radial nerve (small arrow).

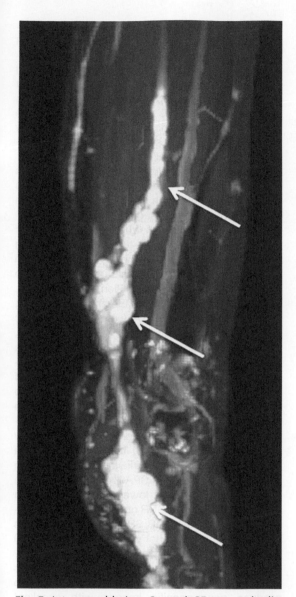

Fig. 5. Intraneural lesion. Coronal, 3D, spectral adiabatic inversion recovery, sampling perfection with application optimized contrasts using varying flip angle evolutions (SPACE, Siemens, Erlangen, Germany) image through the forearm shows a plexiform peripheral nerve sheath tumor of the median nerve (*arrows*).

nerve); (2) high-grade nerve injury with nerve in continuity or neuroma in continuity (abrupt change in nerve caliber with focal nerve enlargement and effaced fascicular appearance) (**Fig. 6**); and (3) nerve root avulsion or nerve transection (complete discontinuity) with end bulb neuroma formation. Stretch injuries usually require conservative management and rehabilitation. Sometimes, neurolysis or nerve decompression may be attempted depending on the clinical situation. Surgery is commonly performed in high-grade nerve injury,

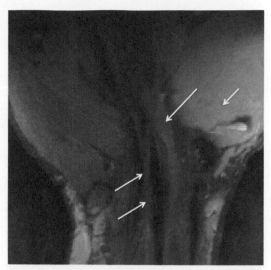

Fig. 6. Neuroma in continuity. Coronal, 3D, diffusion-weighted reversed fast imaging in steady state free precession image shows focally enlarged median nerve (*large arrow*) with diffuse mild hyperintensity from prior iatrogenic injury during the carpal tunnel release in keeping with a neuroma in continuity. Notice thenar muscle denervation edemalike signal (*small arrow*) and normal ulnar nerve (*medium arrows*).

painful neuroma in continuity, nerve avulsion, and transection because the functional return is often incomplete or none in these injuries.[10–13] An important imaging feature of alternating signal alteration of bright-black-bright (triple-B sign) along the length of the nerve is an indicator of severe focal neuropathy that can be seen with nerve transection, very severe entrapment, loss of nerve coaptation, dehiscence/degeneration of nerve graft, or freeze injury related to cryoablation (**Fig. 7**).

Finally, regional muscles serve as an important key indicator of neuropathy. The muscles show edema like T2 signal abnormality in the acute stages (appearing within 24–48 hours), which progresses to fatty infiltration and atrophy in subacute or chronic stages of denervation. The muscle involvement is usually diffuse with a lack of associated perimuscular edema, hemorrhage, or nearby fascial involvement (**Fig. 8**).[4,5,7]

MRN TECHNICAL CONSIDERATIONS

The MRN technique has been separately covered by Chhabra and colleagues in this issue. This article briefly discusses the techniques as they pertain to MRN interpretation. MRN examinations can be broadly divided into anatomic (conventional T2–based) techniques and functional (diffusion-based) techniques.[14–16] The author primarily focuses on routinely performed T2-based

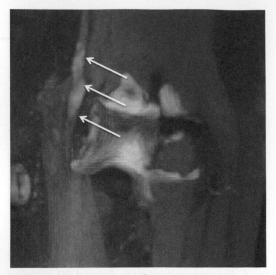

Fig. 7. Triple-B sign. Coronal, maximum intensity projection, 3D, diffusion-weighted reversed fast imaging in steady state free precession image shows severe re-entrapment ulnar neuropathy following prior anterior transposition with moderate enlargement and abrupt signal changes along the length of the nerve from bright-black-bright (*arrows*).

techniques. A good MRN examination should produce nerve selective/specific images with multiplanar isotropic display of the nerve anatomy and lesions, ideally creating images in both axial and longitudinal planes of the peripheral nerves using a combination of high-resolution 2D and 3D spin echo–type imaging techniques on a high-field (ideally 3T) scanner.[17,18] For 2D imaging, the author prefers axial T2 spectral adiabatic inversion recovery imaging because it provides higher signal to noise ratio, less pulsation artifacts, and specific absorption rate favorability than short tau inversion recovery (STIR) imaging while maintaining better

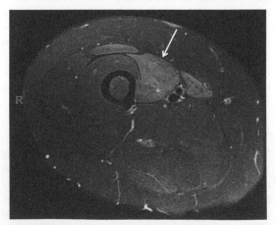

Fig. 8. Muscle denervation edema (*arrow*) caused by femoral neuropathy. Notice lack of fascial edema or hemorrhage.

fat suppression than the fat suppressed T2-W imaging technique. Two-dimensional sagittal STIR imaging is particularly useful in brachial or lumbosacral plexus imaging because it allows individual nerve segments to be easily traced from the root level to cords and peripheral upper limb branches on sequential images. On this sequence, the nerves show symmetric hyperintensity and nearly symmetric sizes for easy comparison among ipsilateral and contralateral segments.[11,19]

Three-dimensional imaging is advantageous over 2D imaging on 3T imaging because it avoids crosstalk (magnetization transfer effects) between the adjacent slices; consequently, thinner axial slices can be nicely reconstructed using isotropic imaging. The 3D spin echo–type isotropic imaging is performed using the sampling perfection with application optimized contrasts using varying flip angle evolutions (SPACE, Siemens, Erlangen, Germany)/Cube (General Electric Healthcare, Waukesha, WI) and VISTA (volumetric isotropic T2-weighted acquisition, Philips, Best, Netherlands) imaging techniques. The 3D images are high definition and high contrast and can be reconstructed in any desired plane without loss of resolution to visualize nerves as small as 2 to 3 mm with sub 1-mm voxels. The 3D images can also be used to produce maximum intensity projection (MIP) of the nerves for longitudinal display of anatomy and pathology, thereby leading to a better understanding of the lesions to the referring physician.[1,5,9,16] The 3D SPAIR SPACE technique is used for upper and lower extremity imaging because of the higher SNR obtained with this technique than with 3D STIR SPACE, which provides better fat suppression for plexus imaging. The 3D diffusion-weighted reversed fast imaging in steady state free precession is also used at the author's institute for extremities because of its ability to produce nerve-specific images with excellent vascular suppression (because of low diffusion moment) while it retains all the advantages of an isotropic 3D MR imaging technique.[20,21] Because injury/entrapment–related nerve pathology usually does not enhance, postcontrast imaging is only indicated in suspected infection, tumor, or diffuse polyneuropathy (CIDP, CMT, MMN, neurocutaneous syndromes, amyloidosis, and lymphoma) to provide possible leads into the diagnosis and biopsy guidance, if such a procedure is being contemplated.

SYSTEMATIC APPROACH TO MRN INTERPRETATION

There is a steep learning curve to MRN interpretation; however, it requires substantial interest on the part of reader to learn the nerve anatomy and systematically evaluate the 2D and 3D imaging sequences for various findings.

The coronal/sagittal (large field of view) images should be evaluated first to rule out a mass lesion/any other locoregional pathology that may confound the diagnosis of neuropathy. This evaluation should be followed by the evaluation of sequential axial T1-W and T2 SPAIR images for a detailed assessment of the nerve architecture, spatial anatomy, and pathology.

Axial T1-W images are most useful to distinguish nerve (fascicular appearance) from vessels (vein [in plane flow], artery [usually flow void]); for finding perineural fibrosis (strandy hypointense tissue deforming/encasing the nerve); to characterize mass lesions (tail sign and split fat sign with PNST, fat within fibrolipomatous hamartoma (FLH), lipoma, hemorrhage in sciatic endometriosis); and for the assessment of intraepineurial fat (Normally, the fascicle size is more or equal to the adjacent intraepineurial fat tissue; with chronic atrophic neuropathy, the fat tissue becomes more prominent than the adjoining fascicles.), nerve caliber, epineurium thickness (normally less than 1- to 2-mm thick uniform lining without focal thickening), nerve course (normally smooth with no focal deviation), regional muscle fatty infiltration, and atrophy.[3,4,6,10,22,23]

Axial T2 SPAIR images are most useful to assess nerve signal (abnormal hyperintensity approaching adjacent vessels); fascicular abnormality (enlargement, disruption, or effacement); nerve caliber; abnormal epineurium thickness (abnormal is equal to or more than 2 mm or focal thickening); characterization of mass lesions (target sign with central T2 hypointensity, fascicular sign, and tail sign of PNST); nerve course; and regional muscle edema–like signal.[5]

Three-dimensional imaging is useful to produce a longitudinal display of the nerves, especially using curved planar reformations and MIP reconstructions. These images are particularly useful to discuss cases with referring physicians, to depict course deviations/focal changes in nerve caliber, and to demonstrate the relationship to the adjacent space-occupying lesions for presurgical planning. Fascicular abnormality is, however, best seen on axial images, which is the mainstay of diagnosis for neuropathy. The isotropic 3D T2 SPACE technique is used for spine interpretation because spine pathology is a major confounder in the clinical diagnosis of plexopathy.[2,19]

A multidisciplinary approach with involvement of referring physicians and readers and the correlation of available clinical examination findings and electrodiagnostic results is ideal to accurately diagnose various lesions on MRN. However, it is not always possible, especially if the examination is performed in the community setting. Therefore, the author outlines a stepwise systematic assessment approach to diagnose the spectrum of peripheral nerve lesions.

Step 1: Regional Muscle Denervation Change

Know the regional muscle innervation patterns and recognize the denervation change because this finding is key to the diagnosis of neuropathy and is present in most motor neuropathies.

Step 2: Rule Out Locoregional or Spine Pathology

Various conditions may mimic symptoms of neuropathy, such as pain, numbness, and weakness. These pathologies may include disk herniation, moderate-severe neural foraminal stenosis with radiculopathy, myelopathy, tendon and ligament pathologies, and so forth.

Step 3: Rule Out a Mass Lesion in the Vicinity of the Nerve

If present, characterize the mass, which could be suggestive of a PNST (typical MR imaging signs: split fat sign, fascicular sign, target sign, tail sign, underlying other manifestations of a neurocutaneous syndrome, variable enhancement); malignant PNST (invasive margins, peritumoral edema, large size >5 cm, necrotic areas, hemorrhage or calcification in the setting of neurofibroma, vascular encasement, heterogeneous enhancement, increased glucose uptake on F18 fluorodeoxyglucose positron emission tomography [FDG PET] scan, with standardized uptake value maximum >3–4, and especially with increasing uptake on delayed scan); neuroma in continuity or end bulb neuroma (nonenhancing lesion that may show fascicular sign, history of injury/limb amputation); perineurioma (young age, slow motor functional loss, nerve enlargement outside the expected entrapment sites, prominent and usually uniform fascicular enlargement [honeycomb appearance], and homogeneous enhancement); FLH (fibrofatty proliferation within a single enlarged nerve segment with or without association with macrodystrophia lipomatosa, coaxial cable/spaghetti appearance caused by fascicular enlargement, variable enhancement); lymphoma (known systemic lymphoma, diffuse nerve enlargement with multifocal masses, fascicular enlargement or disruption with or without interspersed T2 hypointense signal alterations, homogeneous enhancement, increased glucose uptake on F18 FDG PET scan); amyloidoma (underlying chronic condition, such as multiple myeloma, diffuse nerve enlargement with multifocal masses with or without interspersed T2 hypointense signal alterations); or benign and malignant perineural soft tissue mass lesions displacing or encasing the nerve (ganglion [intraneural or extraneural], lipoma, hemangioma, lymphangioma, myositis ossificans, or soft tissue sarcoma) (**Fig. 9**).[24–26]

Step 4: Rule Out Diffuse Polyneuropathy

Multi-compartmental or multifocal nerve involvement may be seen with DM, vasculitis, toxic conditions (such as chemotherapy-related neuropathy), CIDP, CMT, MMN, lymphoma, amyloidosis, leprosy, and neurocutaneous syndromes.

Diabetes neuropathy/vasculitis/toxic condition–related abnormality manifests as increased T2 signal intensity and fascicular prominence of the extremity (commonly lower) and lumbosacral plexus nerves in acute-subacute stages. Chronic axonal degeneration leads to prominent intraepineurial fat surrounding the fascicles and, particularly, in DM or radiation neuropathy (see **Fig. 8**). CIDP leads to mild-moderate nerve enlargement, and the abnormality is commonly bilateral in the classic form and may involve plexuses. However, pure sensory, pure motor, or heterogeneous patterns are also possible. These demyelinating neuropathies may be associated with underlying malignancy, such as myeloma/mononclonal

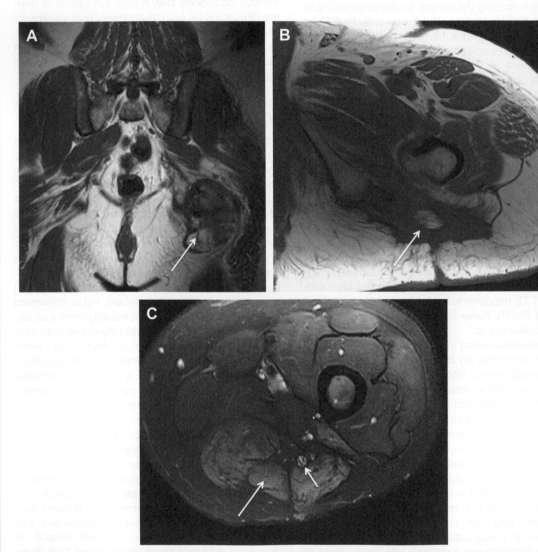

Fig. 9. Nerve encasement by perineural mass lesion and radiation neuropathy. (*A*) Coronal T1-W image shows a hemorrhagic synovial cell sarcoma (*arrow*) encasing the left sciatic nerve. Axial T1-W (*B*) image following sarcoma resection and radiation treatment shows hyperintense fatty sciatic nerve (*arrow*) surrounded by a postoperative seroma. Axial, fat-suppressed, T2-W (*C*) image shows bright sciatic nerve (*small arrow*) from neuropathy and regional muscle denervation changes (*large arrow*).

gammopathy, and a search for the same should be performed. CMT (type 1A) leads to moderate to severe symmetrical bilateral nerve enlargement with frequent involvement of plexuses. Underlying family history of neuropathy is usually present; patients may show other typical clinical features, such as high plantar arches. MMN leads to mild diffuse nerve enlargement and T2 hyperintensity in areas outside the expected confines of entrapment neuropathy. Sometimes, patients may present with double crush syndrome; nerve affected proximally might be predisposed to additional distal entrapment (eg, a patient with MMN findings in the forearm may present with carpal tunnel syndrome caused by vulnerability of the abnormally enlarged median nerve to distal entrapment). Leprosy is seen in patients of Indian/Asian descent, and hypertrophic changes within various cutaneous and extremity motor-sensory nerves may be seen. Nerve calcification and bony changes (licked candy stick) characteristic of leprosy may also be seen. Neurocutaneous syndromes, such as NF and SW, are associated with specific genetic abnormalities, family history, other typical local or systemic stigmata, and multiple PNSTs. These pathologies are separately discussed in another article.[5,9,10,19,22,27]

Step 5: Focal Nerve Abnormality of One or More Regional Nerves

Rule out entrapment or injury. In cases of entrapment, the nerve and fascicular abnormality is most prominent at and immediately proximal to the entrapment site, such as with various tunnel syndromes. With milder case, there is abnormal T2 signal abnormality, and the signal intensity gradually fades distally. With more severe entrapment, the nerve also enlarges proximally and shows fascicular abnormality. Regional muscle denervation changes are a key to the diagnosis of entrapment. One should diligently assess for the cause of entrapment, such as thickened fascia, accessory muscle, local mass lesions, hematoma, tenosynovitis, bony callus, varicosities and paralabral cyst, and so forth. The finding of one nerve entrapment does not preclude the diagnosis of entrapment of another regional nerve. Thus, full regional assessment should be performed for all major peripheral nerves. Also, note that the muscle variations known to predispose to regional nerve entrapment are frequently seen as an isolated finding. It is not uncommon to see these variations on high-resolution MRN images (eg, split piriformis/accessory belly of piriformis may be observed as a normal variant without causing nerve entrapment). Therefore, it becomes

paramount to evaluate for the primary nerve abnormality rather than looking for indirect signs, such as asymmetry of piriformis, to diagnose entrapment. In cases of injury, the nerves should be evaluated for various findings, such as the presence of stretch injury–related signal and size abnormality with nerve in continuity, formation of neuroma in continuity, nerve root avulsion and nerve transection with end bulb neuroma formation, as discussed earlier. In chronic entrapment/chronic injury cases, the nerves may regain normal signal intensity; however, they may show increased intraepineurial fat around relatively small fascicles on high-resolution images. Regional muscle denervation changes are a key finding in neuropathy cases, absent only in about 12% of cases of larger motor neuropathy, such as sciatic neuropathy. For smaller sensory nerves, such as pudendal nerve/calcaneal nerve or Joplin nerve, scarring along the course of the nerve is a major finding indicating entrapment as opposed to the primary nerve abnormality itself. This finding may be used to direct MR-guided perineural therapeutic injections.[3–8,28]

Step 6: Failed Surgical Cases

Previous surgical history may or may not be available at the time of interpretation. The readers should recognize the discontinuity of the retinaculum in previous carpal, cubital, or tarsal tunnel releases or anteriorly transposed ulnar nerve in prior subcutaneous or submuscular transposition.[3] Additionally, a hypointense ring of collagen wrap or serrated edges of the nerve tube placed around the neurolyzed/reconstructed nerve may be observed as an indicator of prior surgery.[12] However, a sincere effort should be made to obtain the surgical note before interpretation. Although increased T2 signal alteration of the nerve may persist in some cases for prolonged periods following these surgeries, the abnormal hyperintense signal should gradually decrease in most cases by 4 to 6 weeks after the surgery. Worsening T2 signal abnormality along with persistent or worsening fascicular abnormality or abrupt course deviation are indicators of persistent neuropathy and surgical failure. When such a procedure is being contemplated, fibrotic nerve tethering/encasement should also be looked for and the degree of nerve involvement in terms of circumference of nerve surrounded by fibrosis should be commented for repeat surgical planning. Other causes of failure, such as recurrent tenosynovitis/ganglion, hematoma, and regrowth of retinaculum/failure of complete resection of retinaculum, if present, should also be reported.[3,5,12,13,28]

Step 7: Myopathy/Myositis

If no nerve abnormality is apparent and only muscle abnormalities are observed, the diagnosis may be myopathy/myositis rather than neuropathy. The former is usually associated with muscle signal alterations/atrophy in more than one nerve distribution. Additionally, there may be associated fascial edema/hemorrhage or focal muscle involvement, which is usually not observed with denervation muscle changes. Because MRN is a highly sensitive technique, the finding of normal nerves in a suspected case of neuropathy should also put the diagnosis of a neurogenic cause of symptoms to rest, especially if supported by negative electrodiagnostic studies.[5]

MRN IMAGING PITFALLS

Several pitfalls should be considered while interpreting MRN examinations. T2-based MRN is an anatomic imaging technique unlike electrodiagnostic study, which is a physiologic study. Therefore, both types of studies may show false positives and negatives for different reasons. Mild increased T2 signal intensity of the nerve should be reported as a nonspecific finding because it may be seen with neuropathy or may merely represent a magic angle artifact.[17,18] The magic angle artifact is common in obliquely oriented nerves, such as sciatic nerves at the greater sciatic notch, femoral nerves in their pelvic course, medial plantar nerve in the hind foot, or common peroneal nerve at the popliteal fossa.[3,10] However, magic angle artifacts usually affect small and fixed areas (55° to the magnetic field) of the nerve, and the finding is usually bilaterally symmetric because of the constant position of the nerves. Therefore, asymmetric hyperintensity not explained by heterogeneous fat suppression or in areas not prone to magic angle artifacts, such as the inguinal region for femoral nerves or the thigh region for the sciatic nerves, should be viewed with suspicion.[5,27] Mild hyperintensity is also commonly observed in asymptomatic patients in nerves predisposed to subclinical traction/friction neuropathy because of their superficial location or around the joints, such as the median nerve in carpal tunnel, ulnar nerve in the Guyon canal or cubital tunnel, medial plantar nerve in the hindfoot, and C8 and T1 nerve roots at the thoracic outlet. Therefore, additional signs of neuropathy, such as moderate-severe T2 hyperintensity, fascicular abnormality, proximal nerve enlargement with flattening at the entrapment site, and denervation muscle changes, should be assessed for good correlation with symptomatic neuropathy. Also, close communication with the referring physicians and correlation with available electrodiagnostic findings are essential for an accurate diagnosis and clarification of minimally abnormal-appearing MR imaging findings, which in isolation should be reported as nonspecific findings.

On 3D STIR SPACE and 2D STIR images of the brachial and lumbosacral plexus, the nerves are normally T2 hyperintense because of good fat suppression, increased fluid sensitivity, and increased dynamic range of contrast. The reader should diligently look for asymmetric T2 hyperintensity and/or enlargement/flattening of the abnormal nerves as compared with normal-appearing nerves on the ipsilateral or contralateral side.[19] A detailed comparison with the 2D findings for subtle nerve signal asymmetry, presence of other signs, such as focal altered contour or displacement, and secondary signs of muscle denervation should be assessed to make a confident diagnosis of abnormality.[29]

Finally, muscle denervation changes should be differentiated from myositis/myopathy. In the denervated muscle, the findings are usually diffuse in the regional area of the nerve and are not associated with fascial edema/enhancement as opposed to infectious myositis or muscle strains. Myopathies are also frequently bilateral and may involve multiple muscle compartments.[30,31]

To conclude, proper imaging technique, knowledge of nerve anatomy and pathologic appearances, and a systematic approach to interpretation on MRN are essential for a radiologist to correctly evaluate these examinations and to make an accurate diagnosis. Regional muscle innervation patterns and several imaging pitfalls should also be kept in mind for appropriate interpretation.

REFERENCES

1. Chhabra A, Andreisek G, Soldatos T, et al. MR neurography: past, present, and future. AJR Am J Roentgenol 2011;197(3):583–91.
2. Mallouhi A, Marik W, Prayer D, et al. 3T MR tomography of the brachial plexus: structural and microstructural evaluation. Eur J Radiol 2012;81(9): 2231–45.
3. Chhabra A, Subhawong TK, Williams EH, et al. High-resolution MR neurography: evaluation before repeat tarsal tunnel surgery. AJR Am J Roentgenol 2011;197(1):175–83.
4. Chhabra A, Chalian M, Soldatos T, et al. High resolution MR neurography of sciatic neuropathy. AJR, Am J Roentgenol 2012;198(4):W357–64.

5. Chhabra A, Lee PP, Bizzell C, et al. 3 Tesla MR neurography–technique, interpretation, and pitfalls. Skeletal Radiol 2011;40(10):1249–60.

6. Bäumer P, Dombert T, Staub F, et al. Ulnar neuropathy at the elbow: MR neurography–nerve T2 signal increase and caliber. Radiology 2011;260(1):199–206.

7. Filler AG, Maravilla KR, Tsuruda JS. MR neurography and muscle MR imaging for image diagnosis of disorders affecting the peripheral nerves and musculature. Neurol Clin 2004;22(3):643–82, vi–vii.

8. Subhawong TK, Wang KC, Thawait SK, et al. High resolution imaging of tunnels by magnetic resonance neurography. Skeletal Radiol 2012;41(1):15–31.

9. Thawait SK, Chaudhry V, Thawait GK, et al. High-resolution MR neurography of diffuse peripheral nerve lesions. AJNR Am J Neuroradiol 2011;32(8):1365–72.

10. Chhabra A, Faridian-Aragh N, Chalian M, et al. High-resolution 3-T MR neurography of peroneal neuropathy. Skeletal Radiol 2012;41(3):257–71.

11. Chalian M, Soldatos T, Faridian-Aragh N, et al. High resolution 3T MR neurography of suprascapular neuropathy. Acad Radiol 2011;18(8):1049–59.

12. Thawait SK, Wang K, Subhawong TK, et al. Peripheral nerve surgery: the role of high-resolution MR neurography. AJNR Am J Neuroradiol 2012;33(2):203–10.

13. Chhabra A, Williams EH, Wang KC, et al. MR neurography of neuromas related to nerve injury and entrapment with surgical correlation. AJNR Am J Neuroradiol 2010;31(8):1363–8.

14. Zhang Z, Song L, Meng Q, et al. Morphological analysis in patients with sciatica: a magnetic resonance imaging study using three-dimensional high-resolution diffusion-weighted magnetic resonance neurography techniques. Spine (Phila Pa 1976) 2009;34(7):E245–50.

15. Eguchi Y, Ohtori S, Yamashita M, et al. Diffusion-weighted magnetic resonance imaging of symptomatic nerve root of patients with lumbar disk herniation. Neuroradiology 2011;53(9):633–41.

16. Vargas MI, Viallon M, Nguyen D, et al. New approaches in imaging of the brachial plexus. Eur J Radiol 2010;74(2):403–10.

17. Chappell KE, Robson MD, Stonebridge-Foster A, et al. Magic angle effects in MR neurography. AJNR Am J Neuroradiol 2004;25(3):431–40.

18. Kästel T, Heiland S, Bäumer P, et al. Magic angle effect: a relevant artifact in MR neurography at 3T? AJNR Am J Neuroradiol 2011;32(5):821–7.

19. Chhabra A, Thawait GK, Soldatos T, et al. High resolution 3T MR neurography of brachial plexus and its branches, with emphasis on 3D imaging. AJNR Am J Neuroradiol 2013;34(3):486–97.

20. Chhabra A, Subhawong TK, Bizzell C, et al. 3T MR neurography using three-dimensional diffusion-weighted PSIF: technical issues and advantages. Skeletal Radiol 2011;40(10):1355–60.

21. Chhabra A, Soldatos T, Subhawong TK, et al. The application of three-dimensional diffusion-weighted PSIF technique in peripheral nerve imaging of the distal extremities. J Magn Reson Imaging 2011;34(4):962–7.

22. Chhabra A, Soldatos T, Durand DJ, et al. The role of magnetic resonance imaging in the diagnostic evaluation of malignant peripheral nerve sheath tumors. Indian J Cancer 2011;48(3):328–34.

23. Petchprapa CN, Rosenberg ZS, Sconfienza LM, et al. MR imaging of entrapment neuropathies of the lower extremity. Part 1. The pelvis and hip. Radiographics 2010;30(4):983–1000.

24. Donovan A, Rosenberg ZS, Cavalcanti CF. MR imaging of entrapment neuropathies of the lower extremity. Part 2. The knee, leg, ankle, and foot. Radiographics 2010;30(4):1001–19.

25. Du R, Auguste KI, Chin CT, et al. Magnetic resonance neurography for the evaluation of peripheral nerve, brachial plexus, and nerve root disorders. J Neurosurg 2010;112(2):362–71.

26. Spinner RJ, Atkinson JL, Scheithauer BW, et al. Peroneal intraneural ganglia: the importance of the articular branch. Clinical series. J Neurosurg 2003;99(2):319–29.

27. Chhabra A, Faridian-Aragh N. 3T MR Neurography of femoral neuropathy. AJNR, Am J Roentgenol 2012;198(1):3–10.

28. Chalian M, Soldatos T, Faridian-Aragh N, et al. 3T Magnetic resonance neurography of tibial nerve pathologies. J Neuroimaging 2013;23(2):296–310.

29. Chhabra A, Lee PP, Bizzell C, et al. High-resolution 3-Tesla magnetic resonance neurography of musculocutaneous neuropathy. J Shoulder Elbow Surg 2012;21(2):e1–6.

30. Mulcahy H, Chew FS. MRI of nontumorous skeletal muscle disease: self-assessment module. AJR Am J Roentgenol 2011;196(Suppl 6):WS57–61.

31. Kim SJ, Hong SH, Jun WS, et al. MR imaging mapping of skeletal muscle denervation in entrapment and compressive neuropathies. Radiographics 2011;31(2):319–32.

MR Imaging of the Brachial Plexus

Amelie M. Lutz, MD[a],*, Garry Gold, MD, MS[b,c,d],
Christopher Beaulieu, MD, PhD[c,e]

KEYWORDS

- MR neurography • Brachial plexus • Brachial plexus neuropathy • Brachial plexus tumors

KEY POINTS

- Continuous improvements in magnetic resonance (MR) scanner, coil, and pulse sequence technology have resulted in the ability to perform routine, high-quality imaging of the brachial plexus.
- Reliable fat suppression on T2-weighted images is an absolute essential for successful brachial plexus MR imaging.
- MRI of the brachial plexus is a valuable diagnostic tool for detection and preoperative staging of mass lesions involving the brachial plexus, in evaluating inflammatory and traumatic brachial plexus changes.

INTRODUCTION

Direct multiplanar imaging capabilities and superior soft tissue contrast have turned magnetic resonance (MR) imaging into the primary imaging tool for evaluation of peripheral nerves, including the brachial plexus.[1,2] There is increasing recognition that dedicated nerve imaging, often called MR neurography (MRN), can add valuable adjunct information to the clinical examination findings of patients with suspected nerve lesions, including brachial plexopathies. Although the term MRN often refers to images such as maximum intensity projections created from source 3-dimensional (3D) T2 images, we refer to dedicated high-resolution MR imaging of the plexus as MRN for the purposes of this article. Indications for brachial plexus MRN include intrinsic and extrinsic tumors, trauma, and inflammatory diseases. Brachial plexus MRN can initially appear somewhat daunting, considering the complexity of the neural structure. However, the nerves

follow a consistent distribution after exiting the intervertebral foramina, such that anyone having an understanding the topographic anatomy and performing careful imaging can do high-quality interpretation of the plexus. In this overview, we present techniques for imaging the brachial plexus, discuss the anatomy, and demonstrate relevant examples of normal and abnormal findings.

ANATOMY OF THE BRACHIAL PLEXUS

The brachial plexus arises from the ventral rami of nerves C5 to C8 and T1 (Fig. 1). The brachial plexus structures travel through the supraclavicular fossa, closely paralleling the course of the subclavian artery (which is the most helpful anatomic landmark on sagittal images), generally forming 3 trunks, each dividing into anterior and posterior divisions forming a total of 6 divisions, which then merge to form 3 cords.[3,4] Individual ventral rami or roots are often best seen on axial images. Roots

[a] Department of Radiology, Stanford University School of Medicine, 300 Pasteur Drive, Stanford, CA 94305, USA; [b] Department of Radiology, Lucas Center, Stanford University School of Medicine, 1201 Welch Rd, Palo Alto 94304, USA; [c] Department of Orthopedic Surgery (by Courtesy), Stanford University School of Medicine, Stanford, CA 94305, USA; [d] School of Bioengineering, Stanford University, Stanford, CA 94305, USA; [e] Department of Radiology, Stanford University School of Medicine, 300 Pasteur Drive, Stanford, CA 94305, USA
* Corresponding author.
E-mail address: alutz@stanford.edu

Neuroimag Clin N Am 24 (2014) 91–108
http://dx.doi.org/10.1016/j.nic.2013.03.024
1052-5149/14/$ – see front matter © 2014 Elsevier Inc. All rights reserved.

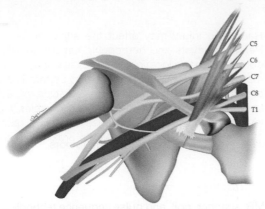

C5
C6
C7
C8
T1

Fig. 1. Important anatomic relationships of the brachial plexus. The plexus arises from C5–C8 nerve roots and passes between the anterior and middle scalene muscles. Identification of the subclavian/axillary artery is the key to localization of the plexus, which generally travels along with the artery.

are also well seen on sagittal images. Because sagittal images are perpendicular to the plane of the plexus, in our practice, this is the favored plane for following the elements from the spine to the axilla. The coronal plane also depicts the plexus elements to good advantage, as the plexus courses within this plane paralleling the subclavian/axillary arteries.

With some experience, and optimized imaging technique, evaluation of the plexus can be relatively straightforward. Although quite detailed evaluation of each level and nerve of the plexus is conceivable, most clinical applications rely on determination of the presence or absence of plexus involvement by tumor or neuritis, with a general anatomic localization. For this latter purpose, we have found that the concept of 5 key sagittal locations correlating with the 5 levels of organization is helpful: roots, trunks, divisions, cords, and branches.

The 5 key sagittal locations are as follows:

1. Intervertebral foramina: Roots (C5–T1). Plexus is formed by ventral rami only (**Fig. 2**A).
2. Scalene muscles, anterior and middle: Trunks (upper trunk, C5–C6; middle trunk, C7; lower trunk, C8/T1). The plexus travels between the anterior and middle scalene muscles and the very short trunks form at approximately the lateral border of the scalene triangle (see **Fig. 2**B).[4]
3. Supraclavicular triangle: Divisions (anterior and posterior). The supraclavicular triangle is above the middle third of the clavicle. The trunks divide into anterior and posterior divisions just

before the brachial plexus passes posterior to the clavicle and go from the lateral aspect of the anterior scalene muscle to the lateral border of the first rib (see **Fig. 2**C).[4]

4. Axilla: Cords (lateral, medial, and posterior). The subclavian artery becomes the axillary artery at the lateral border of the first rib. Cords run from the mid-clavicle to the inferomedial coracoid process, and are named according to location relative to the axillary artery (see **Fig. 2**D). Typical arrangement anterior to posterior on a lateral view is lateral, posterior, and medial cords.
5. Coracoid/pectoralis minor muscle: Branches. Terminal branches include the radial, axillary, musculocutaneous, median, and ulnar nerves (see **Fig. 2**E).

Normal nerve tracts of the plexus are embedded in fat, and are well delineated from neighboring vessels and musculature on T1-weighted sequences (see **Fig. 2**). Individual nerves can be attributed to specific nerve roots with some interindividual variability (eg, the suprascapular and subclavian nerves represent the first branches of the brachial plexus and arise from the upper trunk formed by C5, sometimes also C5 and C6 nerve roots). The suprascapular nerve can often be easily recognized, because it has a relatively large diameter.[3,5] Of note, the long thoracic nerve arises directly from the nerve roots, usually from C5–C7, less commonly also from C4. The signal intensity of the plexus elements is similar to that of muscle on T1-weighted images, and hyperintense to muscle on fat-suppressed T2-weighted sequences. The axillary and subclavian vessels (especially venous structures) can also show considerable high signal within them on fast spin-echo or inversion-recovery–type pulse sequences, and this signal needs to be distinguished from that of the brachial plexus. Saturation bands may help decrease vascular signal, but is not always effective for veins. Mapping out which structures are vascular or not is effectively accomplished with sagittal gradient-echo sequences, which are a part of our routine MRN protocol.

For clinical correlation, an upper brachial plexus injury/lesion involving spinal nerves C5 and C6 results in paralysis of the shoulder muscles and biceps muscle. If the lesion/injury also includes spinal nerve C7, some of the wrist muscles are also impaired. A lower brachial plexus injury/lesion involves spinal nerves C8 and T1, resulting in paralysis of the forearm flexor and the intrinsic muscles of the hand. Injuries to the stellate ganglion or cervical sympathetic trunk may cause Horner syndrome.[3,6,7]

A

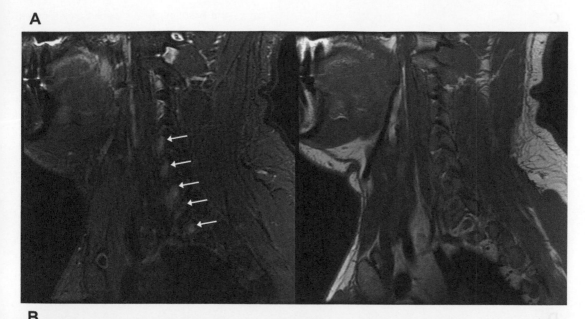

B

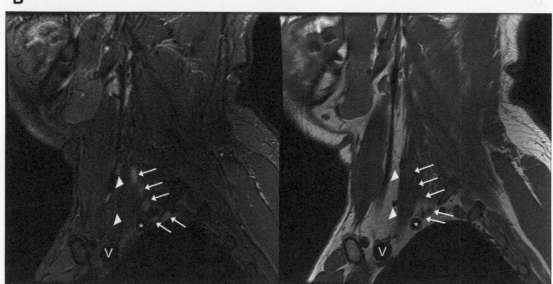

Fig. 2. Normal anatomy of the brachial plexus on sagittal images. Images of sagittal STIR (left, TR, 6000 ms; TE, 45 ms; TI, 170 ms; slice thickness and spacing, 4 and 1 mm, respectively) and T1-weighted FSE (right, TR, 800 ms; TE, 10 ms; slice thickness and spacing, 4 and 1 mm, respectively) demonstrate (*A*) the roots (*white arrows*) of the brachial plexus formed by the ventral rami of C5–T1 just exiting the intervertebral foramina. (*B*) The interscalene region, where the brachial plexus (*white arrows*) travels between the anterior (*white arrowheads*) and middle scalene muscles. This is the level just before the roots merge into the short trunks. Brachiocephalic vein (V) and subclavian artery (*asterisk*).

IMAGING TECHNIQUE

It is slightly controversial whether 1.5-T or 3.0-T field strengths offer the best performance in brachial plexus imaging, but in MRN, there is definitely a trend to use the highest possible field strength for optimal signal-to-noise ratio (SNR) of peripheral nerves at the required fields of view.[1,8–10] Some investigators recommend using 3.0-T scanners,[8,11] although those with 1.5-T scanners can achieve very high-quality imaging with careful technique. The selection of appropriate imaging coils for the brachial plexus is challenging because of the complex anatomy of the supraclavicular region, neck, and shoulders; we are not aware of dedicated coils produced

C

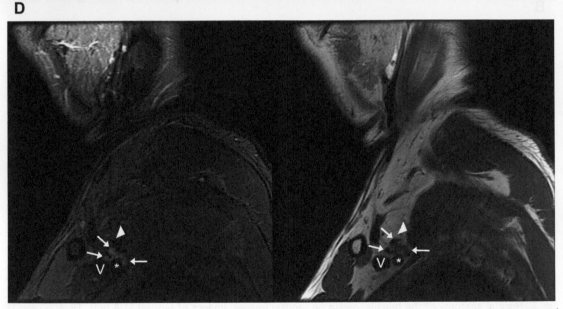

D

Fig. 2. (*C*) The supraclavicular triangle above the middle third of the clavicle where the trunks (*white arrows*) divide into anterior and posterior divisions just before the brachial plexus passes posterior to the clavicle and go from the lateral aspect of the anterior scalene muscle in front of the middle scalene muscle (*white arrowhead*) to the lateral border of the first rib. Subclavian vein (V) and subclavian artery (*asterisk*). (*D*) The divisions merging into cords (lateral, medial, and posterior) at the level where the subclavian artery becomes the axillary artery (*asterisk*) at the lateral border of the first rib. Axillary vein (V).

specifically for brachial plexus imaging. There are also many interfaces with soft tissue and air, creating magnetic field inhomogeneities that can interfere with adequate fat suppression. Although the body coil is capable of imaging a large field of view, the signal to noise of this coil is rarely sufficient to achieve good-quality, high-resolution images covering the brachial plexus from the spine to the axilla. Better options include a torso-type phased-array coil, head-neck-spine phased-array coil, or a specialized neurovascular array coil designed for imaging of the aortic arch and neck vessels. The neurovascular array is our coil of choice for brachial plexus imaging in

E

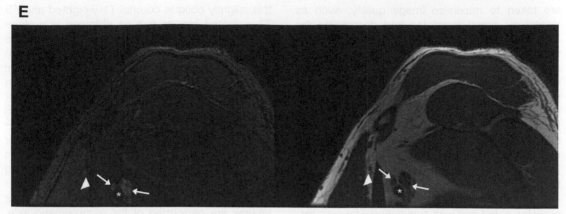

Fig. 2. (*E*) The change from divisions (*white arrows*) into terminal branches at the level of the pectoralis minor muscle just medial to the coracoid (*white arrowhead*), axillary vein (V), and axillary artery (*asterisk*).

almost all cases. Another reasonable coil selection is a flexi-coil or surface coil; the drawback of these coils is that they have limited anatomic coverage without repositioning the coil.[1,12,13]

The classic structural MRN relies predominantly on T2-weighted fat-suppressed (FS) sequences and T1-weighted spin-echo–type sequences. Images are ideally obtained with a high-resolution matrix on a relatively small field of view (**Table 1**). In addition, selective maximum intensity projections of multiple successive sections may be used to lay out the course of a nerve. In our experience, these "neurogram" images are more useful as a communication tool and adjunct image set; primary diagnosis relies on evaluation of source images on all sequences. Reliable fat suppression on

T2-weighted images is an absolute essential for successful brachial plexus MRN. This requisite can actually be very challenging, because conventional spectral ("chemical") saturation techniques that use the differences in resonant frequencies between water and fat fail owing to the multiple air interfaces inside and outside of the chest in the plexus region. Techniques that use differences in T1 relaxation, such as short tau inversion recovery (STIR) and its faster, multi-echo variants, can offer homogeneous fat suppression, but often suffer from relatively lower SNR, longer imaging times, a higher specific absorption rate, and more pulsation artifacts, depending on the technique used. In the authors' experience, however, fast STIR sequences have worked very well when measures

Table 1
Suggested MR imaging protocol for brachial plexus imaging at 3T (neurovascular array coil)

Sequence	Field of View, cm	TR	TE/TI	Slice Thickness, mm/Spacing	Matrix
Cor T1 FSE	22	800	14	3/0.5	512/192
Cor STIR	22	6000	45/170[a]	3/0.5	320/192
Sag T1 FSE	18	800	10	4/1	384/192
Sag STIR	18	6000	45/170	4/1	320/192
Sag GRE	18	25	10[b]	4/1	384/192
Ax T1 FSE	22	800	14	3/1	384/192
Ax STIR	22	6000	45/170	3/1	288/192
If needed:					
Cor T1 IDEAL post Gd	22	900	min full	3/0.5	320/192
Sag T1 IDEAL post Gd	18	900	min full	4/1	320/192

Abbreviations: Ax, axial; Cor, coronal; FSE, fast spin echo; GD, gadolinium; GRE, gradient echo; IDEAL, Iterative decomposition of water and fat with echo asymmetry and least-squares estimation; min full, minimum full; Sag, sagittal; STIR, short tau inversion recovery; TE, echo time; TI, inversion time; TR, repetition time.
[a] Optimal inversion times will vary by scanner field strength and manufacturer. For 1.5 T, we use TI of 140–150 ms. For 3 T, TI is typically set at 170 ms as indicated.
[b] 30° flip angle.

are taken to maximize image quality, such as increasing signal averaging and decreasing the echo time to intermediate values. Consequently, we use predominantly fast inversion recovery imaging with repetition time (TR) of approximately 6000, echo time (TE) approximately 45, and inversion time (TI) approximately 170 ms. This produces robust fat suppression in virtually all cases. Alternatively, we are also using a 3-point Dixon pulse sequence to obtain images with water only, fat only, and combined signal as detailed later in this article. With adequate local or phased-array coils, the image quality can be routinely excellent.

Newer techniques also offer improved fat suppression compared with conventional fat suppression methods: chemical shift imaging, such as the 3-point Dixon-based iterative decomposition of water and fat with echo asymmetry and least-squares estimation (IDEAL) method that applies decomposition of fat and water proton signals according to their chemical shift to isolate these 2 components into 2 separate images,[14,15] as well as hybrid techniques, such as spectral presaturation inversion recovery (SPIR) and spectral presaturation attenuated inversion recovery (SPAIR) that combine both, chemical shift techniques and relaxation rate-dependent techniques.[16,17] The SPAIR technique offers the additional advantages of improved insensitivity to susceptibility limitations or B1 uniformity deficiencies, better SNR than STIR with relative lack of pulsation artifacts, and better SAR attribute.[17]

In traumatic brachial plexus injuries, the application of gadolinium in the acute phase is usually not necessary. The injection of gadolinium contrast agents is usually reserved for neoplastic, inflammatory (infectious, postradiation, autoimmune), and postoperative cases. In chronic plexopathies, gadolinium may demonstrate scar tissue. In plexopathies of unknown origin, it is recommended to check the findings on nonenhanced images to see whether additional contrast-enhanced sequences are required.[10] Although not necessarily adding to the overall diagnostic value for mass detection, selected patients may also undergo 3D contrast-enhanced MR angiography for evaluation of the subclavian, axillary, and brachiocephalic vessels. This may be performed with an ultrafast 3D spoiled gradient echo sequence during dynamic gadolinium injection.[18]

Imaging sequences vary considerably among institutions and for different field strength scanners. The authors' current protocol includes a sagittal localizing image set through the midline to obtain the orientation of the cervical spine. When tolerated, we ideally place the patient's head on a small pad to reduce the normal cervical lordosis. With

this, slightly oblique coronal T1-weighted and FS T2-weighted images can be obtained in a plane that parallels the cervical exit foramina. For those less familiar with the appearance of the plexus on coronal images, it is reasonable to obtain coronal images with a wider field of view of 32 to 40 cm and to evaluate for symmetry. However, for higher-resolution imaging, we decrease the field of view to approximately 24 cm and either center on the cervical spine, or move the coil off center to focus on the plexus unilaterally. This decision is based on radiologist preference. Following coronal images, sagittal T1-weighted, FS T2-weighted, and gradient echo bright blood vascular images are performed of the symptomatic side. Images begin on the contralateral aspect of the cervical spine and continue to the coracoid process on the affected side. The image field of view for these sequences is 20 to 24 cm. Although coronal and sagittal images are adequate to fully evaluate the plexus, the addition of axial images should be considered for those more comfortable with this scan plane or in any case in which detailed evaluation of spinal extent of a focal lesion is needed. Note that we do not consider a brachial plexus examination to include a comprehensive cervical spine study; rather it screens the cervical spine region and focuses on the plexus itself. The exact parameters of the authors' current brachial plexus MR protocol are listed in **Table 1**.

Newer techniques allow for "microstructural" MRN, such as diffusion-weighted imaging (DWI), which can provide information about the integrity of the white matter.[10] But DWI can provide only limited information about the actual direction of the diffusion of water molecules within the nerve, whereas diffusion tensor imaging (DTI) can provide quantitative information about the degree and direction of water diffusion within the nerves of the brachial plexus and, when used for tractography, it can visualize the white matter tract to characterize its integrity.[1,10,11,19] DTI of the brachial plexus is challenging, with some of the main limitations being small size of the nerve fibers, and the localization and course of the brachial plexus between the neck and the shoulder resulting in geometric distortion and artifacts.[19] Recently, however, tractography has been shown to demonstrate the patterns of nerve fibers passing around schwannoma masses, of nerve fibers passing centrally through neurofibromas, and infiltration/disruption of nerve fibers by metastases in the brachial plexus region, which may further help in lesion characterization.[19] Furthermore, another recent study showed good reproducibility of DTI quantitative analysis with only small variations in calculated fractional anisotropy and apparent diffusion coefficient values in the brachial plexus components of normal volunteers.[20] DTI and tractography are not yet in wide routine clinical use, but offer exciting research opportunities. With ongoing technical improvements, the trend toward ever-higher field strengths, and establishing of valid and reproducible standard normal values, they will likely very soon become important tools in the routine evaluation of brachial plexus pathologies.

IMAGE ANALYSIS

In evaluating a brachial plexus study, we use picture archiving and communication system to view anatomically matched T1 and T2 images side-by-side, synchronized in stack mode (see **Fig. 2**). Beginning with coronal images, we identify bony and muscular landmarks and use the flow void of the subclavian/axillary artery to locate the plexus. Once localized, T2-weighted images are reviewed in detail for the caliber, course, and signal intensity of the plexal elements. Care is taken not to confuse bright signal in vessels with nerves. Sagittal images are subsequently analyzed, synchronizing T1, T2FS, and gradient echo (GRE) images in stack mode. Beginning at the spine, the exit foramina lead to the interscalene area and the trunks/divisions, as the nerves descend (C5–C8) or ascend (T1) to travel with the artery. As one proceeds laterally, any deviation, mass, alteration in signal intensity, or discontinuity is sought. The musculature of the shoulder girdle is checked for any denervation-type edema on T2 sequences. Vascular GRE images are used to show patency of the vessels. When obtained, axial images are reviewed primarily for the spinal canal contents and any intraspinal extension of masses. In any case of suspected thoracic outlet syndrome, one should also be conscious to look for angular deviations of the plexus that might reflect fibrous bands, which themselves are too small to resolve. Bony anomalies, such as cervical ribs or fractures of the clavicle or first rib should also be kept in mind, and ideally correlated with radiographs.

PATHOLOGY
Intrinsic Brachial Plexus Tumors

MRN is a valuable tool in the search for preoperative staging of mass lesions involving the brachial plexus, as it often can determine whether a tumor is intrinsic or extrinsic to the brachial plexus components. Commonly reported neurogenic tumors of the brachial plexus are schwannomas, neurofibromas, plexiform neurofibromas, and malignant

peripheral nerve sheath tumors, although benign nerve sheath tumors are more common than malignant ones in this region. Approximately one-third of neurofibromas occur in the setting of neurocutaneous syndromes (all plexiform neurofibromas are usually seen in the context of neurofibromatosis type I), whereas two-thirds of cases occur as isolated tumors.[2,11] The most commonly encountered neurogenic tumors of the brachial plexus are neurofibromas and schwannomas.[21] Peripheral nerve sheath tumors of the brachial plexus may show classic findings on MRN, such as the target, fascicular, and tail signs on T2-weighted images, split fat sign on T1-weighted images, and the bag of worms sign for plexiform neurofibromas[11,22,23]; however, schwannomas can occasionally show cystic necrosis and not develop the target sign, which may then hamper differentiation from malignant nerve sheath tumors. Schwannomas are seen in an eccentric location and tend to be encapsulated, causing fascicular deviation, whereas neurofibromas are not encapsulated and typically invade the nerve causing the appearance of the nerve running through the center of the tumor.[2,11] This differentiation is important for the prognosis, because surgical resection of schwannomas may be feasible without resulting nerve damage.[24] The contrast-enhancement pattern of peripheral nerve sheath tumors is typically very avid.

Reliable differentiation between benign and malignant peripheral nerve sheath tumors is problematic by imaging alone, but features, such as advanced local invasion and poorly defined margins, absence of the target sign on T2-weighted sequences of larger size (>5 cm), and bone destruction, suggest malignancy (**Fig. 3**).[2,11,24] DWI has been shown beneficial in the evaluation of malignant change in plexiform neurofibromas, but in the end biopsy is required when malignant change is suspected within a brachial plexus neoplasm.[11,25]

The most common non-neurogenic primary brachial plexus tumors are desmoid tumors (**Fig. 4**), followed by lipomas.[24] In MRN, desmoid tumors will typically be isointense to muscle on T1-weighted sequences, inhomogeneously hyperintense on T2-weighted sequences (with some low T2 signal because of increased collagen content in parts of the tumors) with infiltrative margins and marked contrast enhancement (see **Fig. 4**).[24] Lipomas are usually well characterized by MRN as fat-isointense lesions, although well-differentiated liposarcomas can show similar imaging characteristics. Another important entity is lymphoma, which cannot only encase the brachial plexus due to enlarged lymph nodes, but can also primarily involve the brachial plexus in rare cases.

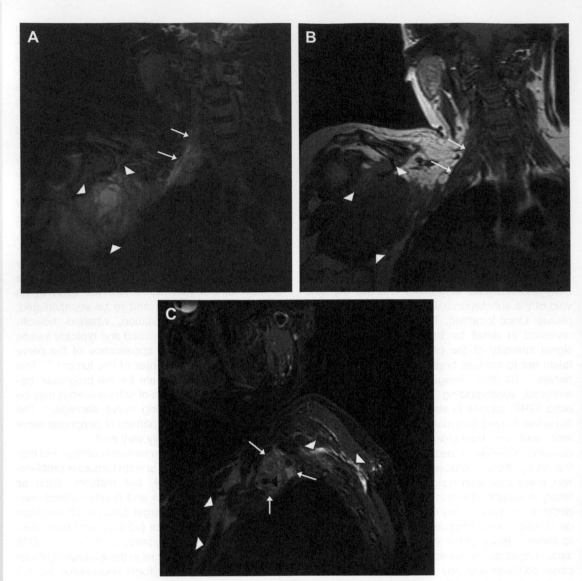

Fig. 3. A 42-year-old female patient with a malignant peripheral nerve sheath tumor of the right brachial plexus. (A) Images of coronal STIR sequence (TR, 6000 ms; TE, 45 ms; TI, 170 ms) and (B) corresponding image of coronal T1-weighted FSE sequence (TR, 800 ms; TE, 14 ms) both demonstrate a large mass with heterogeneous, predominantly T2-hyperintense signal (*white arrowheads*) reaching from the right lateral chest wall to the proximal humerus with proximal spread (*white arrows*) along the brachial plexus to the level of the trunks and roots, as indicated by the enlargement and edema of the more proximal brachial plexus components. (C) Image of a sagittal STIR sequence (TR, 6000 ms: TE, 45 ms; TI, 170 ms) demonstrates encasing of the subclavian artery (*black arrowhead*) by the tumor (*white arrows*), which was occluded slightly more distally and associated soft tissue edema (*white arrowheads*) involving the adjacent muscles including pectoralis major and minor, infraspinatus, teres minor, and latissimus dorsi.

Lymphoma may affect nerve roots and trunks causing increased signal and neural enlargement of selected levels (**Fig. 5**). Primary neurolymphoma may present in MRN with diffuse thickening or multifocal nodularity of the involved neural structures and show diffuse contrast enhancement.[11]

Extrinsic Brachial Plexus Tumors

In extrinsic brachial plexus masses, MRN offers important information on the site and extent of proximity to the neural structures for surgical planning.

Primary neoplasms in close vicinity to the brachial plexus, such as bronchogenic carcinoma/Pancoast tumors of the thoracic apex;

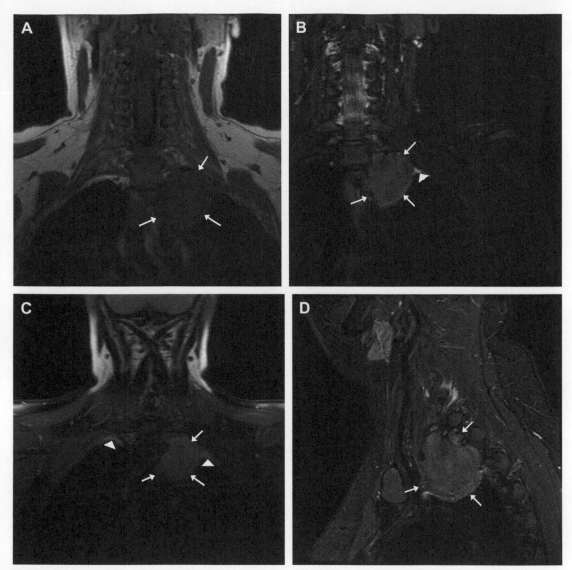

Fig. 4. A 30-year-old female patient with desmoid tumor (*white arrows*) at the left medial lung apex involving the left brachial plexus. Images of (*A*) coronal T1-weighted FSE sequences (TR, 800 ms; TE, 14 ms), of (*B*) coronal STIR sequences and of (*C*) contrast-enhanced T1-weighted fat-saturated FSE sequence demonstrate the tumor (*white arrows*) at the left lung apex with low T1 and high T2 signal and relatively homogeneous contrast enhancement involving primarily the inferior trunk/medial cord. Mild pleural thickening/pleural fluid is noted at the lung apex (*white arrowheads* on images *B, C*). (*D*) Image of a sagittal STIR (TR, 6000 ms: TE, 45 ms; TI, 170 ms) sequence demonstrates the proximal tumor (*white arrows*) extent reaching just distal to the inferior brachial plexus roots.

neurogenic tumors of the vagus nerve, phrenic nerve, and sympathetic trunk (typically, the course of those tumors is in a more vertical direction than for primary brachial plexus tumors); or bone tumors can directly extend into and involve the brachial plexus. But more commonly, metastatic disease, particularly from breast carcinoma (**Fig. 6**), melanoma, head and neck cancer, and lymphoma will involve nodes adjacent to the brachial plexus, causing nerve irritation/

compression or invasion.[2,11] In patients with plexopathy and Horner syndrome, axial images are especially useful to demonstrate a possible paraspinal extension of tumor. In the posttreatment setting, high-resolution coronal and sagittal images are especially beneficial to distinguish whether a patient's symptoms are caused by (recurrent) tumor, postoperative or posttreatment changes with scarring, or compressive neuropathy resulting from regional deformity.

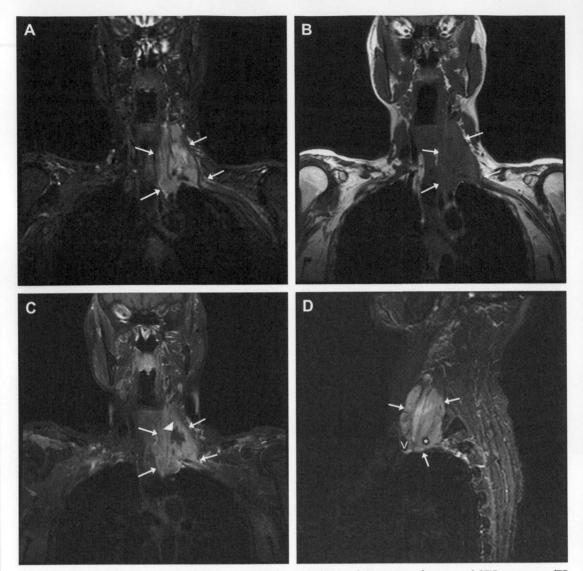

Fig. 5. A 56-year-old female patient with non-Hodgkin lymphoma. (A) Images of a coronal STIR sequence (TR, 6000 ms: TE, 45 ms; TI, 170 ms) and (B) of a coronal T1-weighted FSE sequence (TR, 800 ms; TE, 14 ms) demonstrate a large enhancing mass (*white arrows*) with moderately increased heterogeneous T2 signal and intermediate to low T1 signal intensity in the left neck immediately adjacent to the cervical spine extending out to the midclavicular region encasing the brachial plexus from the roots to the trunks above the subclavian artery. (C) Image of a coronal T1 IDEAL sequence (TR, 900 ms; TE, minimum full) demonstrates an area of low-attenuation centrally within the tumor (*white arrowhead*) that does not enhance after contrast administration, consistent with necrosis. (D) Image of a sagittal STIR sequence (TR, 6000 ms: TE, 45 ms; TI, 170 ms) clearly demonstrates involvement of the brachial plexus by the lymphoma (*white arrows*) and encasement of the subclavian artery (*asterisk*) and vein (V). (*Courtesy of* Kathryn Stevens, MD, Associate Professor of Radiology, Stanford School of Medicine.)

Inflammatory Brachial Plexus Pathologies

In cases of inflammatory brachial plexus pathologies, patients may present with sudden onset of pain, often followed by weakness and paraesthesia, or patients may experience only sensory abnormalities. Sometimes it is difficult to differentiate acute plexitis from a cervical radiculopathy or

even rotator cuff tears clinically, but virtually all cases can be solved by MR imaging.[26]

Inflammation After Radiation Treatment

The most common inflammatory plexopathy occurs following radiation treatment, which may manifest up to 30 months after treatment, usually

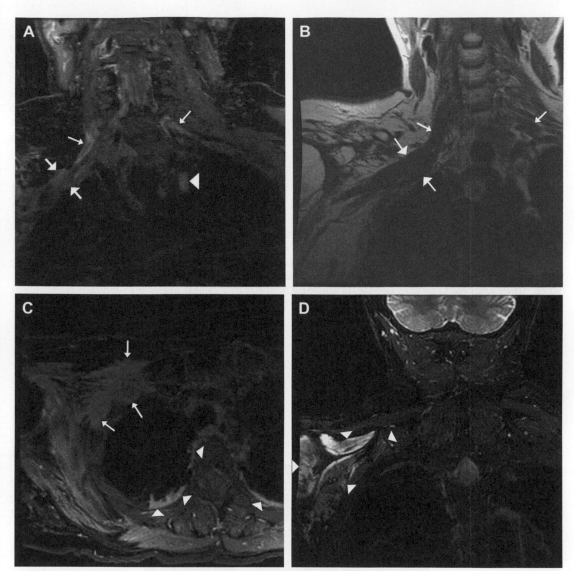

Fig. 6. A 62-year-old female patient with breast cancer metastasis involving the right brachial plexus. (A) Image of a coronal STIR sequence (TR, 6000 ms: TE, 45 ms; TI, 170 ms) and (B) image of a coronal T1-weighted FSE sequence (TR, 800 ms; TE, 14 ms) show marked thickening and increased T2 signal within the roots, trunks, and divisions of the right brachial plexus (*small white arrows*). Mild thickening and edema are also present within the brachial plexus on the left in image (A, B) (*white arrows*). Pleural thickening, as seen on image (B) (*white arrowheads*) indicates status post radiation therapy, which could explain part of the brachial plexus pathology as post-therapeutic changes. But an additional area of nodularity with increased T2 signal (*big white arrows*) is noted at the level of the right divisions in image (A, B, C). The latter finding is confirmed by areas of nodular/masslike enhancement (*white arrows*), as seen on the image of an axial T1-weighted IDEAL sequence post contrast administration. (D) Image of a coronal T1-IDEAL sequence (TR, 900 ms; TE, min full) demonstrates contrast enhancement (*white arrowheads*) as seen along the muscles of the right back and shoulder girdle, most pronounced within the right trapezius muscle and rotator cuff. Along with the edema that was present on T2-weighted images, this finding likely represents the late subacute phase of denervation injury. The fact that these nodular changes of the brachial plexus and the muscle edema were not present on the left side further supports the notion of involvement of the brachial plexus by the underlying malignancy on the right. (*Courtesy of* Kathryn Stevens, MD, Associate Professor of Radiology, Stanford School of Medicine.)

with doses exceeding 6000 cGy.[27] In the post radiation setting, it is essential to differentiate tumor recurrence from inflammatory changes of the brachial plexus. Typical MR imaging findings to expect in radiation-induced brachial plexus inflammation include relatively uniform, symmetric thickening and contrast enhancement of brachial plexus structures along with T2 hyperintensity of the plexus within the irradiated region (Fig. 7). Often, the different neural structures can no longer be separated from each other. Tumor recurrence, on the other hand, will result in a focal or diffuse heterogeneously enhancing mass.[1,2] Because of the often extensive and persistent tissue changes in radiation-induced inflammation, follow-up studies are often needed to reliably differentiate between tumor recurrence and post radiation treatment changes. Over time, fibrotic changes of the brachial plexus and surrounding tissue may prevail.

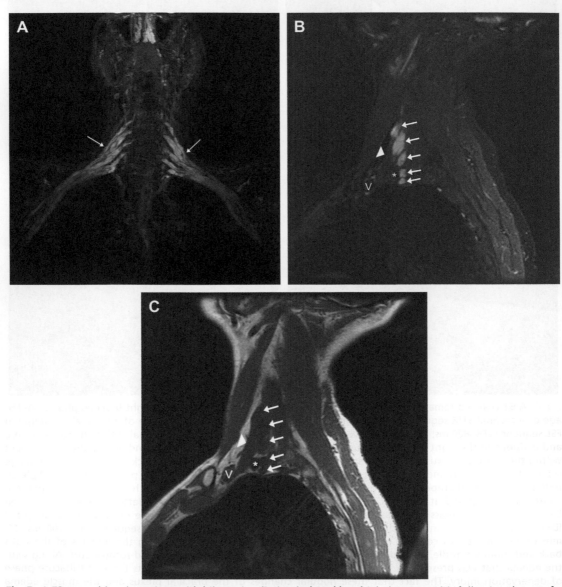

Fig. 7. A 52-year-old male patient with bilateral radiation-induced brachial plexus neuritis following therapy for non-Hodgkin lymphoma. (*A*) Maximum intensity projection of coronal STIR sequences (TR, 6000 ms: TE, 45 ms; TI, 170 ms) demonstrates symmetric, relatively smooth enlargement and edema of the bilateral brachial plexuses (*white arrows*). (*B*) Image of a sag T1-weighted FSE sequence (TR, 800 ms; TE, 10 ms) and (*C*) image of a sagittal STIR sequence (TR, 6000 ms: TE, 45 ms; TI, 170 ms) also show the marked enlargement and edema of the brachial plexus (*white arrows*) at the level of the roots. Also seen are the anatomic landmarks brachiocephalic vein (V), subclavian artery (*asterisk*), and anterior scalene muscle (*white arrowhead*).

Other Inflammatory Plexopathies, Including Immune-Mediated Plexopathies

Brachial plexitis/parsonage turner syndrome

Idiopathic brachial plexitis, also known as Parsonage Turner syndrome, is a usually self-limiting inflammatory disorder of the brachial plexus, more common in men than in women, and may sometimes be bilateral. The exact etiology is still unknown, but autoimmune/inflammatory causes are suggested. Initially, patients typically present with pain in the neck, shoulder, and scapula regions, most pronounced at night. After a few weeks to months, muscle weakness will prevail. Disease durations range from several months up to 3 years, and in a small percentage symptoms may never fully resolve. On MRN, diffuse T2 hyperintensity and enlargement of affected neural structures may be seen, along with muscle edema; muscle atrophy may be seen on T1-weighted images. In fact, a commonly seen presentation on shoulder MR imaging is T2-hyperintensity in various muscles that often does not follow a typical innervation pattern (eg, isolated edema in the teres minor muscle).[11,28]

Chronic inflammatory demyelinating polyneuropathy/Multifocal motor neuropathy/Multifocal inflammatory demyelinating neuropathy/Guillain-Barré Syndrome

Most of the immune-mediated plexopathies are diagnosed clinically according to the distribution of deficits, which allows differentiation of predominant involvement of motor/sensory fibers and the time course, but also based on electrophysiology examination findings, laboratory parameters, such as serum antibodies, and clinical context. Chronic inflammatory demyelinating polyneuropathy (CIDP), an acquired chronic, immune-mediated, multifocal, demyelinating neuropathy, primarily affects the spinal nerves, plexi, and proximal nerve trunks, whereas Guillain-Barré syndrome (GBS) is an acute syndrome and typically involves many nerves in a distal-to-proximal ascending distribution pattern and is most commonly seen in the post respiratory or gastrointestinal tract infection setting, but other triggers, such as vaccinations (including influenza) have also been reported.[26,29] Rarely, GBS may even present in an atypical manner, involving predominantly the upper extremities, mimicking brachial plexus neuritis and entirely sparing the lower extremities.[30] Multifocal motor neuropathy (MMN), an immune-mediated demyelinating neuropathy, results in asymmetrical weakness and atrophy, and affects individual peripheral nerves, more commonly of the upper extremity.[26] On MR imaging, the immune-mediated plexopathies may demonstrate nonspecific inflammatory changes, such as diffuse thickening of the affected nerves with increased signal intensity on T2-weighted images, sometimes associated with contrast-enhancement.[2] The hereditary, Charcot-Marie-Tooth disease can mimic the appearance of CIDP on MR imaging with findings of focal or diffuse peripheral nerve enlargement, limb atrophy, and fatty degeneration of the involved muscles.[26] **Fig. 8** shows an example of CIDP.

Sarcoidosis

Another inflammatory entity that may affect the brachial plexus, although much rarer, is sarcoidosis, usually seen in the context of systemic sarcoidosis. The imaging findings include mild thickening of nerves that may appear nodular and slightly irregular with mild to moderate T2 hyperintensity and mild enhancement after contrast. Sometimes associated subacute denervation changes within the affected muscles with T2 hyperintensity can be seen, but atrophy is rare. Because metastatic malignancy is the main differential diagnosis, short-term follow-up examinations and/or biopsy are often required.[31]

Infection

Direct infectious involvement of the brachial plexus is rare, but pyogenic infection may develop after surgical treatment of either the brachial plexus itself or of nearby structures. Compression of the brachial plexus by adjacent abscess formations is likely more common.[32] *Mycobacterium leprae* is a known entity that can directly involve peripheral nerves, but tends to favor superficial nerves in cooler body regions. MRN findings may demonstrate moderate T2 hyperintensity associated with mild thickening of the affected neural structures in leprosy, but contrast enhancement is rare.[11]

Inflammatory involvement of the brachial plexus is also known to occur secondary to viral infections, such as in herpes zoster flares or herpes virus infections.[33,34]

Brachial plexus trauma

In infants, brachial plexus palsy is often secondary to excessive severe traction force exerted on the brachial plexus during complicated deliveries. Coincidental presence of cervical ribs can even increase the risk to develop brachial plexus palsy from complicated deliveries.[35]

In adults, however, most plexus palsies are due to traumatic injuries, usually resulting from high-velocity trauma, such as motorcycle accidents. Clinical symptoms include and/or range from pain to paralysis of the involved limb. Clinical

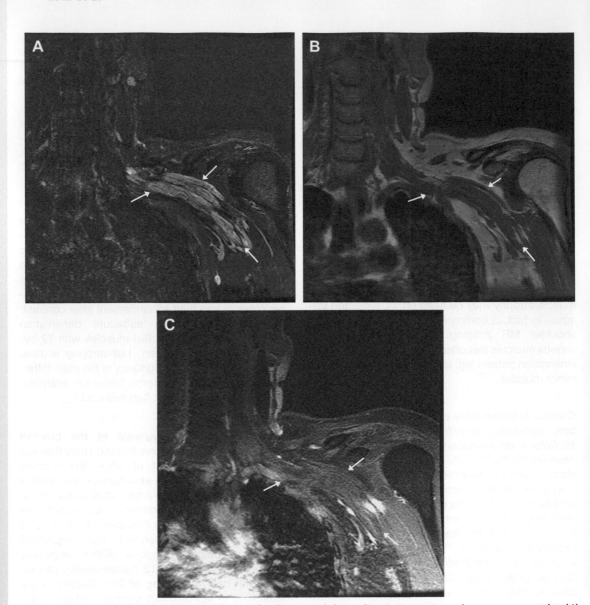

Fig. 8. A 39-year-old female patient with multifocal acquired demyelinating sensory and motor neuropathy. (*A*) Image of a coronal STIR sequence (TR, 600 ms: TE, 45·ms; TI, 170 ms), (*B*) of a coronal T1-weighted FSE sequence, and (*C*) of a coronal T1-weighted fat-saturated multiplanar spoiled gradient-recalled acquisition in the steady state (MPSPGR) sequence (TR, 150 ms; TE, 2 ms) after contrast administration demonstrate prominent enlargement of the entire left brachial plexus elements (*white arrows*) with increased T2 signal and are remarkable for lack of contrast enhancement following administration of a gadolinium contrast agent. The lack of enhancement makes malignancy or acute inflammatory neuritis unlikely and favors a chronic demyelinating process. Biopsy proved the etiology to be multifocal acquired demyelinating sensory and motor neuropathy, a variant of chronic inflammatory demyelinating neuropathy.

examination alone cannot reliably distinguish between the preganglionic and postganglionic injuries, but differentiation between both is important for prognosis and therapeutic management.[6,36,37] Nerves may also be indirectly affected (eg, by compression or injury of nerves by osseous fragments, hematomas, or compressed by large callus formations in a more chronic phase post fracture).[38,39]

Preganglionic injuries often are associated with spinal cord changes, such as contralateral displacement of the cord, T2-hyperintensity consistent with cord edema (acute phase), myelomalacia, syringomyelia (in a more subacute to chronic phase), and susceptibility effects from hemosiderin accumulation.[6] The observed pathologic changes may be extensive on the affected side of the spinal cord or localized to the exit zone of the ventral nerve root. Avulsion injuries with or without formation of pseudomeningocele may also be seen in preganglionic plexus injuries. In addition, indirect signs, such as muscular denervation changes in the posterior cervical paraspinal muscles, especially in the multifidus muscle, may help identify a preganglionic injury, but contrast enhancement of affected paraspinal muscles is considered a more accurate indirect sign of root avulsion injury.[6,26,36]

Postganglionic injuries can present as stretch injuries, with the nerve remaining in continuity, or as an avulsion injury with nerve disruption. In the more common stretch-type injuries, thickening of T1-hypointense to isointense and T2-hyperintense nerves is seen, with the nerve remaining in contiguity, whereas fibrosis with thickening of the nerves is seen in a more chronic phase of the injury. Discontinuity and distal nerve retraction is seen in avulsion-type injuries.[6,26,36] Figs. 9 and 10 demonstrate the difference in imaging appearance between brachial plexus stretch injury versus complete avulsion.

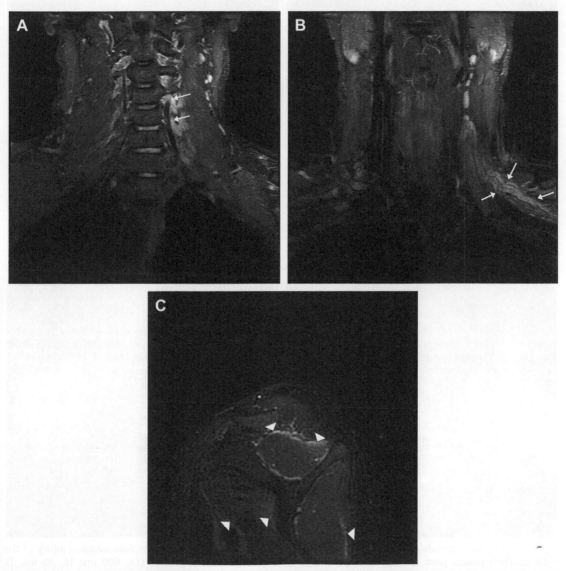

Fig. 9. A 28-year-old male patient with left brachial plexus stretch injury after a motorcycle accident. (*A, B*) Images of coronal STIR sequence (TR, 600 ms: TE, 45 ms; TI, 170 ms) demonstrate mild enlargement and hyperintensity of the entire brachial plexus, most pronounced at C5 and C6, from the roots (*A, white arrows*) to the branches, with perineural edema as well as curvilinear course of the plexus at the level of the divisions and cords (*B, white arrow*). (*C*) Images of sagittal STIR sequence (TR, 600 ms: TE, 45 ms; TI, 170 ms) with ipsilateral perimuscular edema (*white arrowheads*) seen surrounding the entire rotator cuff musculature indicating hyperextension of the left neck/shoulder region during the injury.

Thoracic outlet syndrome

The term thoracic outlet syndrome (TOS) is generally reserved for dynamically induced neural, arterial, or venous compression, which can typically be induced by arm elevation due to congenital or acquired narrowing in any of the 3 compartments of the thoracic outlet region. Often, neurologic symptoms will predominate. Although clinical examinations, including provocative maneuvers and electrophysiologic examinations, still represent the mainstay of diagnostic workup, MR imaging has become the imaging modality of choice, especially in the workup of neural TOS, owing to the significant overlap of clinical symptoms with other disease entities, including Parsonage-Turner syndrome or even unknown tumors. The 3 compartments of the thoracic outlet include the interscalene triangle most medially (the subclavian

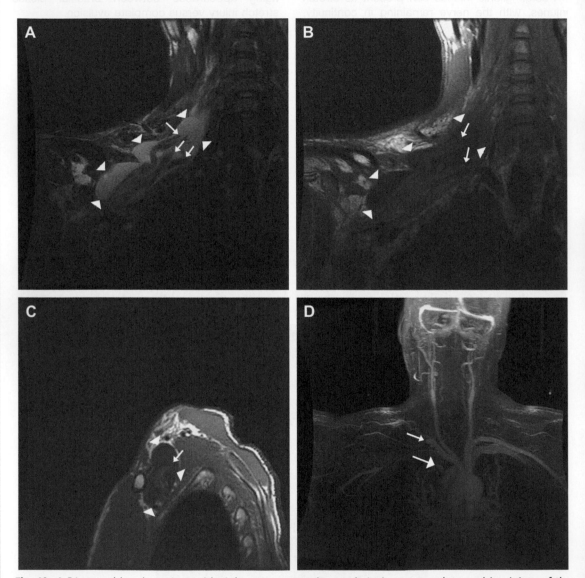

Fig. 10. A 31-year-old male patient with right upper extremity paralysis due to complete avulsion injury of the right brachial plexus post car accident. (A) Image of a coronal STIR sequence (TR, 600 ms: TE, 45 ms; TI, 170 ms), (B) image of a coronal and (C) of a sagittal T1-weighted FSE sequence (TR, 800 ms; TE, 14 ms) show a large supraclavicular hematoma (*white arrowheads*). In this hematoma, serpiginous, thickened cordlike structures can be seen that represent ruptured, edematous components of the brachial plexus (*white arrows*), which had been completely avulsed off the level of the right trunks. (D) Maximum intensity projection of a coronal MFAST MR angiography sequence (TR, 4.2 ms; TE, 0.9 ms) demonstrates complete occlusion of the right subclavian artery (*small white arrow*) and severe compression of the right brachiocephalic/subclavian vein (*large white arrow*), the latter likely in the context of the large adjacent hematoma.

artery travels at the bottom and the trunks of the brachial plexus posteriorly and superiorly, respectively, to the artery), then slightly more laterally the costoclavicular space (the subclavian vein travels through this space anteriorly, the subclavian artery right adjacent posterior to it, and the 3 cords of the brachial plexus are located above and posterior to the vascular structures), and the most lateral the retropectoralis minor space (the subclavian vein travels through this space anteriorly, the subclavian artery right adjacent posterior to it, and the 3 cords of the brachial plexus are located above and posterior to the vascular structures).[40] Compression of brachial plexus structures is known to be most common in the costoclavicular space and in the interscalene triangle, but rarely occurs in the retropectoralis minor space.[40] Acquisition of high-quality images in the sagittal plane is of particular importance in TOS cases. Some institutions obtain images not only in the arm-down, neutral position, but additionally also in hyperabduction of the arm. Comparing these images, the width of the anatomic spaces and the caliber of involved structures can be assessed. Typical etiologies causing TOS range from congenital osseous variants (cervical ribs or elongated transverse processes of C7, exostoses of the rib and clavicle) to acquired osseous anomalies (displacement and/or callus formation of rib and clavicle fractures), from congenital soft tissue variants (fibrous bands, muscle insertion variations and accessory muscles) to acquired soft tissue abnormalities (excessive scarring) and can also include muscular problems from backpacking or weight lifting with excessive weight load, and even bad posture.[40,41] Fibrous bands are typically difficult to image directly, but elevation of the subclavian artery or angular deviation of the plexus elements, as seen on sagittal images, may be an important indirect sign of a tight fibrous band.[40] On coronal FS T2-weighted images, review of multiple images in sequence may show an angular deformity at the lateral border of the scalene muscles.

ACKNOWLEDGMENTS

The authors thank Amy Morris for the design of the anatomic sketch.

REFERENCES

1. Vargas MI, Viallon M, Nguyen D, et al. New approaches in imaging of the brachial plexus. Eur J Radiol 2010;74(2):403–10.

2. van Es HW, Bollen TL, van Heesewijk HP. MRI of the brachial plexus: a pictorial review. Eur J Radiol 2010; 74(2):391–402.

3. Kawai H. Anatomy of the brachial plexus. In: Kawai H, Kawabata H, editors. Brachial plexus palsy. Singapore: World Scientific Publishing Co; 2000. p. 1–24.

4. Rubin JA, Wesolowski JR. Neck MR imaging anatomy. Magn Reson Imaging Clin N Am 2011;19(3): 457–73, vii.

5. Chalian M, Faridian-Aragh N, Soldatos T, et al. High-resolution 3T MR neurography of suprascapular neuropathy. Acad Radiol 2011;18(8):1049–59.

6. Yoshikawa T, Hayashi N, Yamamoto S, et al. Brachial plexus injury: clinical manifestations, conventional imaging findings, and the latest imaging techniques. Radiographics 2006;26(Suppl 1):S133–43.

7. Millesi H. Brachial plexus injuries. In: Jupiter JP, editor. Flynn's hand surgery. Baltimore (MD): Williams & Wilkins; 1991. p. 457–63.

8. Tagliafico A, Succio G, Emanuele Neumaier C, et al. MR imaging of the brachial plexus: comparison between 1.5-T and 3-T MR imaging: preliminary experience. Skeletal Radiol 2011;40(6):717–24.

9. Zhang Z, Song L, Meng Q, et al. Segmented echo planar MR imaging of the brachial plexus with inversion recovery magnetization preparation at 3.0T. J Magn Reson Imaging 2008;28(2):440–4.

10. Mallouhi A, Marik W, Prayer D, et al. 3T MR tomography of the brachial plexus: structural and microstructural evaluation. Eur J Radiol 2012;81(9): 2231–45.

11. Chhabra A, Chalian M, Andreisek G. Brachial plexus. In: Chhabra A, Andreisek G, editors. Magnetic resonance neurography. New Delhi (India): Jaypee; 2011. p. 133–60.

12. Hayes CE, Tsuruda JS, Mathis CM, et al. Brachial plexus: MR imaging with a dedicated phased array of surface coils. Radiology 1997;203(1):286–9.

13. Panasci DJ, Holliday RA, Shpizner B. Advanced imaging techniques of the brachial plexus. Hand Clin 1995;11(4):545–53.

14. Reeder SB, Pineda AR, Wen Z, et al. Iterative decomposition of water and fat with echo asymmetry and least-squares estimation (IDEAL): application with fast spin-echo imaging. Magn Reson Med 2005;54(3):636–44.

15. Reeder SB, McKenzie CA, Pineda AR, et al. Water-fat separation with IDEAL gradient-echo imaging. J Magn Reson Imaging 2007;25(3):644–52.

16. de Kerviler E, Leroy-Willig A, Clement O, et al. Fat suppression techniques in MRI: an update. Biomed Pharmacother 1998;52(2):69–75.

17. Lauenstein TC, Sharma P, Hughes T, et al. Evaluation of optimized inversion-recovery fat-suppression techniques for T2-weighted abdominal MR imaging. J Magn Reson Imaging 2008;27(6):1448–54.

18. Nael K, Villablanca JP, Pope WB, et al. Supraaortic arteries: contrast-enhanced MR angiography at 3.0 T–highly accelerated parallel acquisition for

improved spatial resolution over an extended field of view. Radiology 2007;242(2):600–9.

19. Vargas MI, Viallon M, Nguyen D, et al. Diffusion tensor imaging (DTI) and tractography of the brachial plexus: feasibility and initial experience in neoplastic conditions. Neuroradiology 2010;52(3): 237–45.

20. Tagliafico A, Calabrese M, Puntoni M, et al. Brachial plexus MR imaging: accuracy and reproducibility of DTI-derived measurements and fibre tractography at 3.0-T. Eur Radiol 2011;21(8):1764–71.

21. Bowen BC, Pattany PM, Saraf-Lavi E, et al. The brachial plexus: normal anatomy, pathology, and MR imaging. Neuroimaging Clin N Am 2004;14(1): 59–85, vii–viii.

22. Jee WH, Oh SN, McCauley T, et al. Extraaxial neurofibromas versus neurilemmomas: discrimination with MRI. AJR Am J Roentgenol 2004;183(3):629–33.

23. Thawait SK, Chaudhry V, Thawait GK, et al. High-resolution MR neurography of diffuse peripheral nerve lesions. AJNR Am J Neuroradiol 2011;32(8): 1365–72.

24. Saifuddin A. Imaging tumours of the brachial plexus. Skeletal Radiol 2003;32(7):375–87.

25. Todd M, Shah GV, Mukherji SK. MR imaging of brachial plexus. Top Magn Reson Imaging 2004; 15(2):113–25.

26. Sureka J, Cherian RA, Alexander M, et al. MRI of brachial plexopathies. Clin Radiol 2009;64(2): 208–18.

27. Aralasmak A, Karaali K, Cevikol C, et al. MR imaging findings in brachial plexopathy with thoracic outlet syndrome. AJNR Am J Neuroradiol 2010;31(3): 410–7.

28. Gaskin CM, Helms CA. Parsonage-Turner syndrome: MR imaging findings and clinical information of 27 patients. Radiology 2006;240(2):501–7.

29. Lehmann HC, Meyer Zu Horste G, Kieseier BC, et al. Pathogenesis and treatment of immune-mediated neuropathies. Ther Adv Neurol Disord 2009;2(4): 261–81.

30. Bamberger PD, Thys DM. Guillain-Barre syndrome in a patient with pancreatic cancer after an epidural-general anesthetic. Anesth Analg 2005;100(4):1197–9.

31. Amrami KK, Felmlee JP, Spinner RJ. MRI of peripheral nerves. Neurosurg Clin N Am 2008;19(4):559–72, vi.

32. Aycicek A, Eser O, Sezer M, et al. A neck mass with brachial plexus injury: Pott's disease. Am J Otol 2009;30(5):350–2.

33. Ayoub T, Raman V, Chowdhury M. Brachial neuritis caused by varicella-zoster diagnosed by changes in brachial plexus on MRI. J Neurol 2010;257(1):1–4.

34. Heo DH, Jun AY, Cho YJ. Magnetic resonance neurography findings in herpetic brachial plexopathy. J Neurol 2011;258(1):137–9.

35. Desurkar A, Mills K, Pitt M, et al. Congenital lower brachial plexus palsy due to cervical ribs. Dev Med Child Neurol 2011;53(2):188–90.

36. Doi K, Otsuka K, Okamoto Y, et al. Cervical nerve root avulsion in brachial plexus injuries: magnetic resonance imaging classification and comparison with myelography and computerized tomography myelography. J Neurosurg 2002;96(Suppl 3):277–84.

37. Abbott R, Abbott M, Alzate J, et al. Magnetic resonance imaging of obstetrical brachial plexus injuries. Childs Nerv Syst 2004;20(10):720–5.

38. Lin CC, Lin J. Brachial plexus palsy caused by secondary fracture displacement in a patient with closed clavicle fracture. Orthopedics 2009;32(10). pii:orthosupersite.com/view.asp?rID=43780.

39. Murata K, Maeda M, Yoshida A, et al. Axillary artery injury combined with delayed brachial plexus palsy due to compressive hematoma in a young patient: a case report. J Brachial Plex Peripher Nerve Inj 2008;3:9.

40. Demondion X, Herbinet P, Van Sint Jan S, et al. Imaging assessment of thoracic outlet syndrome. Radiographics 2006;26(6):1735–50.

41. Linda DD, Harish S, Stewart BG, et al. Multimodality imaging of peripheral neuropathies of the upper limb and brachial plexus. Radiographics 2010; 30(5):1373–400.

High-Resolution Magnetic Resonance Neurography in Upper Extremity Neuropathy

Majid Chalian, MD[a], Ashkan Heshmatzadeh Behzadi, MD[a],
Eric H. Williams, MD[a], Jaimie T. Shores, MD[a],
Avneesh Chhabra, MD[b],*

KEYWORDS

- Magnetic resonance imaging • Magnetic resonance neurography • Entrapment neuropathy
- Upper extremity • Neurography • Injury

KEY POINTS

- High field strength allows better 3-dimensional (3D) imaging, therefore 3T MR scanning is preferred.
- The imaging around the joints is best accomplished using joint-specific coils.
- Auto-shimming is essential before 3D diffusion-weighted PSIF (reversed steady-state free precession) and diffusion tensor imaging to avoid ghosting and attain uniform fat suppression.
- Additional long-axis fluid-sensitive 2D images (fat-suppressed proton density or short-tau inversion recovery) are acquired to evaluate the joints and other structures in the imaging field of view.
- Nerve variations and magic angle artifact should be kept in mind to avoid overcalling neuropathy.
- Fascicular abnormality or nerve enlargement are definitive MRN imaging signs of neuropathy.
- The critical findings in grading nerve injury are detection of neuroma and nerve transection.

INTRODUCTION

Nerve entrapment and injury of the upper extremity is more common and can be more complex than that of the lower extremity, with the existence of several entrapment sites along the course of major upper limb nerves.[1] These lesions can be diagnosed based on clinical findings and electrophysiologic studies, such as electromyography and nerve conduction studies. However, these studies are invasive, can be uncomfortable, can be falsely negative, frequently show low positive predictive values, and can be nonlocalizing in patients with mild lesions or in cases of severe axonal injury with low distal compound action potentials.[2–5]

Such studies are normal in cases of neurapraxia (mild nerve injury) and can be normal up to 7 to 14 days after nerve injury, even when the nerve is physically divided. Ultrasonography has been widely used for common sites of entrapment, such as carpal tunnel or cubital tunnel syndromes, because of its low cost, portability, and real-time capability. However, ultrasonographic study requires operator skill, may be limited by local calcifications/dense scarring, does not demonstrate nerve and muscle signal intensity alterations as with magnetic resonance (MR) imaging, and frequently lacks objectivity.[2,3] Therefore there has been much interest in development and use of high-resolution MR imaging techniques capable

Disclosures: A.C. acknowledges the support of GE-AUR, Integra Life Sciences, and Siemens for patient research.
[a] Johns Hopkins University, Baltimore, MD 21218, USA; [b] The University of Texas Southwestern, 5323 Harry Hines Blvd, Dallas, TX-75390-9178, USA
* Corresponding author.
E-mail address: avneesh.chhabra@utsouthwestern.edu

neuroimaging.theclinics.com

of more precisely delineating nerve abnormality and its underlying cause.[4–6] High-resolution MR imaging that provides multiplanar isotropic depiction of the nerves using a combination of 2-dimensional (2D) and 3-dimensional (3D) imaging with and without uniform fat-suppression techniques, also referred to as MR neurography, has been increasingly used for peripheral nerve evaluation.[7–12] MR neurography not only reveals the morphologic characteristics of nerves but also provides information on pathologic processes including nerve inflammation, edema, fibrosis, and fat proliferation.[12] It has been increasingly used in the assessment of lesions affecting peripheral nerves, plexus, and spinal nerve roots.[7,8,13–15] This article reviews the normal 3-T MR neurographic appearance of the upper extremity nerves, and abnormal findings related to injury, entrapment, and other pathologic conditions.

TECHNICAL CONSIDERATIONS IN MR NEUROGRAPHY

Technical considerations in MR neurography are extensively discussed in another article in this issue by Chhabra and colleagues. In brief, some key points should be followed in upper extremity imaging. Higher field strength allows better 3D imaging, therefore 3-T scanning is preferred. The imaging around the joints is best accomplished using joint-specific coils. Contiguous imaging, for example elbow and forearm, should be performed using separate fields of view for elbow and forearm, ideally with separate phased array coils for each. To avoid wraparound artifacts, dead (air) space around the extremity should be avoided or minimized as much as possible to attain the highest possible resolution and contrast. 2D imaging using axial T1-weighted and axial T2 spectral adiabatic inversion recovery (SPAIR) imaging is performed with less thickness than the plexus or lower leg imaging, to keep in-plane resolution between 0.3 and 0.4 mm. The slice thickness is kept at 4 mm, 3 mm, and 2 mm for upper arm, forearm, and wrist, respectively. 3D diffusion-weighted (DW) reversed steady-state free precession (PSIF) imaging is very useful for displaying the anatomy along the long axis of the extremity. 3D SPAIR sampling perfection with optimized contrasts using varying flip-angle evolutions (SPACE) works better in extremities than 3D short-tau inversion recovery (STIR) SPACE, because of its higher signal-to-noise ratio. Auto-shimming is essential before 3D DW PSIF and diffusion tensor (DT) imaging, to avoid ghosting and attain uniform fat suppression.[16,17] Additional long-axis fluid-sensitive 2D images (fat-suppressed proton density or STIR) are acquired to evaluate the joints and other structures in the imaging field of view.

BRACHIAL PLEXUS BRANCHES

The brachial plexus has a complex anatomy, and is formed by the contribution of the ventral branches coming from the 4 lower cervical and first thoracic nerves; it is covered elsewhere in this issue by Lutz and colleagues. The discussion here focuses on brachial plexus branch nerves relevant to the upper extremity. Whereas certain nerves come directly from the plexus, such as the spinal accessory nerve, the most commonly imaged nerves include the 3 peripheral nerves of the upper limb: the median nerve, ulnar nerve, and radial nerve. The radial nerve arises from the posterior cord; the majority of the median nerve arises from the lateral cord while the median nerve and the ulnar nerve receive contributions from the medial cord.[15] It is worth mentioning that brachial plexus abnormality can extend into the peripheral nerves (**Fig. 1**). Proximal plexus abnormality can also cause double-crush syndrome and present with distal peripheral nerve symptomatology at one of the entrapment sites, and this syndrome should be considered in the differential diagnosis, both clinically and during imaging for proper management. For example, thoracic outlet syndrome causing C8 and/or T1 neuropathy may predispose the ulnar nerve to entrapment distally or exacerbate ulnar neuropathy symptoms.

ULNAR NERVE

The ulnar nerve originates from the medial cord of the brachial plexus (C8, T1) with occasional contributions from the C7 nerve root. It courses along the posteromedial compartment of the upper arm in a relatively straight fashion. At the mid-arm level, the nerve penetrates the medial intermuscular septum and courses adjacent to the epimysium of the medial head of the triceps and deep fascia before reaching the cubital tunnel, where it passes between the medial epicondyle of the humerus and the olecranon at the condylar groove. Here, it lies deep to the cubital tunnel retinaculum (CTR), also known as the Osborne fascia, and aponeurosis formed between the 2 heads of the flexor carpi ulnaris.[18–20] The nerve courses straight between superficial and deep compartments of the forearm along its medial side and at the wrist, and passes through a fibro-osseous tunnel known as the Guyon canal (**Fig. 2**).[21,22] The floor of this tunnel is formed by hamate, hypothenar muscles, and flexor retinaculum; the roof is composed of the pisohamate

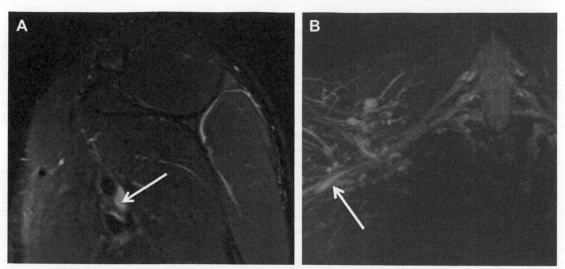

Fig. 1. Radial nerve malignancy in a 24-year-old man with slowly progressive radial neuropathy. Sagittal short-tau inversion recovery (STIR) image (*A*) and maximum-intensity projection (MIP) reconstruction from coronal 3-dimensional (3D) STIR sampling perfection with optimized contrasts using varying flip-angle evolutions (SPACE) (*B*) show the fusiform enlargement of the radial nerve in the axilla (*arrows*) in a biopsy-proven case of primary radial nerve sarcoma.

ligament, volar carpal ligament (the terminal thickened portion of the antebrachial fascia), palmaris brevis muscle, and fibers of the palmar fascia.[21–23] There is typical topographic arrangement of dorsal cutaneous sensory, motor, and sensory fascicles within the nerve in the forearm from medial to lateral. The ulnar nerve enters the Guyon canal after separating off its dorsal cutaneous branch,

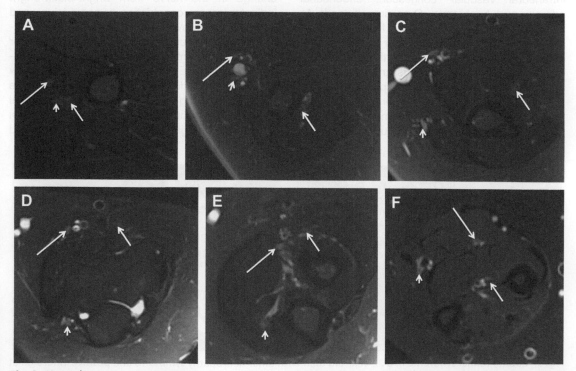

Fig. 2. Normal course and appearance of upper extremity nerves. Sequential axial T2 spectral adiabatic inversion recovery (SPAIR) images through the arm and forearm show the median nerve (*large arrows*), radial nerve and branches (*medium arrows*), and ulnar nerve (*small arrows*). (*A*) Axilla, (*B*) upper arm, (*C*) just distal to spiral groove, (*D*) cubital tunnel, (*E*) proximal forearm, (*F*) distal forearm. Medium arrow in *F* is anterior interosseus nerve.

and splits into the superficial sensory nerve and the deep motor nerve during its course within the canal. The 2 terminal branches of the nerve can be easily visualized: the sensory branch running in proximity to the ulnar artery; and the motor branch, which courses more deeply, adjacent to the medial surface of the hamate hook.[1] The ulnar nerve may be damaged at any place along its course in the upper extremity. In addition, the aforementioned double-crush phenomenon should be considered in cases of ulnar neuropathy.[1,24]

Cubital Tunnel Syndrome

Ulnar nerve entrapment (UNE) at the elbow is the second most common entrapment neuropathy.[1] Cubital tunnel syndrome is defined by ulnar neuropathy beneath or near the CTR.[1,7,25] Various hypotheses of ulnar neuropathy at this site have been hypothesized. Although evidence is limited, it seems that repeated elbow flexion, which can cause a 4- to 5-fold increase of pressure inside the cubital tunnel, and repeated external pressure on the ulnar nerve from chronically resting the elbow on firm surfaces provide possible explanations for neuropathy.[7,26,27] Early stages of peripheral nerve entrapment may be associated with intraneural vascular congestion, endoneurial edema, and hyperemia. Over time it leads to initiation of intraneural fibrosis, focal demyelination, and axonal loss.[7,28–31] Other causes of cubital tunnel narrowing include a thickened CTR/Osborne fascia, an anomalous anconeus epitrochlearis muscle, and a range of space-occupying lesions (eg, tumors, scarring, heterotopic ossification, loose bodies, fracture fragments, and ganglion cysts).[32–35] The clinical features of UNE are heterogeneous, and include intermittent paresthesias and sensory loss in the ulnar nerve distribution, especially the ring or/and small fingers, with or without atrophy; and weakness of the ulnar nerve innervated hypothenar and interosseus muscles and pain, which can be limited to over the cubital tunnel or radiate to the shoulder or wrist. The Tinel sign over the cubital tunnel is frequently present.[36]

Imaging Findings

Electrophysiologic studies are usually used to confirm the diagnosis of UNE, but these studies may be nonlocalizing in patients with mild lesions or in those with severe axonal injury and low amplitudes of distal compound muscle action potential.[36] MR neurography imaging findings reveal abnormal T2 hyperintensity of the nerve approaching adjacent in-plane veins (Fig. 3). Mild hyperintensity of the nerve is commonly seen as an incidental finding, similar to slowing of nerve conduction velocity on electrophysiologic study, and it should be reported as a nonspecific finding to be correlated clinically for neuropathy.[7] Nerve enlargement and fascicular abnormality, with or without distal muscle denervation change, are seen with moderate neuropathy. Abrupt signal change in the nerve from bright-black-bright indicates severe constriction or nerve injury, and correlates with severe neuropathy. Severe entrapment is usually seen with organic mass lesions or with reentrapment in previously anteriorly transposed nerve (Fig. 4).[25] The latter may also show abnormal angulation along the course of the nerve caused by kinking by scarring, along with regional muscle denervation edema in the flexor carpi ulnaris, flexor digitorum profundus of fourth and

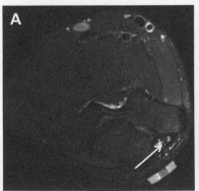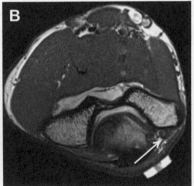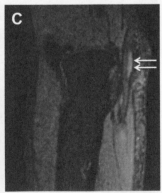

Fig. 3. Cubital tunnel syndrome in a 22-year-old man with ulnar neuropathy symptoms and positive Tinel sign at the cubital tunnel. Axial T2 SPAIR (A) and T1-weighted image (B) show mildly prominent ulnar nerve and prominent hyperintense sensory fascicle (arrows). MIP reconstruction from coronal oblique 3D diffusion-weighted (DW) reversed steady-state free precession (PSIF) sequence (C) shows the abnormal sensory fascicle along the long axis of the nerve (arrows).

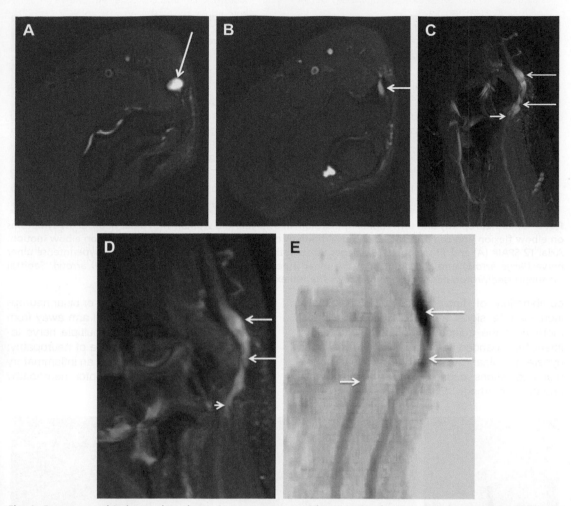

Fig. 4. Recurrent cubital tunnel syndrome in a young man with recurrent ulnar neuropathy symptoms following anterior transposition of the nerve 1 year prior. Sequential axial T2 SPAIR images (*A*, *B*) at the level of the cubital tunnel show abnormally enlarged ulnar nerve with fluid-like hyperintensity proximally, and flattening distally under the thickened pronator fascia and perineural scar (*small arrows*). MIP reconstructions from coronal oblique 3D SPAIR SPACE sequence (*C*), 3D DW PSIF (*D*), and diffusion tensor (DT) imaging (*E*) show the full extent of abnormality (*arrows*). Notice abnormal signal of ulnar nerve (*large arrows*) in comparison with median nerve (*small arrow*) on the DT image. There was abnormally low fractional anisotropy (0.1–0.2) of the ulnar nerve in comparison with the median nerve (0.4).

fifth digits, and interosseous and hypothenar muscles of the hand. Indeed, muscle wasting is more prevalent among patients with cubital tunnel syndrome than in patients with carpal tunnel syndrome.[37] DT imaging selectively shows abnormally hyperintense nerve on the tensor image, with low fractional anisotropy values owing to demyelination and/or axonal degeneration. In addition, MR neurography is useful for the assessment of patients at risk for double-crush injuries, because MR neurography shows the most abnormal findings at and immediately proximal to the site of injury.[38] Although ultrasonography is better for real-time assessment of ulnar nerve subluxation or dislocation, MR neurography can show

secondary findings of ulnar nerve abnormalities, a thickened or absent retinaculum, or a space-occupying lesion, such as an accessory muscle or low muscular insertion of the medial head of the triceps (**Fig. 5**). Surgical release of an entrapped nerve is commonly accompanied by subcutaneous or submuscular transposition anteriorly. Transposed but otherwise normal nerve shows mild increased signal on MR neurography that decreases over time. Reentrapment of the anteriorly transposed ulnar nerve may occur because of overzealous dissection and development of perineural fibrosis, necessitating repeat surgical ulnar nerve release. Findings of MR neurography in symptomatic patients include 1 or a

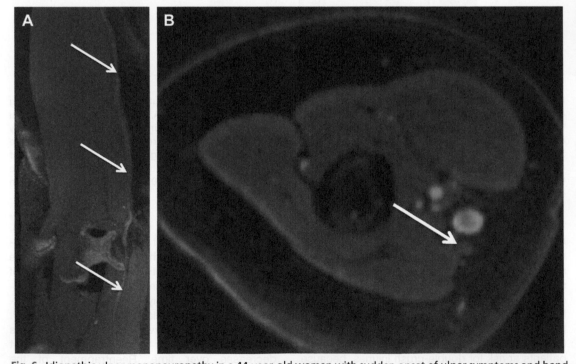

Fig. 5. Ulnar neuropathy and torn cubital retinaculum in a 49-year-old woman with ulnar neuropathy symptoms on elbow flexion and compression, and clinical findings of subluxation out of cubital tunnel on elbow motion. Axial T2 SPAIR (*A*) and T1-weighted (*B*) images through the cubital tunnel show abnormally hyperintense ulnar nerve (*large arrow*) and chronic tear of the ulnar aspect of the cubital retinaculum (*small arrow*). Sagittal fat-suppressed proton-density image (*C*) shows the full extent of abnormality.

combination of findings, such as persistent/increased T2 signal abnormality approaching or more than the adjacent in-plane venous signal intensity, expanded nerve fascicles in the enlarged hyperemic ulnar nerve with or without abnormal angulations caused by perineural fibrosis, and/or hemorrhage. Finally, long-segment nerve abnormality on MR neurography, or ulnar neuropathy in the proximal arm or distal arm away from the site of entrapment and/or multiple nerve lesions, indicates a systemic cause of neuropathy: lymphoma, neurofibromatosis, or an inflammatory condition such as multifocal motor neuropathy (**Figs. 6 and 7**).[39]

Fig. 6. Idiopathic ulnar mononeuropathy in a 44-year-old woman with sudden onset of ulnar symptoms and hand weakness. There was mild improvement initially, followed by persistent weakness for many months. Recent electromyogram suspected lesion in the upper arm above the elbow joint, and MR neurography was ordered. MIP reconstruction from coronal oblique 3D DW PSIF sequence shows the diffuse long-segment ulnar mononeuropathy (*arrows* in *A*). No cause could be discerned. Postcontrast 3D volume-interpolated breath-hold examination (VIBE) image (*B*) shows no abnormal diffuse or focal enhancing lesion.

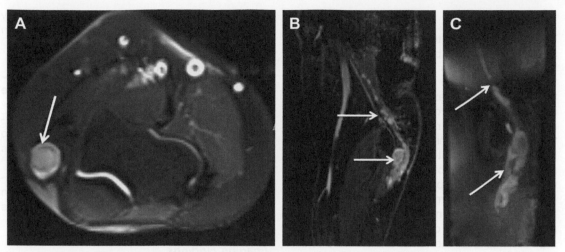

Fig. 7. Segmental schwannomatosis in a 51-year-old woman with ulnar neuropathy symptoms. Axial T2 SPAIR (*A*) image through the cubital tunnel shows a target lesion in the tunnel (*arrow*). MIP reconstructions from coronal oblique 3D SPAIR SPACE sequence (*B*) and 3D DW PSIF (*C*) sequence show multifocal tumors along the course of the ulnar nerve (*arrows*), in keeping with diagnosis of segmental schwannomatosis.

Guyon Canal Syndrome

The Guyon canal is another common potential site of ulnar nerve compression. The location of compression may be classified among 3 zonal locations[40,41]:

> Zone 1: Proximal edge of volar carpal ligament to bifurcation of ulnar nerve, where patients present with combined motor and sensory deficits
>
> Zone 2: From nerve bifurcation to just distal to fibrous arch of hypothenar muscles, where patients may present with pure motor deficit
>
> Zone 3: Distal end of the canal containing superficial sensory branch, where patients may present with pure sensory deficit

Nerve entrapment in zones 1 and 3 are the most common, although most patients have symptoms in more than 1 zone. Entrapment neuropathy can

result from extrinsic compression factors (eg, bicycle riding, judo, tennis), intrinsic space-occupying lesions (ganglion, lipoma, ulnar artery aneurysm, uremic tumoral calcinosis, trauma, and anomalous muscle, such as accessory abductor digiti minimi), or from chronic traction neuropathy caused by regional fracture or use of crutches.[1,34,41,42]

Imaging Findings

The value of MR imaging in Guyon canal syndrome is in the detection of space-occupying lesions within the canal and/or signal intensity and size changes of the nerve itself.[34,41,42] Secondary signs of neuropathy include denervation atrophy/edema of the hypothenar muscles, third/fourth lumbricals, and interossei muscles. Isolated deep-bundle neuropathy may also be diagnosed on high-resolution 3-T MR neurography, which is a difficult diagnosis on electrodiagnostic testing (**Fig. 8**).[3]

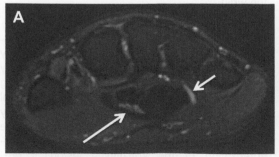

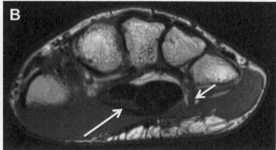

Fig. 8. Carpal tunnel syndrome and deep bundle ulnar neuropathy in a 31-year-old woman with hand pain in both median and ulnar nerve distributions. Axial T2 SPAIR (*A*) and axial T1-weighted (*B*) images show abnormally hyperintense and flattened median nerve in the carpal tunnel (*large arrow*) and deep branch of the ulnar nerve (*small arrow*).

RADIAL NERVE

The radial nerve is the terminal branch of the posterior cord of the brachial plexus (C5–C8, T1). In the arm, it courses posterior to the humerus in the spiral groove and penetrates the lateral intermuscular septum to exit the spiral groove and lie anterior to the lateral condyle beneath the brachioradialis muscle. The radial nerve innervates the triceps muscle, brachioradialis muscle, anconeus muscle, and inferolateral half of the brachialis muscle. At the level of the elbow joint, the radial nerve splits into a superficial sensory branch that courses in the forearm along the brachioradialis muscle, and a deep motor branch that traverses deep to the arcade of Frohse to penetrate the supinator muscle. The radial tunnel refers to an enclosed space from the level of the radiocapitellar joint to the point of the proximal part of the supinator muscle.[18,43] It is bounded by the extensor carpi radialis longus and brevis muscles (anterolaterally), brachialis muscle (medially), capitellum (posteriorly), and the supinator muscle (anteriorly). Its contents include the radial nerve, which divides in the proximal forearm into superficial (primarily sensory) and deep (primarily motor) branches. The superficial branch of the radial nerve descends in the forearm under the brachioradialis and eventually pierces the deep fascia near the back of the wrist (see **Fig. 2**). The deep branch of the radial nerve pierces the supinator muscle, after which it is known as the posterior interosseous nerve (PIN).[18,44–46] At the elbow, the deep branch innervates the extensor carpi radialis brevis muscle and the supinator muscle. The PIN innervates the posterior-compartment muscles including the extensor carpi ulnaris, abductor pollicis longus, extensor digitorum communis, extensor pollicis longus and brevis, extensor indicis proprius, and extensor digiti minimi.[43] The radial sensory nerve courses into the dorsum of the hand and provides cutaneous innervation to the proximal parts of the dorsum of the thumb, index finger, and middle finger.[47]

Radial neuropathy may result from brachial plexopathy, proximal nerve injury in the axilla from crutches or shoulder dislocation, a manifestation of intraneural or extraneural mass lesion, or its related surgery (see **Fig. 1**; **Figs. 9–11**). Compression sites from proximal to distal include thickened lateral intramuscular septum and tight sheath of lateral head of triceps, fibrous bands from the radiocapitellar joint, the tendinous edge of the extensor carpi radialis brevis muscle, prominent radial recurrent vessels, or thickened arcade of Frohse (tendinous proximal edge of supinator).[48,49] Entrapment of the PIN beneath the thickened arcade of Frohse is the most commonly reported lesion, which may develop after repetitive pronation-supination microtrauma.[18]

Posterior Interosseous Nerve Syndrome

Isolated motor neuropathy is the hallmark feature of PIN syndrome (also known as supinator syndrome). Loss of ability to extend the digits accompanied by radial wrist deviation related to weakness of extensor carpi ulnaris represents the typical clinical spectrum of this syndrome.[44] It should also be noted that many cases of refractory "tennis elbow" (ie, lateral epicondylitis) may in fact in part be due to PIN entrapment, as there is clinical overlap in their presentation.[45]

Imaging Findings

The radial nerve is almost never artifactually hyperintense in the arm or elbow. The only areas prone to magic-angle artifacts are in the axilla and PIN as it traverses through the supinator muscle.[3,7,50] At the latter sites, however, the signal intensity of the normal nerve does not approach the adjacent in-plane veins. Patients with neuropathy show abnormal vessel-like PIN hyperintensity at the entrapment or injury site, with or without enlargement of the nerve. It is imperative to evaluate the extensor muscles in clinically suspected cases of PIN neuropathy, as denervation edema in these muscles is the most common MR manifestation of the syndrome (**Fig. 12**).[46]

Radial Tunnel Syndrome

Radial tunnel syndrome, on the other hand, is a distinct clinical but controversial entity, often occurring as the result of repetitive motion injuries to the elbow, and is distinguished by the general absence of motor weakness.[49,50] Patients typically report pain in the region of the proximal extensor and supinator muscles, exacerbated by forearm pronation, extension of the elbow, and flexion of the wrist.[46,47]

Imaging Findings

Although ultrasonography is currently the modality of choice for evaluating the superficial sensory branch or for detection of a commonly offending mass lesion such as a ganglion cyst, technological advances in high-resolution MR neurography allow demonstration of the abnormal nerve appearance, regional joint abnormality, and characterization of the soft-tissue lesion, if present.[50,51] The accurate localization of the nerve compression is a key factor in making a decision on the possibility, and planning, of the surgical

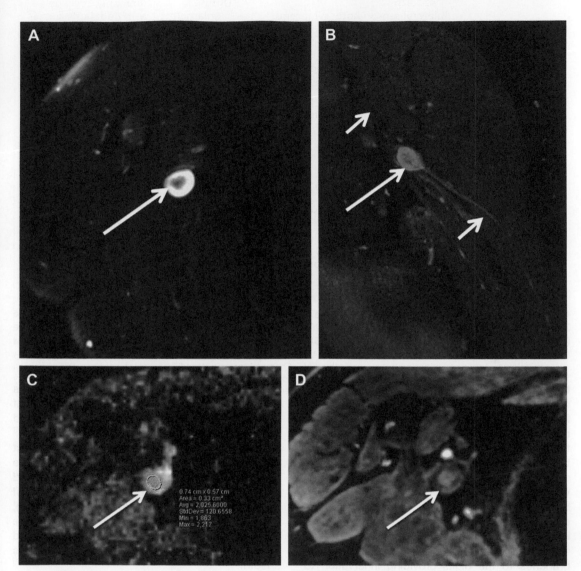

Fig. 9. Radial nerve neurofibroma in a 29-year-old woman with known neurofibromatosis and radial-sided pain. Axial T2 SPAIR (*A*) and MIP reconstruction from coronal 3D SPAIR SPACE (*B*) images show target lesion (*large arrow*) of the radial nerve (*small arrows*). On DT image (*C*), there is a high apparent diffusion coefficient (ADC) value (-2.0×10^{-3} mm/s^2) and there was targetoid contrast enhancement (*D*). The lesion was successfully resected.

approach.[50] MR neurography allows excellent anatomic imaging of radial nerve entrapment with an added capability of demonstrating structural lesions along the course of the affected nerve (**Fig. 13**).

MEDIAN NERVE

The median nerve originates from the medial and lateral cords of the brachial plexus (C6–C8, T1) and courses beside the brachial artery in the anterior-medial compartment of the arm.

Immediately above the elbow, it passes through the antecubital fossa, deep in relation to the bi-ceps aponeurosis and anterior to the brachialis muscle. The nerve lies between the humeral (su-perficial) and ulnar (deep) heads of the pronator teres muscle at the elbow joint, and comes in the anterior compartment of the forearm by passing under the fibrous arch of 2 heads of the flexor dig-itorum superficialis muscle.[18,52] The nerve courses between the flexor digitorum superficialis and pro-fundus muscles in the forearm (see **Fig. 2**).[18,35] The median nerve enters the hand through the carpal

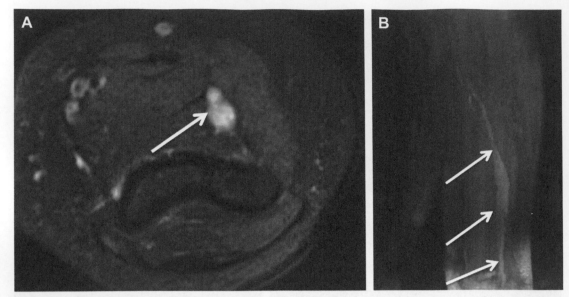

Fig. 10. Segmental schwannoma of the radial nerve in a 20-year-old woman with known neurofibromatosis type 2 and radial-sided pain and weakness. Axial T2 SPAIR (*A*) image shows multiple lesions involving the radial nerve (*arrow*). MIP reconstruction from coronal 3D DW PSIF image (*B*) shows the full extent of these multifocal lesions (*arrows*).

tunnel between flexor pollicis longus and flexor digitorum superficialis tendons, and deep to the flexor retinaculum. In the forearm, the median nerve gives off 2 named branches, the anterior interosseous nerve and the palmar cutaneous branch. A persistent median artery may be demonstrated in 11% to 20% of carpal tunnels, which is often associated with a bifid or high-branching median nerve.[3,53] Multiple branches originate from the median nerve in the hand, including the recurrent motor branch to the thenar muscles (million-dollar nerve), multiple sensory branches to the digits providing innervation to

the palmar aspect of the radial 3 and a half digits and distal dorsal aspect of the radial 2 and a half digits, as well as motor branches to first and second lumbricals.[54]

Apart from the commonly identified entrapment at the carpal tunnel, other sites of median nerve entrapment include supracondylar spur and ligament of Struthers, between the 2 heads of the pronator teres muscle (pronator syndrome), beneath the anterior interosseous membrane (anterior interosseous nerve syndrome), and fascial edge of the flexor digitorum superficialis sheath.[3,35]

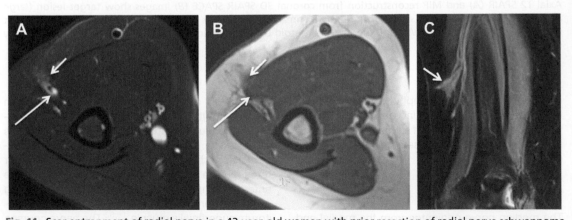

Fig. 11. Scar entrapment of radial nerve in a 43-year-old woman with prior resection of radial nerve schwannoma with persistent pain in the radial nerve distribution. Axial T2 SPAIR (*A*) and T1-weighted (*B*) images show mildly enlarged and markedly hyperintense radial nerve (*large arrows*) with surrounding scarring (*small arrows*). Only irregular enhancing scarring (*arrows*) but no enhancing mass was seen on the postcontrast 3D VIBE imaging (*C*).

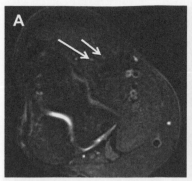
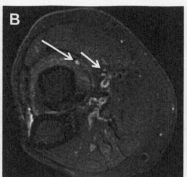
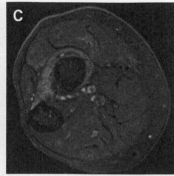

Fig. 12. Posterior interosseous nerve (PIN) entrapment in a 54-year-old woman with radial-sided weakness and wrist drop for a few months. Sequential axial T2 SPAIR images (*A, B*) show normal superficial (*small arrow*) and deep (*large arrow*) radial nerve branches at the elbow, and abnormally hyperintense PIN (*large arrow* in *B*) at the level of supinator. Notice denervation edema-like change and atrophy of supinator muscle (*B, C*).

Pronator Syndrome

Although median neuropathy can result from brachial plexopathy, nerve sheath tumors anywhere along its course (**Fig. 14**), or nerve injury high in axilla or upper arm, pronator syndrome is the most proximal entrapment site for the median nerve.[55,56] Another potential site of compression of the median nerve in the region of the elbow is the ligament of Struthers that connects the supracondylar spur to the medial epicondyle, which can mimic pronator syndrome. The supracondylar spur is usually an incidental finding and occurs in approximately 1% of individuals.[57] Probable reasons for pronator syndrome include hypertrophy of the pronator teres muscle or a fibrous band of the bicipital aponeurosis, compression by an aberrant median artery, crossing branches of the radial artery and vein, hematoma, local fracture-subluxation or related iatrogenic injury (**Fig. 15**), or a soft-tissue mass.[1,57–59]

Pronator syndrome is associated with pain and paresthesia in the volar aspects of the elbow, forearm, and hand, affecting the first through third digits and lateral half of the ring finger.[43] Patients with pronator syndrome also may have numbness of the palm caused by compression of the palmar cutaneous nerve. In addition, symptom reproduction during resisted forearm pronation suggests median nerve compression by the pronator teres, and symptom reproduction during resisted elbow flexion and supination suggests biceps aponeurosis as the cause of compression.[43–45,55,56]

Imaging Findings

MR neurography demonstrates the nerve T2 signal change appearing at the site of entrapment with gradual signal normalization along its distal course. It should be noted that magic-angle artifact is common as the nerve dives under the pronator teres muscle. However, neuropathy leads

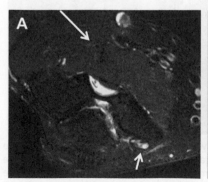
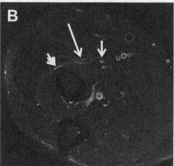
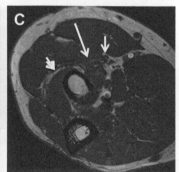

Fig. 13. Recurrent radial tunnel syndrome with PIN entrapment in a 44-year-old man with painful forearm and elbow following prior radial tunnel release. Axial T2 SPAIR (*A*) image shows normal radial nerve (*large arrow*) and abnormal ulnar nerve (*small arrow*) at the level of elbow, consistent with cubital tunnel syndrome. Axial T2 SPAIR (*B*) and T1-weighted (*C*) images at proximal forearm show the postoperative scarring (*large arrows*), mildly hyperintense superficial radial nerve (*small arrows*), and markedly abnormal PIN (*double small arrows*).

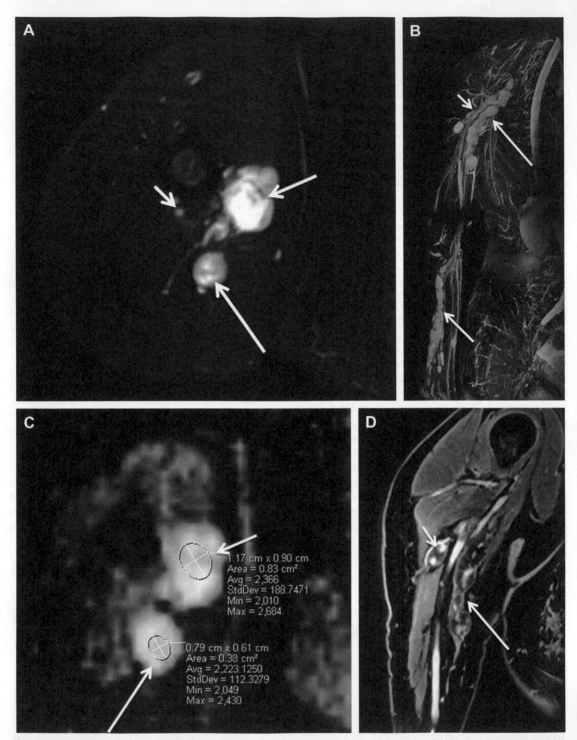

Fig. 14. Segmental schwannomatosis in a 36-year-old woman with arm weakness and pain. Axial T2 SPAIR image (*A*) through the upper arm shows well-defined lesions involving the radial nerve (*small arrow*), median nerve (*medium arrow*), and ulnar nerve (*large arrow*). MIP reconstruction from coronal oblique SPAIR SPACE sequence (*B*) shows the string of schwannomas along the long axis of these nerves in the upper arm and forearm. Axial DT image (*C*) through the upper arm shows a high ADC value (2.2–2.3 × 10⁻³ mm/s²) in the median and ulnar nerve lesions. Notice patchy central targetoid appearance of enhancement among the lesions on postcontrast 3D VIBE imaging, classic for benign peripheral nerve sheath tumors (*D*).

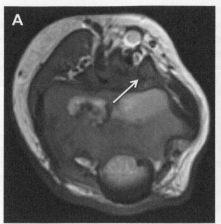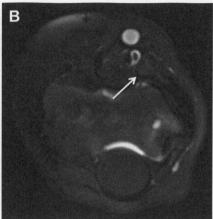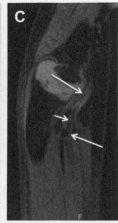

Fig. 15. Median nerve neuroma in continuity (Sunderland grade IV injury) in a 4-month-old child with prior supracondylar fracture and surgery, presenting with median nerve distribution pain, sensory changes, and weakness. Axial T1-weighted (*A*) and T2 SPAIR (*B*) images at the level of the elbow show abnormally enlarged median nerve with heterogeneous nerve signal and thickened epineurium (*arrow*). MIP reconstruction from oblique sagittal 3D DW PSIF sequence (*C*) shows the abnormally enlarged median nerve (*large arrows*) and normal proximal anterior interosseus nerve (*small arrow*).

to abnormally increased signal approaching the adjacent vessels, as well as change in nerve caliber. Regional muscle denervation changes shown on MR neurography additionally confirm the neuropathy findings. Sometimes double entrapment may be perceived, with the nerve entrapped proximally at the flexor digitorum superficialis sheath as well as distally at the carpal tunnel (double-crush syndrome). In these patients, surgery for carpal tunnel syndrome (CTS) alone may not alleviate the symptoms.[58,59] The median nerve may get reentrapped at the pronator teres release site or in the carpal tunnel.

On MR neurography, moderate to severe T2 hyperintensity, nerve-caliber changes across the site of entrapment, and fascicular abnormality along with perineural encasing fibrosis confirms median nerve reentrapment and persistent neuropathy.[35,55]

Anterior Interosseous Nerve Syndrome

Anterior interosseous nerve (AIN) syndrome is also referred to as Kiloh-Nevin syndrome. The AIN, similar to PIN in that it is a predominantly a motor nerve, is the largest branch of the median nerve. It courses between the 2 heads of the pronator teres muscle and reaches the anterior aspect of the interosseous membrane to travel beside the anterior interosseous artery (see **Fig. 2**). The AIN provides motor innervation to the radial belly of the flexor digitorum profundus (FDP), flexor pollicis longus (FPL), and pronator quadratus (PQ) muscles. It also provides sensory innervations to the

wrist. Compression of the nerve results in weakness of pinching, even though the weakness of PQ (pronation) may be compensated for by the concurrent action of the pronator teres.[60–63] There are many causes of AIN palsy: fibrous bands from the deep (more common) or superficial head of the pronator teres to the brachialis fascia, fractures of the forearm bones or supracondylar fracture, local pressure after sleeping on the affected arm or resulting from a poorly applied cast, exercise and weightlifting, and viral neuritis.[47,62–68]

Imaging Findings

On MR imaging of AIN neuropathy, changes in muscle denervation are easily observed in a typical distribution, involving FPL, FDP, and PQ muscles.[67–69] Although PQ is always the first muscle involved in AIN neuropathy, it should be noted that isolated signal change or atrophy in the PQ muscle is commonly seen as an asymptomatic finding. On high-resolution MR neurography, AIN itself can easily be differentiated from adjacent veins and abnormal signal, and size changes are appreciated in cases of neuropathy (see **Fig. 15**).[70] The radiologist should be conscious that other patterns of muscle edema in AIN injury (eg, involvement of the flexor carpi radialis) may mirror variability of innervation, and that the accessory muscle belly of FPL (Gantzer muscle) is also supplied by the AIN, and may itself cause AIN neuropathy or show denervation change in AIN syndrome.[71]

Carpal Tunnel Syndrome

Median neuropathy caused by entrapment within the carpal tunnel is the most common neuropathy of the upper extremity, with an annual incidence of 50 to 150 cases per 100,000.[72,73] The carpal tunnel is a fibro-osseous canal formed by carpal bones and a rigid fibrous transverse carpal ligament. The median nerve branches into a recurrent motor branch, which supplies the thenar muscles and multiple sensory branches that provide innervation to the 3 radial digits and the radial half of the fourth digit.[8,72–74]

The pathophysiology of CTS involves a combination of mechanical trauma, increased intratunnel pressure, and ischemic injury to the median nerve, leading to perineurial and epineurial edema and hyperemia, followed by demyelination and axonal loss.[72,73] When ischemia lasts for an extended time, irreversible fibrosis of the median nerve develops.[74] Clinically, the patients complain of nocturnal pain, hand clumsiness, tingling, numbness, and paresthesia in the distribution of the median nerve. Sensory loss typically precedes the motor deficit. Patients with long-standing disease may have wasting of the soft tissues in the thenar eminence. Clinically, there is a positive Phalen test (increased paresthesia after 1 minute of passive wrist flexion) and Tinel sign (paresthesia in nerve territory after gentle tapping over carpal tunnel).[72–74]

Imaging Findings

Although electrophysiology studies are frequently performed for wrist neuropathies, false-negative rates can be as high as 10% to 30% and positive predictive values can be as low as 33%, which clearly indicate a need for improved diagnosis.[48] Nerve-conduction studies are especially less accurate early in the course of the disease when complaints are mild.[75,76] MR imaging has been reported to be positive in more than 90% of cases,[77] and MR findings have been shown to predict surgical benefit for patients with CTS independently of the nerve-conduction studies. However, isolated MR signs of abnormal nerve T2 hyperintensity have low reported specificities of

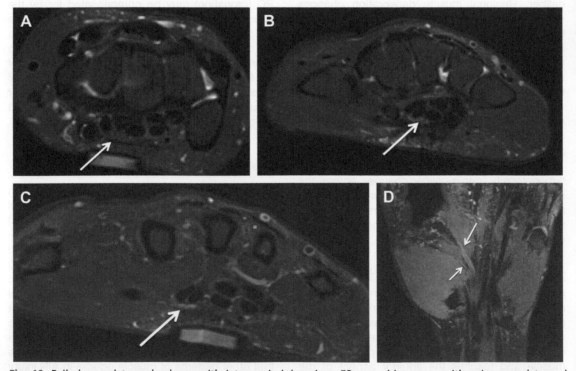

Fig. 16. Failed carpal tunnel release with iatrogenic injury in a 52-year-old woman with prior carpal tunnel release presenting with numbness in the C6 distribution. Sequential axial T2 SPAIR images (*A–C*) through the wrist and proximal hand. Note the normal appearance of the median nerve in the proximal carpal tunnel (*arrow in A*), and abnormal nerve hyperintensity and flattening in the distal tunnel (*arrow in B*). The abnormality extends into the radial branch of the median nerve (*arrow in C*). Coronal MIP reconstruction from 3D DW PSIF sequence (*D*) shows the full extent of abnormality-enlarged and hyperintense index finger branch (*large arrow*), and the million-dollar branch (first thenar muscle branch, *small arrow*).

less than 40%, which has limited more widespread adoption of imaging for the diagnosis of CTS in the clinical setting.[48,77,78] Other signs such as flattening of the median nerve in the carpal tunnel, proximal enlargement, volar bowing of the retinaculum, extension of T2 hyperintensity distally in the median nerve branches, and effacement of deep fat pad in the carpal tunnel increase the specificity of the diagnosis of CTS. MR neurography also shows tenosynovitis, internal wrist derangement, and changes in regional muscle denervation in a noninvasive fashion. 3-T MR neurography depicts the individual bundle abnormality of a bifid nerve, and nerve abnormalities can also be shown in the longitudinal plane of the nerve. Release of flexor retinaculum is commonly performed in cases that fail conservative treatment.[72–74,79,80] Martin-Gruber anastomosis, representing anomalous connections between median and ulnar nerves in the proximal forearm, can lead to variation or confusion in electrodiagnostic findings, and MR neurography can help clarify the neuropathic abnormalities in such confusing cases.[81] Recently, DT imaging has been shown to be another useful tool that may aid in detection of median neuropathy and, potentially, in nerve regeneration.[82,83] Finally, postrelease reentrapment of median nerve, reformation or incomplete release of retinaculum, or iatrogenic injury to the median nerve can be detected using high-resolution MR neurography (Fig. 16).

SUMMARY

MR neurography is an excellent tool for the evaluation of upper extremity peripheral nerve anatomy, neuropathic findings, and associated changes in regional muscle denervation that aids in more accurate therapeutic strategy by enhancing presurgical planning and postsurgical follow-up.

REFERENCES

1. Kim S, Choi JY, Huh YM, et al. Role of magnetic resonance imaging in entrapment and compressive neuropathy—what, where, and how to see the peripheral nerves on the musculoskeletal magnetic resonance image: part 2. Upper extremity. Eur Radiol 2007;17(2):509–22.
2. Beekman R, Van Der Plas JP, Uitdehaag BM, et al. Clinical, electrodiagnostic, and sonographic studies in ulnar neuropathy at the elbow. Muscle Nerve 2004;30:202–8.
3. Subhawong TK, Wang KC, Thawait SK, et al. High resolution imaging of tunnels by magnetic resonance neurography. Skeletal Radiol 2012;41(1):15–31.
4. Bashir WA, Connell DA. Imaging of entrapment and compressive neuropathies. Semin Musculoskelet Radiol 2008;12:170–81.
5. Spratt JD, Stanley AJ, Grainger AJ, et al. The role of diagnostic radiology in compressive and entrapment neuropathies. Eur Radiol 2002;12:2352–64.
6. Filler AG, Howe FA, Hayes CE, et al. Magnetic resonance neurography. Lancet 1993;341:659–61.
7. Bäumer P, Dombert T, Staub F, et al. Ulnar neuropathy at the elbow: MR neurography—nerve T2 signal increase and caliber. Radiology 2011; 260(1):199–206.
8. Chanlalit C, Vipulakorn K, Jiraruttanapochai K, et al. Value of clinical findings, electrodiagnosis and magnetic resonance imaging in the diagnosis of root lesions in traumatic brachial plexus injuries. J Med Assoc Thai 2005;88(1):66–70.
9. Aagaard BD, Maravilla KR, Kliot M. Magnetic resonance neurography: magnetic resonance imaging of peripheral nerves. Neuroimaging Clin N Am 2001;11:131–46.
10. Dailey AT, Tsuruda JS, Goodkin R, et al. Magnetic resonance neurography for cervical radiculopathy: a preliminary report. Neurosurgery 1996;38:488–92.
11. Grant GA, Britz GW, Goodkin R, et al. The utility of magnetic resonance imaging in evaluating peripheral nerve disorders. Muscle Nerve 2002;25:314–31.
12. Chhabra A, Chalian M, Soldatos T, et al. 3-T high-resolution MR neurography of sciatic neuropathy. AJR Am J Roentgenol 2012;198(4):W357–64.
13. Kuntz CT, Blake L, Britz G, et al. Magnetic resonance neurography of peripheral nerve lesions in the lower extremity. Neurosurgery 1996;39:750–6.
14. Moore KR, Blumenthal DT, Smith AG, et al. Neurolymphomatosis of the lumbar plexus: high-resolution MR neurography findings. Neurology 2001;57:740–2.
15. Chhabra A, Thawait GK, Soldatos T, et al. High-resolution 3T MR neurography of the brachial plexus and its branches, with emphasis on 3D imaging. AJNR Am J Neuroradiol 2012;34(3):486–97.
16. Martinoli C, Gandolfo N, Perez MM, et al. Brachial plexus and nerves about the shoulder. Semin Musculoskelet Radiol 2010;14(5):523–46.
17. Chhabra A, Lee PP, Bizell C, et al. 3 Tesla MR neurography technique, interpretation, and pitfalls. Skeletal Radiol 2011;40(10):1249–60.
18. Miller TT, Reinus WR. Nerve entrapment syndromes of the elbow, forearm, and wrist. AJR Am J Roentgenol 2010;195(3):585–94.
19. Siqueira MG, Martins RS. The controversial arcade of Struthers. Surg Neurol 2005;64(Suppl 1):S17–20.
20. von Schroeder HP, Scheker LR. Redefining the "arcade of Struthers". J Hand Surg Am 2003;28: 1018–21.
21. Gross MS, Gelberman RH. The anatomy of the distal ulnar tunnel. Clin Orthop Relat Res 1985; 196:238–47.

22. Moneim MS. Ulnar nerve compression at the wrist. Ulnar tunnel syndrome. Hand Clin 1992;8:337–44.

23. Britz GW, Haynor DR, Kuntz C, et al. Ulnar nerve entrapment at the elbow: correlation of magnetic resonance imaging, clinical, electrodiagnostic, and intraoperative findings. Neurosurgery 1996; 38:458–65.

24. Panegyres PK, Moore N, Gibson R, et al. Thoracic outlet syndromes and magnetic resonance imaging. Brain 1993;116:823–41.

25. Shi Q, MacDermid JC, Santaguida PL, et al. Predictors of surgical outcomes following anterior transposition of ulnar nerve for cubital tunnel syndrome: a systematic review. J Hand Surg Am 2011;36(12):1996–2001.

26. Gelberman RH, Yamaguchi K, Hollstien SB, et al. Changes in interstitial pressure and cross-sectional area of the cubital tunnel and of the ulnar nerve with flexion of the elbow: an experimental study in human cadavers. J Bone Joint Surg Am 1998;80(4):492–501.

27. Wilbourn AJ, Ferrante MA. Ulnar neuropathy. In: Dyck PJ, editor. Peripheral neuropathy. 4th edition. Philadelphia: Elsevier Saunders; 2005. p. 1478–83.

28. Gupta R, Steward O. Chronic nerve compression induces concurrent apoptosis and proliferation of Schwann cells. J Comp Neurol 2003;461(2): 174–86.

29. Mackinnon SE, Dellon AL, Hudson AR, et al. Chronic human nerve compression: a histological assessment. Neuropathol Appl Neurobiol 1986; 12(6):547–65.

30. Posner MA. Compressive ulnar neuropathies at the elbow. I. Etiology and diagnosis. J Am Acad Orthop Surg 1998;6(5):282–8.

31. Rempel DM, Diao E. Entrapment neuropathies: pathophysiology and pathogenesis. J Electromyogr Kinesiol 2004;14(1):71–5.

32. O'Driscoll SW, Horii E, Carmichael SW, et al. The cubital tunnel and ulnar neuropathy. J Bone Joint Surg Br 1991;73:613–7.

33. Campbell WW, Pridgeon RM, Riaz G, et al. Variations in anatomy of the ulnar nerve at the cubital tunnel: pitfalls in the diagnosis of ulnar neuropathy at the elbow. Muscle Nerve 1991;14:733–8.

34. Beltran J, Rosenberg ZS. Diagnosis of compressive and entrapment neuropathies of the upper extremity: value of MR imaging. AJR Am J Roentgenol 1994;163:525.

35. Andreisek G, Crook DW, Burg D, et al. Peripheral neuropathies of the median, radial, and ulnar nerves: MR imaging features. Radiographics 2006;26:1267–87.

36. Vucic S, Cordato DJ, Yiannikas C, et al. Utility of magnetic resonance imaging in diagnosing ulnar neuropathy at the elbow. Clin Neurophysiol 2006; 117:590–5.

37. Mallette P, Zhao M, Zurakowski D, et al. Muscle atrophy at diagnosis of carpal and cubital tunnel syndrome. J Hand Surg Am 2007;32:855–8.

38. Smith TM, Sawyer SF, Sizer PS, et al. The double crush syndrome: a common occurrence in cyclists with ulnar nerve neuropathy—a case-control study. Clin J Sport Med 2008;18:55–61.

39. Thawait SK, Chaudhry V, Thawait GK, et al. High resolution MR neurography of diffuse peripheral nerve lesions. AJNR Am J Neuroradiol 2011; 32(8):1365–72.

40. May DA, Disler DG, Jones EA, et al. Abnormal signal intensity in skeletal muscle at MR imaging: patterns, pearls, and pitfalls. Radiographics 2000; 20(Spec No):S295–315.

41. Stoller DW, Li AE, Lichtman DW, et al. Chapter 10: the wrist and hand. In: Stoller DW, editor. MRI in orthopaedics and sports medicine. Baltimore (MD): Lippincott Williams & Wilkins; 2007. p. 1798–802.

42. Pećina M, Krmpotić-Nemanić J, Markiewitz AD. Tunnel syndromes. 3rd edition. Boca Raton (FL): CRC Press; 2001.

43. Tsai P, Steinberg DR. Median and radial nerve compression about the elbow. Instr Course Lect 2008;57:177–85.

44. Bencardino JT, Rosenberg ZS. Chapter 12: entrapment neuropathies of the upper extremity. In: Stoller DW, editor. MRI in orthopaedics and sports medicine. Baltimore (MD): Lippincott Williams & Wilkins; 2007. p. 1946–63.

45. Wilhelm A. Tennis elbow: treatment of resistant cases by denervation. J Hand Surg Br 1996;21: 523–33.

46. Ferdinand BD, Rosenberg ZS, Schweitzer ME, et al. MR imaging features of radial tunnel syndrome: initial experience. Radiology 2006;240: 161–8.

47. Dang AC, Rodner CM. Unusual compression neuropathies of the forearm. Part I. Radial nerve. J Hand Surg Am 2009;34:1906–14.

48. Bordalo-Rodrigues M, Rosenberg ZS. MR imaging of entrapment neuropathies at the elbow. Magn Reson Imaging Clin N Am 2004;12:247–63.

49. Bolster MAJ, Bakker XR. Radial tunnel syndrome: emphasis on the superficial branch of the radial nerve. J Hand Surg Eur 2009;34:343–7.

50. Faridian-Aragh N, Chalian M, Soldatos T, et al. High-resolution 3T MR neurography of radial neuropathy. J Neuroradiol 2011;38(5):265–74.

51. Stokvis A, Van Neck JW, Van Dijke CF, et al. High-resolution ultrasonography of the cutaneous nerve branches in the hand and wrist. J Hand Surg Eur 2009;34:766–71.

52. Lee MJ, LaStayo PC. Pronator syndrome and other nerve compressions that mimic carpal tunnel syndrome. J Orthop Sports Phys Ther 2004; 34:601–9.

53. Bayrak IK, Bayrak AO, Kale M, et al. Bifid median nerve in patients with carpal tunnel syndrome. J Ultrasound Med 2008;27(8):1129–36.

54. Kabakci NT, Kovanlikaya A, Kovanlikaya I. Tractography of the median nerve. Semin Musculoskelet Radiol 2009;13(1):18–23.

55. Thawait GK, Subhawong TK, Thawait SK, et al. Magnetic resonance neurography of median neuropathies proximal to the carpal tunnel. Skeletal Radiol 2012;41(6):623–32.

56. Rehak DC. Pronator syndrome. Clin Sports Med 2001;20:531–40.

57. Lordan J, Rauh P, Spinner RJ. The clinical anatomy of the supracondylar spur and the ligament of Struthers. Clin Anat 2005;18:548–51.

58. Johnson RK, Spinner M, Shrewsbury MM. Median nerve entrapment syndrome in the proximal forearm. J Hand Surg Am 1979;4:48–51.

59. Chhabra A, Andreisek G. Magnetic resonance neurography. Chapter 2. 1st edition. Delhi (India): Jaypee Publishers; 2012. p. 23–35.

60. Wertsch JJ, Melvin J. Median nerve anatomy and entrapment syndromes: a review. Arch Phys Med Rehabil 1982;63:623–7.

61. Eversmann WW. Proximal median nerve compression. Hand Clin 1992;8:307–15.

62. Schantz K, Riegels-Nielsen P. The anterior interosseous nerve syndrome. J Hand Surg Br 1992;17:510–2.

63. Seror P. Anterior interosseous nerve lesions. Clinical and electrophysiological features. J Bone Joint Surg Br 1996;78:238–41.

64. Joist A, Joosten U, Wetterkamp D, et al. Anterior interosseous nerve compression after supracondylar fracture of the humerus: a metaanalysis. J Neurosurg 1999;90:1053–6.

65. Nicholls MA, Lawton JN, Lawrence SJ. Radiologic case study. Radial shaft fracture, anterior interosseous nerve injury, and the presence of a foreign body within the soft tissues of the proximal forearm. Orthopedics 2003;26:111–2.

66. Chin DH, Meals RA. Anterior interosseous nerve syndrome. J Hand Surg Am 2001;1:249–57.

67. Dunn AJ, Salonen DC, Anastakis DJ. MR imaging findings of anterior interosseous nerve lesions. Skeletal Radiol 2007;36:1155–62.

68. Gyftopoulos S, Rosenberg ZS, Petchprapa C. Increased MR signal intensity in the pronator quadratus muscle: does it always indicate anterior interosseous neuropathy? AJR Am J Roentgenol 2010; 194:490–3.

69. Grainger AJ, Campbell RS, Stothard J. Anterior interosseous nerve syndrome: appearance at MR imaging in three cases. Radiology 1998;208:381–4.

70. Chhabra A, Subhawong TK, Bizzell C, et al. 3T MR neurography using three-dimensional diffusion-weighted PSIF: technical issues and advantages. Skeletal Radiol 2011;40(10):1355–60. http://dx.doi.org/10.1007/s00256-011-1162-y.

71. al-Qattan MM. Gantzer's muscle: an anatomical study of the accessory head of the flexor pollicis longus muscle. J Hand Surg Br 1996;21:269–70.

72. Bickel KD. Carpal tunnel syndrome. J Hand Surg Am 2010;35:147–52.

73. Martin BI, Levenson LM, Hollingworth W, et al. Randomized clinical trial of surgery versus conservative therapy for carpal tunnel syndrome. BMC Musculoskelet Disord 2005;18(6):2.

74. Omer GE Jr. Median nerve compression at the wrist. Hand Clin 1992;8:317–24.

75. Chang MH, Wei SJ, Chiang HL, et al. Comparison of motor conduction techniques in the diagnosis of carpal tunnel syndrome. Neurology 2002;58: 1603–7.

76. Wilder-Smith EP, Seet RC, Lim EC. Diagnosing carpal tunnel syndrome: clinical criteria and ancillary tests. Nat Clin Pract Neurol 2006;2: 366–74.

77. Jarvik JG, Yuen E, Haynor DR, et al. MR nerve imaging in a prospective cohort of patients with suspected carpal tunnel syndrome. Neurology 2002;58:1597–602.

78. Verdugo RJ, Salinas RA, Castillo JL, et al. Surgical versus non-surgical treatment for carpal tunnel syndrome. Cochrane Database Syst Rev 2008;(4):CD001552.

79. Ibrahim I, Khan WS, Goddard N, et al. Carpal tunnel syndrome: a review of the recent literature. Open Orthop J 2012;6:69–76.

80. Cudlip SA, Howe FA, Clifton A, et al. Magnetic resonance neurography studies of the median nerve before and after carpal tunnel decompression. J Neurosurg 2002;96:1046–51.

81. Lee KS, Oh CS, Chung IH, et al. An anatomic study of the Martin-Gruber anastomosis: electrodiagnostic implications. Muscle Nerve 2005;31: 95–7.

82. Guggenberger R, Markovic D, Eppenberger P, et al. Assessment of median nerve with MR neurography by using diffusion-tensor imaging: normative and pathologic diffusion values. Radiology 2012;265(1):194–203.

83. Guggenberger R, Eppenberger P, Markovic D, et al. MR neurography of the median nerve at 3.0T: optimization of diffusion tensor imaging and fiber tractography. Eur J Radiol 2012;81(7): e775–82.

Magnetic Resonance Neurography of the Pelvis and Lumbosacral Plexus

Holly Delaney, MB BCh*, Jenny Bencardino, MD*,
Zehava Sadka Rosenberg, MD

KEYWORDS

• Neurography • Magnetic resonance imaging • Pelvis • Lumbar plexus • Neuropathy

KEY POINTS

- The diagnosis of pelvic neuropathy is challenging for both radiologists and clinicians. Detailed knowledge of pelvic neural anatomy and of clinical syndromes and denervation patterns that commonly affect the pelvic nerves is crucial to the correct interpretation of magnetic resonance (MR) neurography studies. Advances in MR technology now enable high-resolution imaging of the lumbosacral plexus and its pelvic neural branches, with reliable visualization of many of the nerves commonly implicated in pelvic neuropathy.
- Appropriate use and interpretation of dedicated pelvic MR neurography may show pathologic changes within the peripheral nerves as well as elucidate the underlying disorder.
- In the case of negative MR neurography studies, other musculoskeletal disorders that may explain the patient's clinical presentation may be shown. Recognition of potential pitfalls in MR neurography that may result in false-positive findings by the reporting radiologist is also crucial.
- The diagnostic performance of some of the MR findings that indicate neuropathy is yet to be established. Interpretation of MR neurography findings is best performed in conjunction with the clinical picture and in collaboration with the referring physician.

INTRODUCTION

Neurogenic pain arising from lumbosacral plexus and the nerves of the pelvis poses a particular diagnostic challenge for the clinician and radiologist alike, given the complexity of the anatomy, the frequent coexistent disorders and potential symptom generators, and the difficulty in obtaining high-resolution imaging while using a large field of view. Classic symptoms of pain corresponding with a particular nerve distribution are not always present and patients may have vague symptoms that can be attributed to a multitude of other disorders.[1] The situation becomes even more confusing with involvement of multiple nerves, as seen in lumbar plexopathy. Lumbar discogenic pain and other disorders, such as hip osteoarthrosis, commonly coexist.

Until recently, imaging of peripheral nerves was limited from a technical standpoint, with no established gold standard imaging method to reliably visualize peripheral nerves and show disorders. With technical advances in magnetic resonance (MR) imaging, and particularly with the advent of dedicated high-resolution MR neurography, even small-caliber peripheral nerves and their associated disorders can now reliably be shown. Radiologists nevertheless may lack confidence and experience in reading dedicated high-resolution

Disclosures: The authors have nothing to disclose.
Department of Radiology, New York University Hospital for Joint Diseases, 301 East 17th Street, 6th Floor, New York, NY 10003, USA
* Corresponding authors.
E-mail addresses: holly.delaney@nyumc.org; jenny.bencardino@nyumc.org

MR neurography examinations. By reviewing the basic principles and techniques of neural imaging, revisiting the relevant anatomy and highlighting common disorders, this article is intended to demystify this imaging technique along with its applications and interpretations, enabling the reader to apply it in daily clinical practice.

MR NEUROGRAPHY: TECHNICAL CONSIDERATIONS

MR neurography is a tissue-specific imaging technique optimized for evaluating peripheral nerves, their internal fascicular morphology, alterations in neural signal and caliber, and associated space-occupying and other compressive lesions.[2] Three-dimensional (3D) imaging is of critical importance in tracing the course of peripheral nerves, in identifying points of compression or disruption, and for preoperative planning. In general, MR neurography may either be T2 based or diffusion based. Diffusion-based MR imaging, especially diffusion tensor imaging, allows functional assessment of the nerves, but remains a novel technique, with specific hardware and software requirements to enhance the otherwise low signal/noise ratio (SNR) from these small nerves, limiting its application in routine clinical practice.

The Magnet

The strength of the magnet is an important consideration, with impact on both image quality and speed of acquisition.[3] In general, there is superior performance of MR neurography at 3 T compared with 1.5 T, which has led us to only perform the technique using 3-T platforms. It is the advent of high-tesla imaging and its widespread availability that has facilitated the development of state-of-the-art MR neurography and made it a reality in daily clinical practice. Compared with 1.5-T MR imaging, 3-T MR imaging provides increased (nearly double) SNR, which in part is related to improved coil design, better gradient performance, and wider bandwidths. This improvement translates into higher spatial resolution and thinner slice sections with improved fluid conspicuity, as well as superior contrast/noise ratio, which improves anatomic characterization and lesion detection.[4] Increased conspicuity of fluid and more uniform fat-suppression techniques result in better depiction of fascicular appearance of the nerves. There is also less inhomogeneity of the magnetic field. More robust hardware facilitates the application of multiple radiofrequency saturation pulses required for adequate vascular suppression. Furthermore, the application of parallel imaging allows faster acquisition times. It is difficult to produce quality T2-weighted 3D images on lower

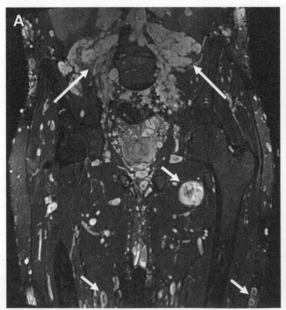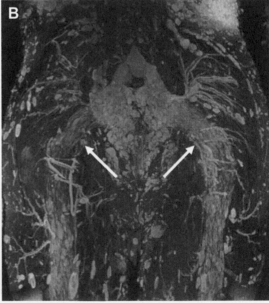

Fig. 1. Neurofibromatosis (NF). A 32-year-old man with bilateral leg pain and weakness. Coronal 3D spectral adiabatic inversion recovery (STIR) sampling perfection with application optimized contrasts by using different flip angle evolutions (SPACE) (*A*) and coronal MIP 3D STIR-SPACE (*B*) MR images through the lower abdomen and pelvis show plexiform lesions in the pelvis (*large arrows*) and numerous hyperintense peripheral nerve sheath tumors, few with target sign (*small arrows*) involving various segments of lumbosacral plexus in keeping with the clinical diagnosis of NF type I. (*B*) Diffuse enlargement of bilateral sciatic nerves with multifocal masses (*large arrows*). (*Courtesy of* Dr Avneesh Chhabra, MD, Dallas, Texas.)

field strength magnets because of time and hardware limitations. 3D gradient echo sequences often have to be used, and images thus generated are frequently nonisotropic with poor SNR and soft tissue contrast and are prone to susceptibility artifacts.[4] In contrast, high-quality isotropic 3D proton density and T2-weighted images can be acquired with relative ease and speed at 3 T and serve as an invaluable adjunct to two-dimensional (2D) images.

The Sequences

T1-weighted imaging

High-resolution T1-weighted imaging is excellent for depicting normal anatomy of the peripheral nerves and surrounding structures. Thin sections (maximum slice thickness of 4 mm), are necessary for adequate resolution of anatomic detail and fascicular morphology. Peripheral nerves appear as linear T1-hypointense structures, following an

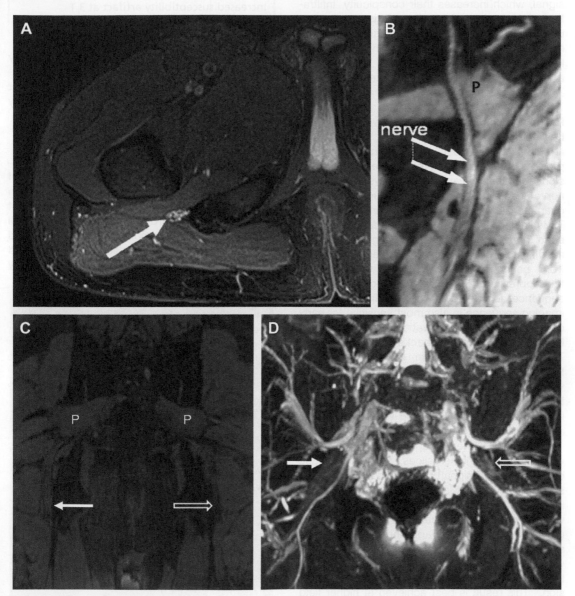

Fig. 2. 3D MR neurography. A 27-year-old man with right sciatic neuropathy following heroin coma with prolonged supine immobilization and secondary external compression just below the level of the piriformis muscle (P). Axial high-resolution fast spin (FS) T2 (*A*), coronal 3D MIP DW PSIF (*B*), coronal 3D DW PSIF (*C*), and coronal MIP 3D SPAIR SPACE (*D*) show focal increased signal and enlargement of the infrapiriformis portion of the right sciatic nerve (*solid arrows*) relative to the left (*open arrows*). Note superior suppression of vascular signal in the PSIF sequence as well as better depiction of abnormal T2 bright signal changes of the sciatic nerve at the site of compression.

expected anatomic distribution. Differentiation from adjacent vessels is often possible, especially with the larger nerves, with arteries appearing as flow voids and veins appearing T1 hyperintense because of inflow phenomenon.[5] With larger nerves or at higher resolution imaging, the individual fascicles may be resolved.[2] Peripheral nerves are outlined by T1-hyperintense perineural fat, with a characteristic reverse tram track appearance of alternating T1-hyperintense and T1-hypointense signal, which increases their conspicuity. Infiltration of the perineural fat and soft tissues is often best depicted on T1-weighted imaging. The presence of muscle fatty replacement in the setting of long-standing denervation is also seen to best advantage on this imaging sequence.

T2-weighted imaging

Pathologic changes within the nerve are seen to best advantage on T2-weighted imaging.[6] In addition, many mass lesions and pathologic processes that commonly result in neural compression (eg, paralabral and ganglion cysts, peripheral nerve sheath tumors, fluid-filled bursae) are best characterized and are most conspicuous on T2-weighted imaging. With standard fast spin echo (non–fat suppressed) T2-weighted imaging, it is difficult to discern abnormal increased T2 signal from perineural and intraneural fat, therefore fat-suppressed T2-weighted imaging is the optimal sequence for detecting neural disorders. This imaging sequence is also most sensitive for early changes of muscle denervation signal alterations. However, there are drawbacks to fat-suppressed T2-weighted imaging with more artifact from hyperintense vascular structures and partial volume averaging.[7] Vascular structures, which typically accompany the nerve, appear hyperintense and may be confused with neural signal abnormality or perineural edema.

Dedicated MR neurography uses increased T2 weighting with thinner slices, to both increase conspicuity of T2 signal change and achieve higher spatial resolution.[7] Maximizing the conspicuity of increased T2 signal in nerves is achieved in 3 ways: (1) using sequences with long echo times (TEs) (90–130 ms), (2) applying radiofrequency saturation pulses to suppress signal from adjacent vessels, and (3) using frequency-selective or adiabatic inversion recovery imaging–type fat suppression.[6] This result is best achieved at higher field strength, emphasizing the importance of technological advances in the development of high-resolution neural imaging. This technique results in increased T2 weighting, minimizes spurious signal from adjacent vessels and fat, and is more sensitive for showing neural signal abnormality.[8]

Newer techniques used in 3D imaging, namely steady-state free precession and diffusion techniques, result in superior suppression of vascular signal in T2-weighted sequences, particularly when imaging the extremities.[9]

3D Imaging

Isotropic 3D imaging is an essential component of state-of-the-art MR neurography. Nerves often follow oblique courses and are not seen to best advantage on standard axial, coronal, and sagittal imaging planes. 3D multiplanar reconstructed (MPR), curved planar reconstructed (CPR), and maximal intensity projected (MIP) images greatly

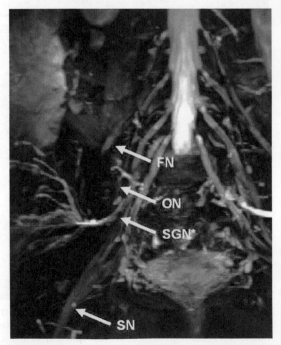

Fig. 3. Coronal MIP 3D STIR-SPACE image showing the sciatic nerve (SN), obturator nerve (ON), and femoral nerve (FN), and superior gluteal neurovascular bundle (SGN*).

facilitate the visualization of nerves and are particularly useful for preoperative planning. Decreased magic angle artifact and partial volume averaging on 3D imaging allow more accurate depiction of disorders. Furthermore, caliber and signal change in nerves, which may be subtle or attributed to volume averaging on axial imaging, are seen to better advantage in the longitudinal plane, allowing better assessment of the extent of the abnormality. Certain disorders, such as plexiform neurofibromata, particularly lend themselves to 3D imaging for depiction of the disease burden in one image (Fig. 1). Compression of peripheral nerves by disc protrusions, space-occupying lesions, and anatomic fibro-osseous tunnels is also more accurately delineated on 3D imaging. Focal interruption of a nerve can be particularly challenging to show on axial imaging, and 3D reconstructions may prove crucial in this scenario. Variations in muscular volume and anatomy may also be better assessed on 3D imaging.

Several techniques may be used in 3D imaging. SPACE (sampling perfection with application optimized contrasts by using different flip angle evolutions, Siemens, Erlangen, Germany) sequence is an isotropic single-slab acquisition, mainly spin echo–type sequence that allows MPR, CPR, and MIP reconstructed images to map out the peripheral nerves and associated disorder in the longitudinal plane. This imaging may be obtained in spectral adiabatic inversion recovery (SPAIR) or short tau inversion recovery sequence (STIR) contrasts, thus providing T2 weighting and optimizing sensitivity for detecting neural disorders. STIR imaging

is preferred for imaging of the lumbosacral and brachial plexus because of superior fat suppression, whereas SPAIR imaging is preferred for imaging of the extremities. More recent developments include the 3D diffusion-weighted (DW) reversed fast imaging with steady-state free precession (PSIF) sequence, which is a heavily T2-weighted technique, combining selective suppression of vascular flow signal with multiplanar capabilities. The PSIF sequence holds great promise, particularly in the imaging of the extremities. Attempts to suppress vascular flow signal with the application of saturation bands usually fails in peripheral locations, either because of the slow or in-plane flow within the peripheral vessels, or because of the variable oblique courses of peripheral neurovascular bundles. PSIF, because of its sensitivity to flow-related dephasing of the transverse magnetization, causes vessels in the imaging field of view to lose their signal intensity. Vascular signal suppression is also enhanced by the small diffusion moment applied to this sequence (Fig. 2).[9]

The Field of View

Large field of view is most commonly used in pelvic neurography protocols, and it occurs at the expense of resolution but allows side-to-side comparison and evaluation of multiple nerve distributions on a single study. In our experience, the nerves most commonly affected in pelvic neuropathy can be reliably shown when a dedicated MR neurography protocol is performed. In large patients, and when a particularly large field of view is required, 3D STIR-SPACE imaging may

Table 1
Lumbosacral plexus muscular innervations by nerve root

	T12	L1	L2	L3	L4	L5	S1	S2	S3	S4	S5
Obturator internus						*	*				
Obturator externus			*	*	*						
Pectineus			*	*	*						
Psoas major	*	*	*	*	*						
Iliacus	*	*	*	*	*						
Iliopsoas			*	*	*						
Gluteus minimus						*	*				
Gluteus medius						*	*				
Gluteus maximus						*	*				
Piriformis						*		*			
Adductor brevis			*	*	*						
Adductor longus				*	*						
Adductor magnus				*	*						
Levator ani								*	*	*	

be preferable to 3D SPAIR-SPACE imaging given the superior and more robust fat suppression.

Pitfalls and Technical Limitations

Magic angle effect, a well-described phenomenon in imaging of tendons, also occurs when imaging peripheral nerves. This effect results in spurious increased signal when the nerve lies in a plane 55° to the main vector of the magnet. Unlike tendons, this effect may persist in nerves, even at longer TEs (>66 milliseconds) and therefore higher TEs must be used to overcome it.[10,11] The interpreting radiologist was traditionally advised to be particularly aware of this phenomenon when reporting increased intraneural T2 signal in MR neurography studies; however, recent literature concludes that magic angle effect is a rare source of false-positive interpretation on MR neurography, particularly in nerves that run parallel to the main vector of the magnet.[12]

Despite the use of suppressive radiofrequency pulses, hyperintense vascular signal is often present on MR neurography examinations, especially

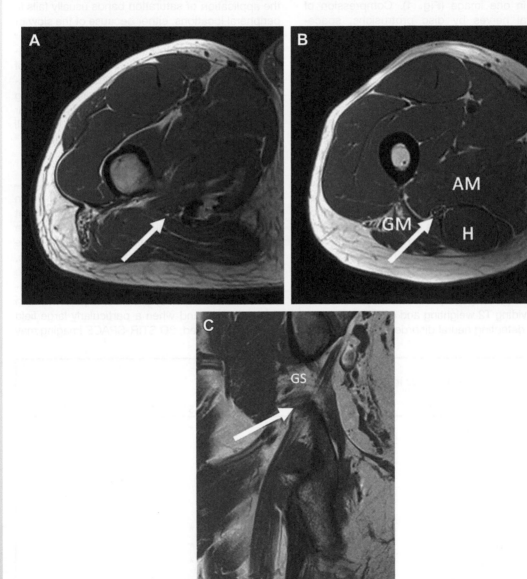

Fig. 4. Normal sciatic nerve. (A) Axial T1 MR images, just below the greater trochanter (A) and at the proximal thigh (B) show the normal fascicular anatomy of the sciatic nerve. Axial T1 image (B) shows the sciatic nerve descending in the thigh between the adductor magnus (AM), gluteus maximus (GM), and hamstring (H) muscles (arrow, B). Coronal T1 image (C) shows the sciatic nerve (arrow) exiting the pelvis at the level of the greater sciatic notch (GS).

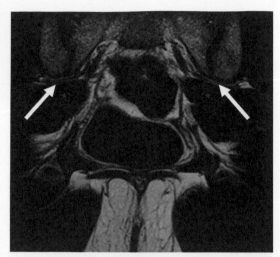

Fig. 5. Normal superior gluteal nerve. Coronal T2-weighted image shows bilateral superior gluteal nerves (*arrows*) curving under the roof of the greater sciatic foramen above the piriformis muscles (*asterisks*). Note the proximity to the inferior sacroiliac joints and potential for entrapment in sacroiliac joint disorders.

at high TE, which is a particular source of confusion in small nerves when it occurs in the accompanying vascular bundle and may be misinterpreted as neural or perineural signal abnormality. Inhomogeneous fat suppression is another potential source of error, particularly in the pelvis, given the large field of view and the high number of patients who have hip or lumbar instrumentation, which further degrades the local magnetic field thus worsening fat suppression. Increased susceptibility and chemical shift artifact, also seen at 3 T, may be counteracted by shortening the ET, performing parallel imaging, and increasing the bandwidth.[13] Nonetheless, 1.5-T imaging may be preferable when evaluating nerves

in close proximity to a metal prosthesis. Specific absorption rate limits are reached earlier at 3 T compared with 1.5 T because there is increased energy deposition for radiofrequency excitation at 3 T. However, this difference is usually balanced by faster image acquisition and shorter examination time and does not usually pose a clinical problem. Other potential drawbacks of 3D imaging include longer imaging times, and time spent producing and interpreting multiplanar reformatted images (**Box 1**).

ANATOMIC CONSIDERATIONS
Lumbosacral Plexus

The lumbosacral plexus is composed of a lumbar and sacral plexus (**Fig. 3**). The lumbar plexus is formed from the ventral rami of L1 to L4 and a small contribution from the 12th thoracic nerve. The plexus descends dorsally or within the psoas muscle. Branches emerging from the lateral border of the psoas muscle include the iliohypogastric, ilioinguinal, genitofemoral, lateral femoral cutaneous, and femoral nerves, whereas branches emerging from the medial border of the psoas muscle include the obturator nerve and lumbosacral trunk. A minor branch of L4 combines with the ventral ramus of L5 to form the lumbosacral cord or trunk. The latter descends over the sacral ala and joins the S1 to S3 nerve roots on the anterior aspect of the piriformis muscle to form the sacral plexus.[14] Thus the sacral plexus is formed from L4 to S4 ventral rami. The sciatic, inferior, and superior gluteal and pudendal nerves constitute its sacral branches. Lumbosacral plexus muscular innervations by nerve root are listed in **Table 1** and the most clinically important motor and sensory innervations of multiple

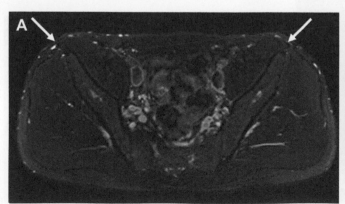

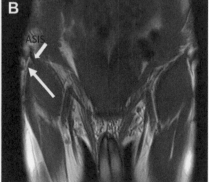

Fig. 6. Normal lateral femoral cutaneous nerve. Axial T2 FS image (*A*) shows the bilateral lateral femoral cutaneous nerves (*arrows*) adjacent to the anterior superior iliac spine. Coronal proton density (PD) image (*B*) shows the right lateral femoral cutaneous nerve (*long arrow*) at the level of the anterior superior iliac spine (ASIS). Note the close relationship with the origin of the sartorius muscle (*short arrow*).

peripheral nerves of the lower limb and pelvis are discussed in more detail later.

Sciatic Nerve

The sciatic nerve is the largest peripheral nerve in the body and is reliably shown on computed tomography (CT) and MR imaging.[15] It is formed from the L4 to S3 nerve roots and may descend anterior to (most commonly), above, or within the piriformis muscle. After exiting the pelvis through the greater sciatic foramen, it descends in the thigh between the adductor magnus and the gluteus maximus muscles (**Fig. 4**). The sciatic nerve is composed of the medial tibial and the lateral common peroneal divisions, which provide motor innervation to the posterior thigh muscles and all motor function below the knee (anterior, lateral, posterior, and deep muscular compartments). It gives all sensory innervation to the lower limb with the exception of medial sensory innervation of the thigh and leg, which is provided by the obturator and femoral nerves.

Superior and Inferior Gluteal Nerves

The superior gluteal nerve is formed from the posterior roots of L4, L5, and S1. It exits the pelvis, curving under the roof of the greater sciatic foramen above the piriformis muscle, and then passes between the gluteus minimus and gluteus medius muscles before giving off superior and inferior branches (**Fig. 5**). The superior branch terminates in the gluteus minimus muscle and the inferior branch terminates in the tensor fascia lata. The

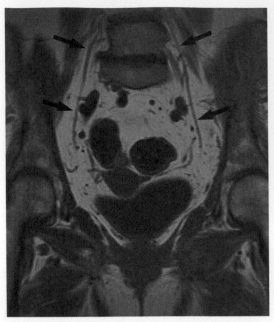

Fig. 8. Normal obturator nerve. Coronal T1 image shows the normal obturator nerves (*arrows*), outlined by pelvic fat, descending the pelvic side walls in a near vertical orientation.

superior gluteal nerve acts to abduct the thigh at the hip by providing motor innervation to the gluteus minimus, gluteus medius, and tensor fascia lata muscles.

The inferior gluteal nerve formed from the posterior roots of L5, S1, and S2 provides motor innervations to the gluteus maximus, which, with the aid of the hamstrings, acts to extend the thigh. It exits the pelvis through the sciatic notch passing below the piriformis muscle and lies medial to the sciatic nerve before its terminal branch provides motor innervation to the gluteus maximus

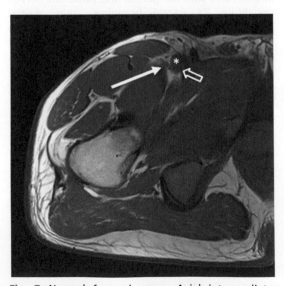

Fig. 7. Normal femoral nerve. Axial intermediate-weighted image depicts the relationship of the femoral nerve (*arrow*), artery (*asterisk*), and vein (*open arrow*) in the groin.

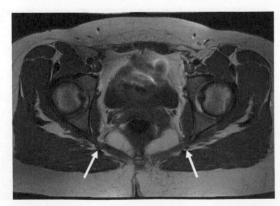

Fig. 9. Normal pudendal nerve. Axial T1 image shows normal appearance of the bilateral pudendal nerves (*arrows*) posterior to the ischial spine and deep to the gluteus maximus muscle.

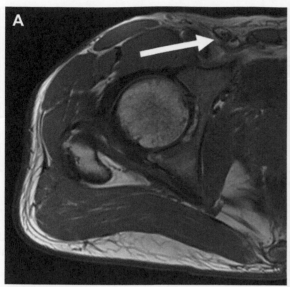 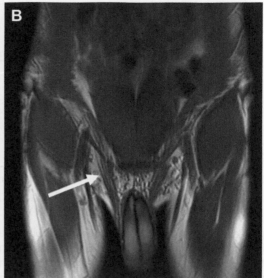

Fig. 10. Normal genitofemoral nerve. Axial PD image (*A*) and coronal PD image (*B*) in a male patient shows the external spermatic branch of the genitofemoral nerve, running alongside the spermatic cord (*arrow*), within the inguinal canal. This branch supplies the cremaster muscle, spermatic cord, scrotum, and adjacent thigh, and is responsible for the cremasteric reflex.

muscle. The superior and inferior gluteal nerves have no sensory contribution.

Lateral Femoral Cutaneous Nerve

The lateral femoral cutaneous nerve arises from L2 and L3, descends lateral to the psoas muscle, crosses the iliacus muscle deep to its fascia, and passes either through or underneath the lateral aspect of the inguinal ligament to the lateral thigh where it divides into anterior and posterior branches (Fig. 6). It innervates the skin on the lateral aspect of the thigh and, as its name implies, is purely sensory.

Femoral Nerve

The femoral nerve is formed by the L2, L3, and L4 nerve roots and descends between the iliacus and psoas muscles before exiting the pelvis under the inguinal ligament, in a canal between the iliopsoas

muscle and the iliopectineal fascia (Fig. 7). It gives off a motor branch to the iliacus and the psoas muscles before dividing into anterior and posterior divisions and forming the saphenous nerve. The femoral nerve controls hip flexion and knee extension by providing motor innervation to the iliacus, psoas, pectineus, sartorius, and quadriceps femoris muscles. Sensory innervation is of the medial thigh, anteromedial knee, medial leg, and foot.

Obturator Nerve

The obturator nerve is formed by the L2 to L4 ventral rami. It descends into the pelvis, running along the iliopectineal line, exiting the pelvis via the obturator canal at the superior aspect of obturator foramen. Within the pelvis, it assumes a near vertical orientation anterior to the psoas muscle and is well shown on coronal imaging (Fig. 8). It divides into an anterior branch, which

Table 2					
Modified standard pelvis imaging protocol					
MR Imaging Sequence	Plane	FOV (cm)	Slice Thickness (mm)	TR (ms)	TE (ms)
T1	Axial	34	5	400–800	min
T2	Axial	34	3	3000	130
T2 FS	Axial	34	3	3000	110
T1	Coronal	34	3	400–800	min
T2 FS	Coronal	34	3	4460	120

Abbreviations: FOV, field of view; min, minimum; TR, recovery time.

Table 3
Dedicated pelvic MR neurography protocol

MR Imaging Sequence	Plane	FOV (cm)	Slice Thickness (mm)	TR (ms)	TE (ms)
T1	Axial	38	3	640	6.3
T2 FS	Axial	38	3	5420	63
PD	Coronal	38	3	4000	39
3D SPACE-SPAIR	Axial	38	0.8	1000	92
3D PSIF	Axial	38	1.1	12.19	2.38
T1 FS C+[a]	Axial	38	3	400–800	min

Siemens Verio 3T MR imaging scanner, Erlangen, Germany.
[a] Optional.

passes anterior to adductor brevis and supplies the hip, and a posterior branch, which passes within the obturator externus muscle, and between adductor brevis and magnus muscles. The anterior branch gives motor innervation to the hip, gracilis, adductor brevis and longus muscles, and occasionally the pectineus muscle, whereas the posterior branch supplies the obturator externus and a portion of the adductor magnus muscles. Sensory innervation is to the medial thigh and knee.

Pudendal Nerve

The pudendal nerve is formed by the ventral rami of S2 and all of the rami of S3 and S4. It passes between the piriformis and the coccygeus muscles and leaves the pelvis through the greater sciatic foramen. After crossing the ischial spine, it reenters the perineum through the lesser sciatic foramen and travels in the Alcock canal along the lateral wall of the ischiorectal fossa (**Fig. 9**). The major branches are the inferior rectal nerve, the perineal nerve, and the dorsal nerve of the penis or clitoris. Motor innervation is of the bulbospongiosus and ischiocavernosus muscles and the external urethral and rectal sphincters, whereas sensory innervation is of the perineum, scrotum, and anus.

Iliohypogastric Nerve

The iliohypogastric nerve is formed mainly from the anterior division of L1, with a small contribution from T12, and runs anteriorly and inferiorly along the lateral border of the psoas major and quadrates lumborum muscles. It pierces the transversus abduminus muscle and runs within the lateral abdominal wall, above the iliac crest, before dividing into its lateral and anterior cutaneous branches. Its terminal branch runs parallel to the inguinal ligament and exits the aponeurosis of the external oblique muscle. The nerve provides motor innervation to the abdominal wall musculature and sensory innervation to the skin above the inguinal ligament and superior lateral gluteal region.

Ilioinguinal Nerve

The ilioinguinal nerve is formed from the anterior division of L1, sometimes with a small contribution from T12. It runs a similar course to the iliohypogastric nerve, running inferiorly along the quadrates lumborum before piercing the lateral abdominal wall and running medially to the inguinal ligament. It contributes to motor innervations of the abdominal wall musculature, and gives sensory branches to the pubic symphysis, femoral triangle, labia majora, or root of the penis and scrotum.

Genitofemoral Nerve

The genitofemoral nerve is formed by the anterior divisions of L1 and L2 nerve roots and pierces the psoas major muscle at the L3/L4 level before dividing into 2 branches that run along the anterior margin of the psoas muscle. The medial genitalis,

Table 4
Direct and indirect signs of neuropathy on MR imaging

Direct	Indirect
Increased size	Infiltration of perineural fat
Increased T2 signal	Perineural edema
Irregular shape	Muscular denervation edemalike signal
Abnormal fascicular morphology	Muscular atrophy (chronic)
Abnormal course	Deformities (pes cavus, hammer-toe)
Enhancement	

Table 5
MR imaging appearances of normal and abnormal peripheral nerves

Feature	Normal	Abnormal
Size	Similar to adjacent artery, decreases distally	Focal or diffuse enlargement, larger than adjacent arteries
Signal intensity	Isointense to skeletal muscle on T1-weighted and T2-weighted imaging	Hyperintense on T2-weighted imaging, similar to adjacent veins
Fascicular pattern	Preserved on T1-weighted and T2-weighted imaging	Enlargement or disruption/blurring of fascicles
Course	Smooth without focal deviation, outlined by fat	Focal or diffuse deviation, discontinuity
Enhancement	Absent (except for deficient blood-nerve barrier, dorsal root ganglion)	Present in tumor, infection, inflammation because of disruption of blood-nerve barrier
Perineural fat planes	Preserved and clean	Effaced

Courtesy of Dr Avneesh Chhabra, MD, Dallas, Texas.

or external spermatic, branch in men enters the inguinal canal and runs along with the spermatic cord to supply the cremaster muscle, spermatic cord, scrotum, and adjacent thigh, and is responsible for the cremasteric reflex (**Fig. 10**). In women, it runs with the round ligament of the uterus and gives sensory innervations of the labia majora and adjacent thigh. The lateral, or femoral, branch runs lateral to the femoral artery and posterior to the inguinal ligament into the proximal thigh, where it pierces the sartorius muscle and supplies the proximal lateral aspect of the femoral triangle. It is a purely sensory nerve.

IMAGING PROTOCOL

Imaging of the pelvic nerves may be performed with modifications to standard pelvic musculo-skeletal imaging protocols or with dedicated pelvic neurographic sequences. The latter encompass high-resolution 2D imaging as well as isotropic 3D imaging, with MPR reformatted images, which are a particularly useful problem solving tool and serve as an excellent adjunct to 2D imaging. Protocols currently used in our institution (Siemens Verio 3T MR imaging scanner, Erlangen, Germany) are detailed in **Tables 2** and **3**, but vary from institution to institution, according to the hardware and software available, radiologist preference, and clinical indication.

IMAGING FINDINGS

MR imaging plays a crucial role in evaluating patients with neurogenic pain and in characterizing potential causes. With recent technical advances in MR imaging, and particularly the advent of MR neurography, direct and indirect signs of neuropathy may be shown even in the absence of a detectable compressive cause (**Tables 4** and **5**). Diagnostic criteria for neural disorders include increased size of the nerve (larger than the adjacent artery), increased intraneural T2 signal, and abnormal fascicular morphology, including focal enlargement or loss of definition of the internal fascicles. Nerves may have an abnormal course with infiltration of the perineural fat when involved in scarring, and abnormal shape when focally enlarged or involved by tumor. Normal nerves should not enhance, except in those locations where the blood-nerve barrier is absent (dorsal root ganglion). Enhancement is most commonly seen in the setting of tumor or inflammation.[13]

Indirect signs of neuropathy, particularly muscle denervation patterns, are also useful secondary signs of pelvic neuropathy (**Table 6**). Increased T2 signal in the setting of muscular denervation does

Table 6
Differential diagnosis of abnormal muscle signal on MR imaging

Focal/Patchy	Diffuse
Infectious myositis	Denervation
Delayed-onset muscle soreness	Postinfectious/inflammatory (Parsonage-Turner syndrome)
Trauma (contusion)	Diabetes mellitus
Muscular strain	Disuse atrophy
Polymyositis/myopathy	Polymyositis/myopathy
Tumor	

not represent true edema, and is best termed edemalike signal or denervation signal alteration. This condition may progress to muscular fatty replacement, best detected on T1-weighted imaging, and eventually to muscle atrophy. Edemalike signal without fatty replacement is potentially reversible, if the underlying neuropathy resolves. There are multiple differential considerations for increased intramuscular T2 signal (see **Table 6**). Denervation edemalike signal is characterized by diffuse homogeneous involvement of the entire muscle, sharp margins, lack of associated fascial

and perifascial fluid or inflammation, and conformation to a particular nerve distribution. However, occasional variant innervation configurations and plexopathy may confuse the pattern of muscle denervation changes.

PATHOLOGY
General Concepts

A wide variety of disorders can result in abnormal imaging findings of the pelvic nerves and musculature, ranging from infectious and inflammatory

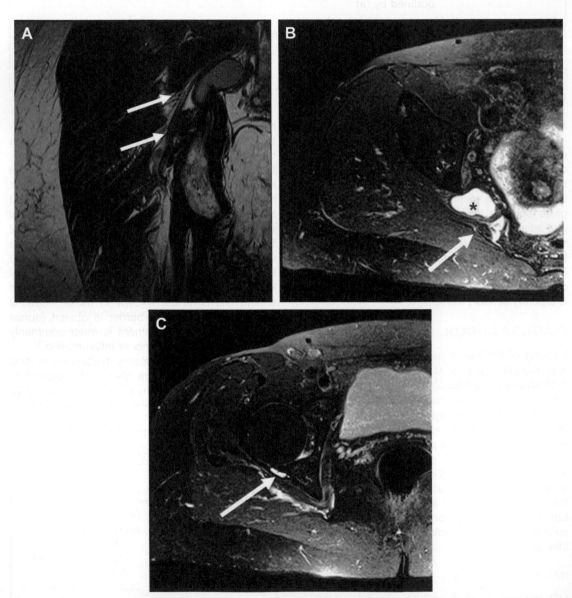

Fig. 11. Sciatic nerve compression by a paralabral cyst. Coronal PD image (*A*) of the right hip shows the right sciatic nerve (*arrows*) draped over the cyst (*asterisk*). Sequential axial T2 FS images depict posterior and lateral displacement of the sciatic nerve by the cyst (*arrow, B*). Note communication of the cyst with the hip joint at the posterior chondrolabral junction (*arrow, C*).

lesions, systemic diseases such as polymyositis, to benign and malignant space-occupying processes. Disorders that result in painful neuropathic symptoms usually have local causes, and can be divided into 3 major categories: (1) space-occupying lesions, (2) posttraumatic lesions, and (3) iatrogenic lesions. Space-occupying lesions may be benign or malignant. Almost any pelvic mass can potentially result in neural compression; however, certain lesions have a predilection for causing neural compression because of their anatomic location. Certain pelvic nerves may be susceptible to compression at particular anatomic bony or fibrous

canals. Other nerves may be placed at risk during certain surgical procedures, or may be susceptible to traumatic injury because of their proximity to commonly fractured or avulsed osseous or tendinous structures. Common benign lesions that may potentially cause a compressive neuropathy include ganglion cysts, perineural cysts, and fluid-filled bursae. Paralabral cysts of the hip should be specifically noted, because they may decompress anteriorly, resulting in obturator nerve compression, or posteriorly, compromising the sciatic or superior gluteal nerve (**Figs. 11** and **12**).[16,17] Communication with the hip joint should always be considered when

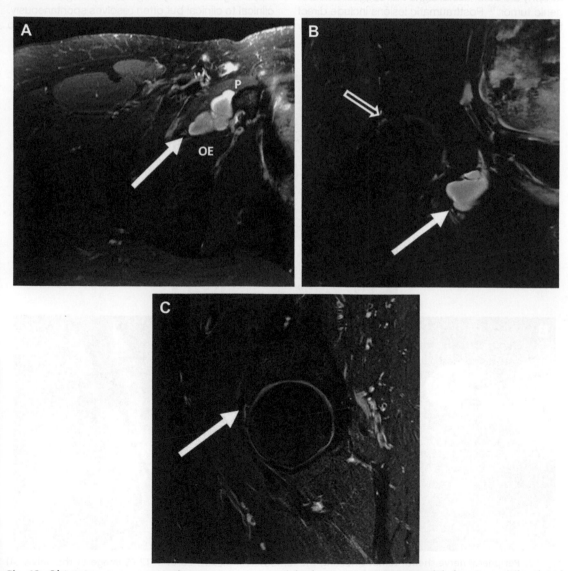

Fig. 12. Obturator nerve compression secondary to paralabral cyst. Axial T2 FS image (*A*) shows a multiloculated cyst (*arrow*) interposed between the pectineus (P) and obturator externus (OE) muscles, along the course of the anterior branch of the obturator nerve. Note subtle homogeneously increased T2 signal within the pectineus muscle consistent with denervation (*asterisk*). Coronal T2 FS images (*B and C*) shows extension of the cyst (*arrow*) toward the hip joint and associated tear of the labrum (*open arrow*).

a cystic lesion in these locations is encountered, particularly because paralabral cysts may grow to a large size and appear to be remote from the hip. Malignant lesions encompass any malignant pelvic soft tissue masses, including gynecologic and rectal tumors, and bone and lymph node metastases. Nerve sheath tumors may be benign or malignant, but are more commonly benign, and have characteristic imaging appearances, manifested by markedly hyperintense T2 signal, sometimes associated with a target sign, and avid enhancement (Fig. 13).[18] The orientation along the long axis of a peripheral nerve and the presence of distal muscular atrophy are other useful signs that suggest a neurogenic tumor.[19] Posttraumatic lesions include direct traumatic injury, in which the more superficially located femoral and sciatic nerves are at greater risk. Nerve impingement may also occur in the setting of healed fractures, remote avulsion injuries, and heterotopic ossification. The obturator nerve is particularly susceptible in the setting of pubic rami and pelvic fractures, whereas the superior gluteal nerve may be injured after hip fracture.[20] Traumatic hamstring tendon avulsion from the ischial tuberosity may result in sciatic neuropathy. The anterior branch of the obturator nerve may be affected by adductor brevis tendinopathy.[21] Traction-related indirect nerve injury, particularly to the sciatic, femoral, and obturator nerves during abdominal, hip, and genitourinary surgery, may range from subclinical to clinical but often resolves spontaneously. Direct iatrogenic injury of pelvic nerves may also

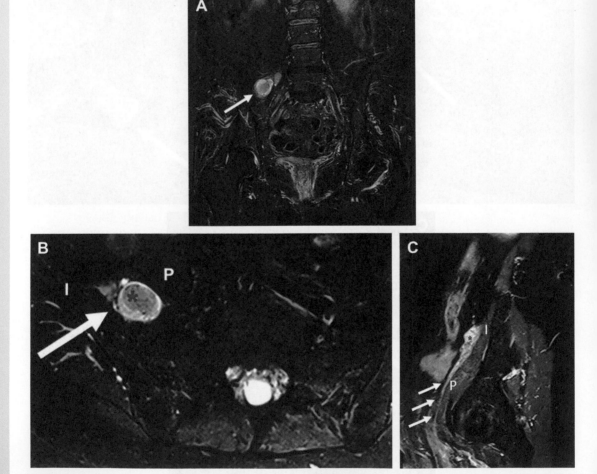

Fig. 13. Peripheral nerve sheath tumor affecting the lumbosacral plexus. Coronal T2 FS image of the pelvis (A) shows multiple lobulated lesions along the right lumbosacral plexus nerve roots (arrow). Axial T2 FS (B) shows one of the lesions (arrow) between the psoas (P) and iliacus (I) muscles, along the L4 contribution to the femoral nerve. Note the target sign–central hypointensity (asterisk), consistent with a peripheral nerve sheath tumor. Sagittal T1 FS postcontrast images (C) showing enhancement of the lesions (asterisk) as they extend along the expected course of the lumbosacral plexus and proximal femoral nerve (arrows).

occur during pelvic surgery, with the obturator nerve being particularly susceptible during genitourinary surgery (eg, hysterectomy and prostatectomy) (Fig. 14).[22] The femoral nerve may be injured following vascular intervention in the groin, either directly while accessing the femoral artery, or indirectly by hematoma or pseudoaneurysm complicating the procedure. Neuropathy of the superior gluteal nerve is a recognized, common complication of total hip arthroplasty (Fig. 15),[23,24] and there have been case reports of femoral and obturator neuropathy caused by cement extrusion.[25] Like any

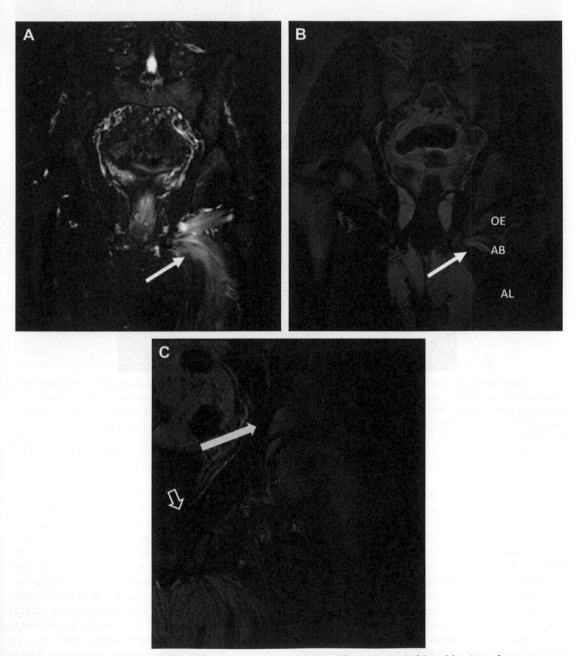

Fig. 14. Iatrogenic obturator nerve injury in a 61-year-old man with weakness in hip adduction after prostatectomy. Coronal STIR (A) and T1 (B, C) images of the pelvis show fatty atrophy and diffuse homogeneous edemalike signal (arrows) involving the left OE, adductor longus (AL), and adductor brevis (AB) muscles. Scar tissue encases the left obturator nerve (C, arrow). Note also susceptibility artifact (open arrow) at the bladder neck consistent with prior prostatectomy.

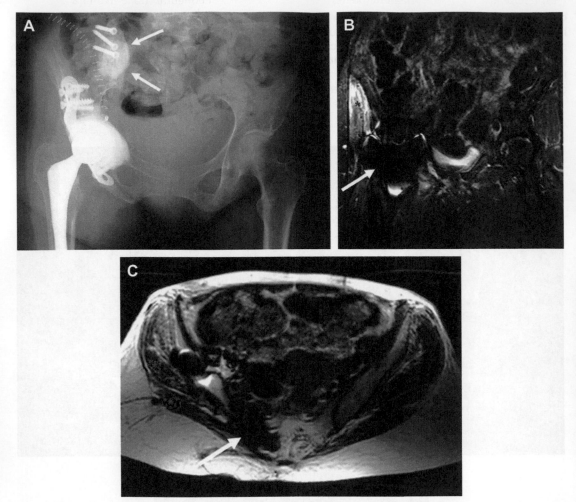

Fig. 15. Superior and inferior gluteal nerve entrapment following total hip arthroplasty (THA) and sacroiliac screw placement in a 52-year-old woman with lung carcinoma and pelvic osseous metastases. Pelvic radiograph (*A*) shows right THA, with augmentation plate and screws, as well as cement and sacroiliac screws (*arrows*). Coronal STIR image of the pelvis (*B*) shows denervation edemalike changes of the right gluteus maximus and medius muscles (*asterisks*). Note hardware artifact from right THA (*arrow*). Axial T1 image (*C*) shows fatty atrophy of the right gluteus minimus, medius, and maximus muscles (*asterisks*). Note proximity of surgical hardware and metastasis in the right sacrum and ilium (*arrow*) along the expected course of the superior gluteal nerve.

peripheral nerve, the nerves of the pelvis and lumbosacral plexus may also become affected by neuritis or neuropathy in the absence of a compressive lesion or injury. This condition may be infectious or inflammatory in origin, and is most commonly seen in the setting of systemic disease, following viral infections (chronic inflammatory demyelinating polyradiculoneuropathy) and pelvic irradiation. Neuropathy with secondary muscular denervation in the clinical setting of diabetes mellitus is a well-recognized phenomenon (diabetic amyotrophy), and has a particular predilection for the lumbosacral plexus.[3] Hereditary neuropathies may also occur, most notably Charcot-Marie-Tooth disease or hereditary motor and sensory neuropathies (HMSN) (**Figs. 16** and **17**).

Lumbosacral neuropathic syndromes
Lumbosacral plexus Lumbosacral plexopathy can be subdivided into structural causes such as tumor, hemorrhage, postsurgical, traumatic, and iatrogenic, and nonstructural causes such as amyotrophic neuralgia, radiation, vasculitis, diabetes, infections, and hereditary pressure palsies. Like any plexopathy, it may result in a confusing clinical picture. Symptoms and objective clinical signs are often related to multiple spinal levels and multiple nerve distributions and do not conform to any recognizable syndrome, which may result in delayed diagnosis. Trauma, commonly secondary to high-speed deceleration, with pelvis or hip fractures and dislocation, typically causes stretch-related or traction-related

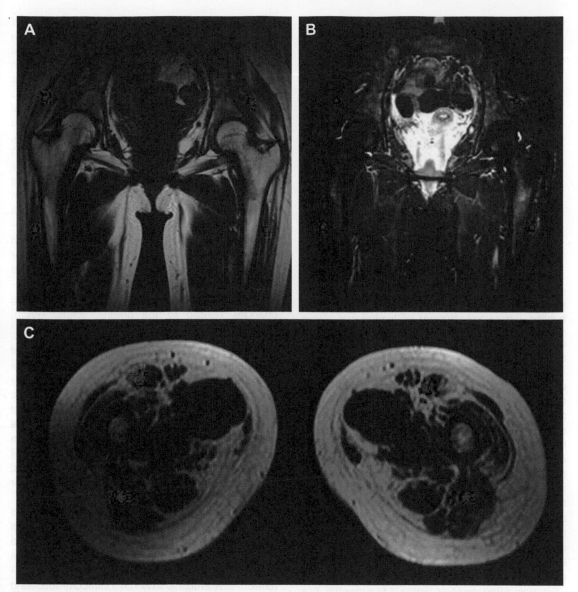

Fig. 16. Hereditary sensory and motor polyneuropathy in 14-year-old girl. Coronal T1 and STIR images with large fields of view (*A*, *B*) show diffuse fatty atrophy of the gluteal and vastus lateralis musculature (*asterisks*). Note lack of edemalike T2 hyperintense signal on STIR images, indicating end-stage denervation. Axial T1 image (*C*) of the proximal thighs shows diffuse fatty atrophy and replacement of the vastus lateralis and intermedius muscles, as well as of the rectus and biceps femoris muscles (*asterisks*). The symmetry and presence of atrophy without edemalike signal supports a long-standing systemic process.

partial plexopathy and, less commonly, nerve avulsions. The lumbar component of the lumbosacral plexus may be involved in retroperitoneal disorders, including psoas abscess and hematoma. Inflammatory conditions such as retroperitoneal fibrosis, and malignant disease such as lymphoma or retroperitoneal lymph node metastases, may infiltrate the lumbosacral plexus. Radiation plexopathy is not often seen with current standard external beam pelvic irradiation regimens, but may be seen in the setting of brachytherapy or intraoperative radiation therapy. Unlike tumor-related plexopathy, which usually causes severe pain, radiation plexopathy is often painless, progresses slowly, appearing on average 5 years after the initial insult. The sacral distribution of the lumbosacral plexus may be involved in disorders of the sacroiliac joints, such as inflammatory arthritis, or of the sacrum and presacral space, including primary and secondary bone tumors (metastases, chordoma) or rectal carcinoma. Hereditary neuropathies may affect the lumbosacral

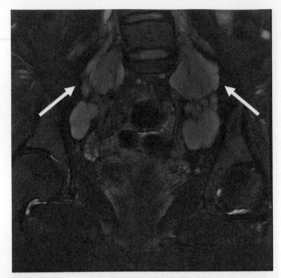

Fig. 17. CMT in a 27-year-old woman with bilateral leg weakness. Coronal FS T2-weighted image shows marked diffuse enlargement of lumbosacral plexus nerves bilaterally (*arrows*) in keeping with history of CMT disease. (*Courtesy of* Dr Avneesh Chhabra, MD, Dallas, Texas.)

plexus. CMT or HMSN is a rare disease that most commonly affects the brachial and lumbosacral plexuses, resulting in degeneration and marked enlargement of the affected nerves, and presenting clinically with sensory loss and muscle wasting and weakness of the distal extremities.[13] Although this is a clinical diagnosis, MR neurography shows moderate to marked nerve enlargement and may help to direct the site of biopsy. Symmetric or asymmetric diabetic neuropathy or plexopathy (diabetic amyotrophy) presenting in older patients with long-standing disease is a common cause of lumbosacral plexopathy. It typically presents with proximal muscle weakness and atrophy. When severe, pain often resolves within a few months, but is often mild or absent. Sensory loss is less severe than with peripheral neuropathy.[13] If present, denervation muscle signal alteration patterns in lumbosacral plexopathy are not helpful and may correspond with multiple muscle groups related to multiple peripheral nerves, which may result in diagnostic confusion with a systemic or primary myopathic disorder such as polymyositis.

Peripheral neuropathic syndromes of the pelvis and hip

Superior and inferior gluteal nerves The clinical syndrome of superior gluteal nerve injury is manifested by weakness in abduction, with a gait limp and a positive Trendelenburg sign. The superior gluteal nerve is commonly injured following pelvic orthopedic surgery.[26] The superior branch may

be injured or compressed following placement of iliosacral screws, whereas the inferior branch may be injured during a lateral or anterolateral approach to hip replacement. Electromyogram abnormalities are shown in 77% of patients after total hip arthroplasty (THA) but usually resolve within 1 year.[13] Muscle denervation–related signal alterations and end-stage muscle atrophy may be seen within the gluteus minimus, gluteus medius, and tensor fascia lata muscles and following THA (**Fig. 19**). The inferior gluteal nerve may also be injured during THA and iliosacral screw placement (see **Fig. 15**), and results in weakness in thigh extension. Injury often occurs in conjunction with superior gluteal nerve injury.[23] Denervation edemalike pattern and atrophy may be seen within the gluteus maximus muscle. Both the superior and inferior gluteal nerves may also be entrapped secondary to infectious or inflammatory processes, fracture, or posttraumatic productive changes related to the greater sciatic notch, sacrum, and sacroiliac joints (**Fig. 18**).

Lateral femoral cutaneous nerve Entrapment of the lateral femoral cutaneous nerve classically results in the clinical syndrome of meralgia paresthetica, characterized by burning, numbness, pain, and paresthesias down the proximal lateral aspect of the thigh. Predisposing causes include obesity, pregnancy, ascites, tight belts, and an anomalous course of the nerve. Compression of the nerve by disc hernia, retroperitoneal tumors, and external pressure around the anterior superior iliac spine are among the most common causes.[27] Injury during elective spine surgery is a recognized complication in up to 20% of patients and is caused by compression of the nerve against the anterior superior iliac spine, traction of the psoas muscle, or harvesting of iliac crest bone graft material.[28] MR imaging may have difficulty following the nerve along its course, except when surrounded by a large amount of fat, but may help identify focal thickening, perineural scarring, or osseous deformity at the site of entrapment, typically following avulsion injury of the sartorius muscle at its origin from the anterosuperior iliac spine (see **Fig. 19**).

Femoral nerve Injury to the femoral nerve results in weakness of knee extension (quadriceps muscle) and hip flexion (iliopsoas muscle) as well as sensory loss of the anteromedial knee, medial leg, and foot.

The nerve is commonly injured in the iliacus compartment secondary to an iliopsoas muscular disorder, or at the groin. Iatrogenic causes are most common and include femoral artery puncture for catheterization or bypass surgery, with

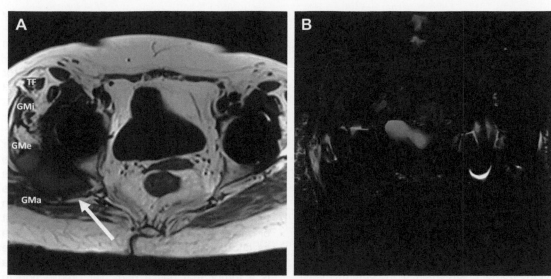

Fig. 18. Pseudotumor resulting in superior and inferior gluteal nerve entrapment in a 75-year-old woman status post right THA, with right leg weakness and palpable mass. Axial PD image (*A*) shows a complex mass centered on the right hip, consistent with pseudotumor (*arrow*). Note fatty atrophy of the gluteus maximus (GMa), gluteus medius (GMe), gluteus minimus (GMi), and tensor fascia lata (TF) muscles and edema like signal (*asterisk*) on coronal T2 FS image (*B*) consistent with compression of the superior and inferior gluteal nerves.

compression of the nerve by hematoma or pseudoaneurysm,[29] or pelvic, hip, and gynecologic surgery. Hysterectomy is a well-known cause of femoral nerve injury. Other common causes include iliopsoas hematoma, iliopsoas abscess, or bursitis. On MR imaging, the intrapelvic femoral nerve may show increased signal and size and course

deviation caused by mass effect. Abnormalities of the nerve at the thigh are more difficult to detect. The iliopsoas muscle may show denervation signal alterations following injury of the intrapelvic femoral nerve, whereas the pectineus, sartorius, and quadriceps muscles may be affected if injury occurs distal to the inguinal ligament. The femoral nerve is

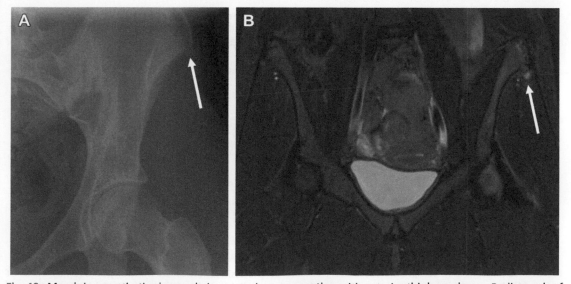

Fig. 19. Meralgia paresthetica in a male lacrosse player presenting with anterior thigh numbness. Radiograph of the pelvis shows apophyseal avulsion injury (*arrow*) at the anterior superior iliac spine (*A*). Coronal STIR MR image (*B*) confirms avulsion and partial-thickness tearing of the sartorius muscle at the anterior superior iliac spine (*arrow*), likely resulting in entrapment or compression/injury to the lateral femoral cutaneous nerve.

frequently involved in diabetic amyotrophy and pathologic changes may also be seen in the setting of HMSN.[3]

Obturator nerve Injury to the obturator nerve results in weak thigh adduction and sensory loss of the medial thigh and knee. As with the femoral nerve, the most common causes are iatrogenic and may occur in several settings. The nerve may be stretched following prolonged lithotomy, or retraction during THA, or it may be directly injured or transected during gynecologic or genitourinary surgery (eg, total hysterectomy and radical prostatectomy) (see **Fig. 14**).[20] The obturator nerve may be entrapped within the obturator canal, formed by the margins of the obturator foramen and a ligamentous band called the obturator membrane, through which the obturator nerve, artery, and vein pass to exit the pelvis. Enlargement of the obturator externus bursa is another recognized cause of obturator nerve compression. The obturator nerve is susceptible to injury at the level of the pubic symphysis because of its proximity to this structure, and the anterior branch may be entrapped secondary to disorders of the pubic bones including fracture, osteitis pubis, and adductor brevis tendinopathy (**Fig. 20**). Denervation-related signal alterations may occur within the adductor muscles, although the adductor brevis muscle may have dual innervation by both anterior and posterior branches and is spared if only one of the branches is involved. Enlargement and increased intraneural signal of the obturator nerve can sometimes be difficult to distinguish from adjacent vessels.

Pudendal nerve Pudendal nerve entrapment may result in symptoms of perineal and genital numbness and fecal and urinary incontinence, which are characteristically exacerbated by the sitting position.[30] This disorder occurs within the pudendal or Alcock canal, a space within the obturator fascia lining the lateral wall of the ischiorectal fossa that transmits the pudendal vessels and nerves, resulting in a clinical entity known as Alcock canal syndrome. This syndrome has a propensity to occur in cyclists because of chronic compression by the saddle (cyclist's syndrome), or in occupations requiring prolonged sitting. The pudendal nerve may also be stretched during childbirth, although this rarely results in permanent neurologic deficit or pain. Sacral or ischiorectal space tumors such as chordoma and rectal carcinoma may involve the pudendal nerve, and sacrococcygeal teratoma is a tumor that has a particular predilection to involve the pudendal nerve. MR imaging helps to delineate perineural scarring or space-occupying lesions at the site of entrapment (**Fig. 21**).

Intrapelvic sciatic nerve The well-known clinical syndrome of sciatica is most commonly caused by lumbar disc disorders. Patients typically presents with sharp shooting pain radiating from the buttock along the back of the thigh, in the distribution of the sciatic nerve. Patients may present with foot drop, mimicking common peroneal neuropathy. The sciatic nerve is commonly entrapped around the hip and within the sciatic notch. It may also be compressed by the piriformis muscle, resulting in piriformis syndrome. The perineal

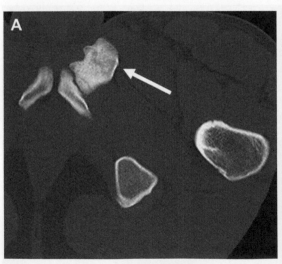 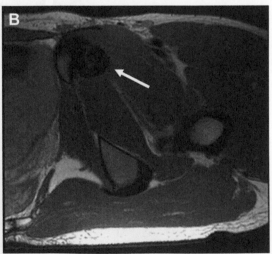

Fig. 20. Obturator nerve compression secondary to heterotopic ossification of the inferior pubic ramus. Axial CT image (*A*) shows robust heterotopic ossification along the medial margin of the inferior pubic ramus (*arrow*), likely related to remote adductor tendon avulsion injury. Axial PD MR image (*B*) shows corresponding hypointense mass adjacent to the inferior pubic ramus and AB origin (*arrow*) in close relationship to the expected location of the posterior division of the obturator nerve.

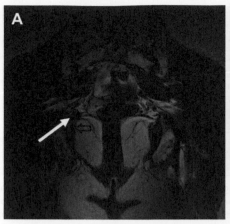
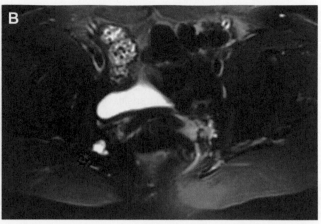

Fig. 21. Pudendal neuropathy secondary to a likely perineural cyst. Coronal T1 image of the pelvis (*A*) shows a fluidlike lobulated structure (*closed arrow*) intimately related to the right pudendal neurovascular bundle (*open arrow*). Axial T2 FS image (*B*) also shows the proximity of the lesion with the neurovascular bundle and ischial spine (*asterisk*). No communication with the hip joint was shown. The lesion did not enhance on postcontrast images (not shown).

component is more commonly affected than the tibial component because it is more superficially located with less supporting connective tissue, and is fixed at 2 separate points. The sciatic nerve may be stretched during THA, or compressed by postoperative fluid collection or hematoma (**Fig. 22**). Paralabral cysts may decompress posteriorly, resulting in sciatic nerve compression.

Hamstring injury may affect the adjacent nerve. Perineural cysts and neurogenic tumors are also commonly in this location. Injury to the sciatic nerve may result in denervation edemalike pattern in the distal lower limb including the muscles of the knee, leg, and foot. The hamstring muscles are less commonly affected because of the high takeoff of the branch that supplies the proximal thigh.

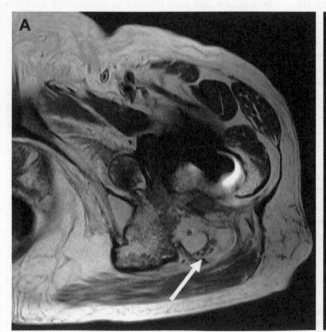
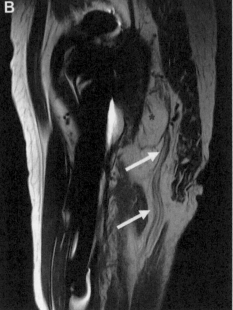

Fig. 22. Sciatic nerve compression caused by postoperative periarticular fluid collection in a woman who underwent left THA 1month ago. Axial (*A*) and sagittal (*B*) PD images show complex posterior periprosthetic fluid collections (*asterisks*). There is secondary posterior displacement and increased signal of the sciatic nerve (*arrows*).

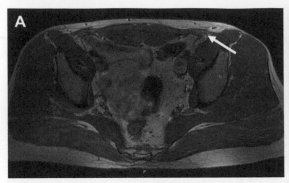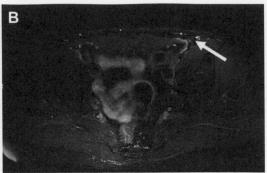

Fig. 23. Genitofemoral neuralgia in a 44-year-old man with left inguinal pain following prior hernia repair. Axial T1-weighted (A) and corresponding axial T2 SPAIR (B) MR images show the entrapped and enlarged left genito-femoral nerve in the inguinal area (arrows). There is focal fibrosis at the site of prior surgery (A). (*Courtesy of Dr Avneesh Chhabra, MD, Dallas, Texas.*)

More detailed information regarding the sciatic nerve can be found in the article elsewhere in this issue by Chhabra and colleagues.

Iliohypogastric nerve Iatrogenic disruption or damage of the iliohypogastric nerve following surgery is the most common cause of injury and usually results in pain and dysesthesia radiating to the hypogastric area. This condition may be seen following transverse abdominal wall incisions or suture placement, iliac bone harvesting, and inguinal hernia repair.[31] Muscle tears related to sports injuries and abdominal wall expansion during pregnancy are other potential causes. The nerve is not always visualized during MR neurography, and local anesthetic injection near the anterosuperior iliac spine may be helpful to confirm the diagnosis.[32]

Ilioinguinal nerve The ilioinguinal nerve is also most commonly injured during surgery, following transverse abdominal incision or suture placement, iliac graft harvesting, inguinal lymph node dissection, femoral vascular intervention, or orchi-ectomy.[33] Muscle tears related to sports injuries and abdominal wall expansion during pregnancy are other potential causes. Patients present with pain and dysesthesia radiating from the site of injury to the inguinal area, labia majora, or scrotum. The nerve is not always visualized during MR neurography, and local anesthetic injection may be helpful to confirm the diagnosis.

Genitofemoral nerve The genitofemoral nerve is most commonly injured during surgery, particularly during hernia repair (**Fig. 23**) or gynecologic procedure but also related to abdominal incision and suture placement and lymph node biopsy or dissection. Previous appendicitis or psoas abscess can also damage the nerve. Retroperitoneal hematoma and pregnancy may also result in compression of the nerve. The clinical presentation is of pain radiating from the surgical site below the inguinal ligament to the anterior thigh, labia majora, or scrotum. The nerve may not reliably be visualized during MR neurography; the portion traveling within the inguinal canal and along the spermatic cord is more readily shown. Local anesthetic injection may be helpful to confirm the diagnosis (**Box 2**).

SUMMARY

There are multiple potential causes for neurogenic pelvic pain and denervation syndromes. Clinical localization of symptoms as well as knowledge of the pelvic neural anatomy is of critical importance in the search for an underlying cause. Recent advances in imaging with appropriate use and interpretation of dedicated pelvic neurography may show pathologic changes within the peripheral nerves as well as elucidate the underlying

---

Box 2
Pointers in detecting potential causes for pelvic neuropathy

Lumbosacral plexus involvement frequently results in a confusing clinical picture.

Denervation changes in the muscles can be subtle but help to isolate the affected nerve.

Paralabral cysts can decompress in any direction and can involve different anterior or posterior nerves: always look for communication with the hip joint.

Look for evidence of prior trauma-related or surgery-related lesions in the absence of an obvious compressive lesion.

Sciatic, femoral, obturator, and superior gluteal nerve disorders are commonly seen after THA.

Obturator and pudendal nerves may be stretched or injured during surgery or childbirth.

disorder or cause. Muscle denervation changes are useful secondary signs of pelvic neuropathy, particularly in the absence of a detectable compressive cause on MR imaging. Pelvic neurography imaging is subject to certain pitfalls, which the radiologist should be cognizant of when interpreting these examinations. It is crucial that these examinations are not reported in isolation and that a diagnosis of pelvic neuropathy is only made from relevant imaging findings in the appropriate clinical setting.

REFERENCES

1. Perry CP. Peripheral neuropathies causing chronic pelvic pain. J Am Assoc Gynecol Laparosc 2000; 7(2):281–7.
2. Maravilla K, Bowen B. Imaging of the peripheral nervous system: evaluation of peripheral neuropathy and plexopathy. AJNR Am J Neuroradiol 1998;19: 1011–23.
3. Chhabra A, Faridian-Aragh N. High-resolution 3T MR neurography of femoral neuropathy. AJR Am J Roentgenol 2012;198:3–10.
4. Chhabra A, Lee PP, Bizzell C. 3 Tesla MR neurography - technique, interpretation, and pitfalls. Skeletal Radiol 2011;40(10):1249–60.
5. Chhabra A, Andreisek G, Soldatos T. MR neurography: past, present, and future. AJR Am J Roentgenol 2011;197:583–91.
6. Filler A, Maravilla K, Tsuruda J. MR neurography and muscle MR imaging for image diagnosis of disorders affecting the peripheral nerves and musculature. Neurol Clin 2004;22:643–82.
7. Filler A. MR neurography and diffusion tensor imaging: origins, history & clinical impact. Nature Precedings. London: Nature Publishing Group, Macmillan Publishers; 2009. p. 2877.
8. Lewis A, Layzer R, Engstrom J, et al. Magnetic resonance neurography in extraspinal sciatica. Arch Neurol 2006;63:1469–72.
9. Chhabra A, Soldatos T, Subhawong TK. The application of three-dimensional diffusion-weighted PSIF technique in peripheral nerve imaging of the distal extremities. J Magn Reson Imaging 2011;34:962–96.
10. Chappell K, Robson MD, Stonebridge-Foster A, et al. Magic angle effects in MR neurography. AJNR Am J Neuroradiol 2004;25:431–40.
11. Petchprapa C, Rosenberg Z, Sconfienza LM, et al. MR imaging of entrapment neuropathies of the lower extremity. Part 1. The pelvis and hip. Radiographics 2010;30:983–1000.
12. Kastel T, Heiland S, Baumer P, et al. Magic angle effect: a relevant artifact in MR neurography at 3T? AJNR Am J Neuroradiol 2011;32:821–7.
13. Chhabra A, Andreisek G. Magnetic resonance neurography. 1st edition. New Delhi, India: Jaypee Brothers Medical Publishers; 2012.
14. Moore K, Tsuruda J, Dailey A, et al. The value of MR neurography for evaluating extraspinal neuropathic leg pain: a pictorial essay. AJNR Am J Neuroradiol 2001;22:786–94.
15. Gupta S, Nguyen HL, Morello HA, et al. Various approaches for CT-guided percutaneous biopsy of deep pelvic lesions: anatomic and technical considerations. Radiographics 2004;24:175–89.
16. Yukata K, Arai K, Yoshizumi Y. Obturator neuropathy caused by an acetabular labral cyst: MRI findings. AJR Am J Roentgenol 2005;184(3):112–4.
17. Sherman P, Matchette M, Sanders T. Acetabular paralabral cyst: an uncommon cause of sciatica. Skeletal Radiol 2003;32:90–4.
18. Woettler K. Tumors and tumor-like lesions of peripheral nerves. Semin Musculoskelet Radiol 2010;14(5): 547–58.
19. Stull MA, Moser RP Jr, Kransdorf MJ. Magnetic resonance appearance of peripheral nerve sheath tumors. Skeletal Radiol 1991;20(1):9–14.
20. Sorenson E, Chen J, Daube J. Obturator neuropathy: causes and outcome. Muscle Nerve 2002; 25(4):605–7.
21. Busis NA. Femoral and obturator neuropathies. Neurol Clin 1999;17(3):633–53.
22. Cardosi R, Cox C, Hoffman M. Postoperative neuropathies after major pelvic surgery. Obstet Gynecol 2002;100(2):240–4.
23. Navarro RA, Schmalzried TP, Amstutz HC, et al. Surgical approach and nerve palsy in total hip arthroplasty. J Arthroplasty 1995;10:1–5.
24. Oldenburg M, Muller RT. The frequency, prognosis and significance of nerve injuries in total hip arthroplasty. Int Orthop 1997;21:1–3.
25. Zwolak P, Eysel P, Michael JW. Femoral and obturator nerves palsy caused by pelvic cement extrusion after hip arthroplasty. Orthop Rev 2011;3:e6.
26. Kenny P, O'Brien CP, Synnott K. Damage to the superior gluteal nerve after two different approaches to the hip. J Bone Joint Surg Br 1999;81:979–81.
27. Murata Y, Takahashi K, Yamagata M. The anatomy of the lateral femoral cutaneous nerve with special reference to the harvesting of iliac bone graft. J Bone Joint Surg Am 2000;82:746–7.
28. Mirovsky Y, Neuwirth M. Injuries to the lateral femoral cutaneous nerve during spine surgery. Spine 2000; 25(10):1266–9.
29. Ahmad F, Turnery SA, Torrie P. Iatrogenic femoral artery pseudoaneurysms. A review of current methods of diagnosis and treatment. Clin Radiol 2008;63: 1310e–6e.
30. Hough D, Wittenberg K, Pawlina W, et al. Chronic perineal pain caused by pudendal nerve

entrapment: anatomy and CT-guided perineural injection technique. AJR Am J Roentgenol 2003;181: 561–7.

31. Whiteside JL, Barber MD, Walters MD. Anatomy of ilioinguinal and iliohypogastric nerves in relation to trocar placement and low transverse incisions. Am J Obstet Gynecol 2003;189(6):1574–8.

32. Madura JA, Madura JA 2nd, Copper CM, et al. Inguinal neurectomy for inguinal nerve entrapment: an experience with 100 patients. Am J Surg 2005; 189(3):283–7.

33. Recht M, Grooff P, Ilaslan H, et al. Selective atrophy of the abductor digiti quinti: an MRI study. AJR Am J Roentgenol 2007;189(3):123–7.

High-Resolution Magnetic Resonance Imaging of the Lower Extremity Nerves

Alissa J. Burge, MD[a], Stephanie L. Gold, BA[a],
Sharon Kuong, MD[b], Hollis G. Potter, MD[c],*

KEYWORDS

• MRI • Nerves • Lower extremity • Neurography

KEY POINTS

- Magnetic resonance (MR) imaging of the peripheral nerves is accomplished by using a combination of pulse sequences allowing detection of changes in both nerve signal and architecture.
- Characteristic MR imaging findings allow differentiation of neuropathic conditions related to entrapment, trauma, iatrogenic injury, extrinsic mass effect, and tumors/tumorlike lesions of the nerves.
- In the setting of suspected neuropathy, MR imaging findings complement clinical evaluation and electrodiagnostic testing, facilitating accurate and timely diagnosis, and promoting appropriate management.

INTRODUCTION

Magnetic resonance (MR) imaging of the nerves, also known as MR neurography (MRN), is increasingly being used as a noninvasive means of diagnosing peripheral nerve disease. Patients often present with vague symptoms, including poorly defined pain and possible functional impairment, producing a complex clinical picture. In the past, patients with perceived neurologic symptoms were referred for electromyography (EMG); however, MR imaging is increasingly being selected over other imaging modalities because of its superior soft tissue contrast, its capacity to identify and describe neural injuries, and its ability to demonstrate additional causes of nerve impairment, as well as secondary findings, such as muscle edema or denervation.[1] MR imaging using high-resolution 2-dimensional (2D) fast spin-echo

(FSE) techniques combined with fluid-sensitive sequences in the plane perpendicular to the long axis of the peripheral nerve can reveal traumatic or iatrogenic injuries, entrapment, inflammation, and tumorlike lesions affecting the nerves of the lower limb. Although the treatment for peripheral neuropathies varies based on the type of injury, region, and underlying disease, early diagnosis is essential to restore normal sensory and motor function. Studies have demonstrated that MRN findings can significantly influence the clinical management of patients with lower limb neuropathies, helping to determine which causes would benefit from surgical intervention.[1–3] This article focuses on MRN of the lower limb, discussing the imaging techniques, normal anatomy, and pathologic conditions affecting the major nerves in the hip, thigh, knee, ankle, and foot.

Conflict of Interest Statement: The institution has received research support from General Electric Healthcare.
[a] Department of Radiology and Imaging, Hospital for Special Surgery, 535 East 70th Street, New York, NY 10021, USA; [b] Department of Radiology, Precision Medical Imaging, Fallon Clinic, 135 Gold Star Boulevard, Worcester, MA 01606, USA; [c] Department of Radiology and Imaging, Hospital for Special Surgery, Weill Cornell Medical College of Cornell University, 535 East 70th Street, New York, NY 10021, USA
* Corresponding author.
E-mail address: potterh@hss.edu

NORMAL ANATOMY AND IMAGING TECHNIQUE
General Imaging Technique

Imaging of the peripheral nerves is best performed at 1.5 or 3.0 T field strengths, with the type of coil used, the imaging planes acquired, and the scan parameters determined by the body part being imaged. Complete evaluation requires the ability to detect alterations in both nerve signal and morphology; therefore, some combination of pulse sequences providing high-resolution morphologic depiction and sensitive detection of mobile water is necessary. At the authors' institution, general extremity imaging consists of 3-plane intermediate 2D moderate echo time FSE images plus fluid-sensitive imaging (short tau inversion recovery [STIR] or T2 with fat saturation) obtained in a single plane optimal to the structure being imaged. When specifically evaluating peripheral nerves, this general protocol is augmented by the addition of axial STIR images oriented perpendicular to the long axis of the nerve in question (Fig. 1). Additional oblique coronal and sagittal images may further disclose the long axis of the nerve and the transition at points of compression. The standard matrix in the frequency direction is 512 with a phase matrix of 320 to 384. Although the field of view varies based on the body part being scanned, off-set images of the affected limb are preferred to minimize pixel size and maximize in plane resolution. Thin slices without an interslice gap further improve through plane resolution.

Other authors have described dedicated neurographic imaging protocols using sequences specifically tailored to the evaluation of peripheral nerves. Chhabra and colleagues[4] advocate a protocol based on a combination of T2 and diffusion-weighted imaging (DWI) neurographic sequences, which includes T1 FSE, T2 adiabatic inversion recovery (IR), proton density (PD), 3-dimensional (3D) IR, and 3D diffusion-weighted reversed fast imaging with steady state precession (DW-PSIF) hybrid pulse sequences; the addition of 3D sequences with isotropic voxel sets allows multiplanar reformation, whereas the addition of hybrid DWI provides nerve-selective images with suppression of adjacent vascular structures.[3–5] The administration of an intravenous gadolinium-based contrast agent is rarely warranted outside of the setting of suspected enhancing soft tissue mass lesion.

More advanced imaging techniques include diffusion tensor imaging (DTI), a technique which exploits the anisotropic properties of axonal fiber

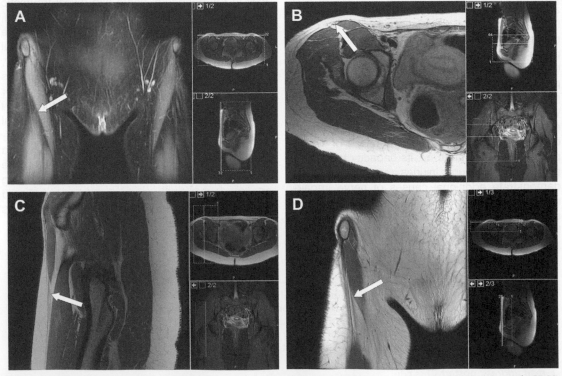

Fig. 1. Imaging planes for the lateral femoral cutaneous nerve (*white arrows*). (*A*) Coronal STIR. (*B*) Axial FSE PD. (*C*) Sagittal FSE PD. (*D*) Thin coronal FSE PD.

tracts and nerves, allowing the creation of fiber tract maps, as well as the calculation of quantitative parameters such as absolute diffusion coefficient (ADC). Although conventional DWI measures restriction in the Brownian motion of water by using the addition of a pair of diffusion gradient pulses before and after the 180° pulse, DTI requires the application of at least 6 diffusion gradients to detect and quantify directional diffusion along the longitudinal axes of axons.[6] The ADC is a quantitative descriptor of diffusivity and fractional anisotropy; neuropathic conditions often result in decreased fractional anisotropy (increased ADC), whereas axons recovering from an insult often exhibit increased fractional anisotropy (decreased ADC). Although DTI provides clinically useful information, the technique is technically demanding, still somewhat experimental, and not yet adapted for routine clinical use.[3,7] New gadolinium-based MR imaging contrast agents have demonstrated potential for neurographic application in animal models. For example, gadofluoride M appears to be useful in assessing demyelination and remyelination in peripheral nerves, selectively accumulating in nerves undergoing Wallerian degeneration, and dispersing when remyelination occurs.[3]

Imaging at higher field strength is often advantageous in terms of image quality, although in certain situations, it may be detrimental. Although 3.0-T imaging results in increased signal-to-noise ratio (SNR) and superior contrast-to-noise ratio, increased field strength also results in exaggeration of certain artifacts, as well as increased energy deposition. In particular, metallic susceptibility artifact is markedly increased at 3.0 T, and patients with orthopedic implants or other hardware are universally scanned at 1.5 T at the authors' institution. Additional considerations include alterations in tissue relaxation parameters; at higher field strengths, T1 relaxation time is prolonged, whereas T2 decay time is shortened. Imaging protocols performed at 3.0 T therefore may require longer time to repetition (TR) and shorter time to echo (TE).[4]

Magic angle artifact affects highly ordered anisotropic structures, such as tendons and nerves, on pulse sequences with short to moderate TE when the structure in question is oriented at 55° relative to the main magnetic field (Bo). The morphology of these structures, with their highly ordered parallel fibers, augments dipole-dipole interactions involving protons within bound water, resulting in rapid dephasing, which manifests as low signal intensity on images. The strength of these dipole interactions varies with the orientation of the structure relative to Bo; at 55° to Bo, dipole interactions are minimized, resulting in relative T2 prolongation and signal hyperintensity. Although this phenomenon can be overcome by increasing the echo time (>40 ms) when imaging other morphologic structures such as tendons, the perceived high signal intensity in the nerve can persist despite slightly longer echo times and is simultaneously visualized on commonly used IR images.[1] However, whereas magic-angle artifact may occur on neurographic imaging, Kastel and colleagues[8] demonstrated that it rarely results in false-positive interpretation of studies, because significant magic-angle effect occurs only at angles above 30°, and that true neuropathic lesions generally result in a much greater degree of hyperintensity than can be accounted for by magic angle alone.[1,8,9] Careful scrutiny of the nerve of interest for associated morphologic changes while remaining cognizant of the potential for magic angle phenomenon allows the interpreting radiologist to avoid false-positive interpretation in the setting of a hyperintense nerve.

MR Imaging Characteristics of Normal Nerves

In the evaluation of MR images for peripheral nerve neuropathies, it is important to have a solid understanding of the normal appearance of nerves, including their size, course, and signal intensity. On T1-weighted images, normal nerves demonstrate a fascicular appearance with intermediate signal intensity, often described as being isointense to the surrounding skeletal muscle. On STIR or fat-suppressed T2-weighted images, a normal nerve can appear slightly hyperintense as compared with the adjacent muscle tissue.[3] Normal nerves appear to be similar in size compared with adjacent arteries (decreasing in size as one moves distally) and there is minimal to no disruption or enlargement of the fascicles. The perineural fat planes should appear preserved and the nerve should be surrounded by a hyperintense halo of perineural fat.[3] If intravenous contrast (ie, gadolinium) is administered, normal peripheral nerves will show no enhancement. Finally, normal nerves should course smoothly and be free of sharp angulation (**Fig. 2**).[3]

Normal Anatomy

To properly image the nerves of the lower limb, a review of the relevant anatomy is helpful. Sensory and motor innervation of the hip, thigh, lower leg, and foot originates in the lumbosacral plexus, which is divided into 2 parts: the lumbar plexus (T12, L1–4) and the sacral plexus (L4–5, S1–4). The lumbar plexus includes the branches of the genitofemoral, obturator, lateral femoral cutaneous, and femoral nerves, with the anterior

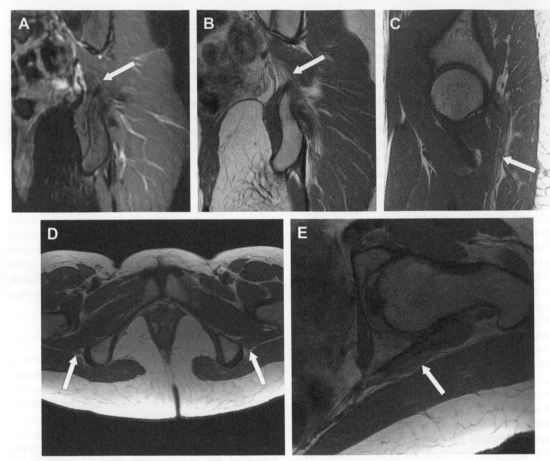

Fig. 2. Imaging characteristics of the normal sciatic nerve (*white arrows*). (*A*) Coronal STIR demonstrating normal signal characteristics on fluid-sensitive imaging. (*B–E*) coronal, sagittal, axial body coil, and axial surface coil images demonstrating normal sciatic morphology.

division innervating the flexors and the posterior division innervating the extensors. The sacral plexus includes the superior and inferior gluteal nerves, as well as the pudendal, sciatic, peroneal, and tibial nerves.[10]

Obturator nerve

The obturator nerve arises from the ventral L2–L4 rami, exiting the pelvis through the obturator canal and splitting into anterior and posterior branches.[1] The nerve innervates the anterior portion of the gracilis muscle as well as the adductor muscles of the thigh.[10] In the pelvis, the nerve runs along the iliopectineal line and descends vertically on the obturator internus before entering the obturator canal and bifurcating. The anterior branch descends anterior to the obturator externus and adductor brevis.[11] The posterior branch descends between the adductor magnus and adductor brevis, innervating the obturator externus and adductor magnus while providing sensation to

the medial aspect of the knee joint.[1] An accessory obturator nerve has been identified in 10% to 30%[12] of individuals, arising from L3 or L4. When present, it innervates the hip joint and often replaces the femoral branch in the pectineus.[11]

On MR imaging, the obturator nerve is well visualized in all 3 imaging planes, possibly because of the nerve's size and abundant perineural fat. Identification of the anterior and posterior branches is easiest on axial images; the anterior branch is located in a thin area of fat, posterior to the adductor longus and anterior to the adductor brevis, whereas the posterior branch is seen within the obturator externus.[1]

Femoral nerve

The femoral nerve is the largest branch of the lumbar plexus and provides both motor and sensory functions. The femoral nerve has extensive cutaneous distribution, starting at the anterior lateral thigh and moving distally to the medial leg and foot.[11] Arising from the ventral L2–L4 rami, the femoral nerve lies between the psoas major and iliacus muscles. The nerve descends inferolaterally through the psoas muscle, traveling in what is commonly known as the iliacus compartment and emerging posterior to the inguinal ligament.[1,11] Once in the femoral triangle, the nerve splits into multiple branches. The anterior branch has both cutaneous and muscular divisions, innervating the pectineus and sartorius muscles and controlling hip flexion and knee extension. The posterior branch of the femoral nerve is best known for its innervation of the quadriceps muscles and subsequent division to form the saphenous nerve.[1]

On MR imaging, the femoral nerve can be visualized in all 3 imaging planes. The femoral nerve appears as a subtle projection off of the surface of the muscle on axial images and can be seen on coronal images as it courses under the inguinal ligament.[1] The femoral nerve can also be identified by its close proximity to the femoral artery and vein throughout the hip and thigh.

Lateral femoral cutaneous nerve

The lateral femoral cutaneous nerve (LFCN) of the thigh arises from the ventral L2 and L3 rami. It is a somatosensory nerve that provides sensation to the lateral thigh and knee. Although the course of the nerve is variable, it commonly emerges anterior to the iliac crest and lateral to the psoas major, descending obliquely toward the anterior superior iliac spine.[1,11] Once distal to the inguinal ligament, the LFCN divides into smaller branches that pierce the fascia lata and innervate the skin of the thigh.[1,13] At the authors' institution, the LFCN is one of the few nerves of the lower limb that requires an additional imaging sequence for proper visualization. A thin (~1 mm) coronal package of the anterior thigh is performed to ensure adequate visualization of the LFCN, as the nerve courses horizontally in the anterior compartment. Although the nerve can be followed in the axial plane intrapelvically, it is well visualized in the coronal and sagittal planes within the thigh.

Sciatic nerve

The sciatic nerve is the thickest nerve in the body, dividing into 2 distinct parts in the distal thigh: the tibial and common peroneal (fibular) nerves. Formed by the nerve fibers of the ventral L4 rami and sacral S1–S3 rami, the sciatic nerve lies anterior to the piriformis muscle. The nerve enters the thigh at the inferior border of the gluteus maximus and continues to descend posterior to the adductor magnus. Although contained by a common epineurium, the nerve splits into the tibial (anterior) and common peroneal (posterior) nerves at roughly the popliteal fossa.[1,11] Similar to the obturator nerve, the sciatic nerve is easily identified on MR imaging in all 3 imaging planes because of its large size and abundant perineural fat content. High-resolution axial FSE images demonstrate 2 distinct nerve fascicles bound by a common sheath (see **Fig. 2**).

Saphenous nerve

The saphenous nerve is formed from the posterior branch of the femoral nerve and travels along the medial aspect of the distal thigh. In the leg, the saphenous nerve descends posteromedially, descending between the sartorius and gracilis muscles and supplying sensation to the infrapatellar region. The nerve continues down the medial aspect of the leg, traveling with the great saphenous vein. It descends anterior to the medial malleolus, and innervates the medial aspect of the foot.[10,11,14] On MR imaging, the saphenous nerve is most commonly evaluated on axial PD or axial IR images through the clinically relevant area.

Tibial nerve

The tibial nerve (L4–L5, S1–S3) arises from the medial portion of the sciatic nerve. It originates at the approximate level of the popliteal fossa and travels through the posterior compartment of the leg, descending between the heads of the gastrocnemius muscle.[15] The tibial nerve provides motor innervation to the deep and superficial posterior compartments, including muscles such as the plantaris, gastrocnemius, soleus, popliteus, posterior tibialis, flexor digitorum longus, and flexor hallucis longus.[10,15] Distally, the tibial nerve becomes increasingly superficial, traveling medial to the Achilles tendon as it enters the ankle, at which point it is termed the posterior tibial nerve. The nerve descends between the flexor digitorum longus and flexor hallucis longus, before entering the foot. On the postero-inferior side of the medial malleolus, the tibial nerve gives rise to the medial calcaneal nerve(s) nerve before bifurcating to form the medial and lateral plantar nerves, the latter of which gives rise to the inferior calcaneal nerve.[11,15] On MR imaging, the tibial nerve is best visualized on axial images through the leg and ankle joint. The posterior tibial nerve courses in close proximity to the tibial artery and vein, providing an easy way to trace the nerve on axial images. In the foot, the terminal branches of the tibial nerve are seen on axial images around and through the tarsal tunnel and on short-axis oblique coronal images more distally.[15]

Common peroneal (fibular) nerve

The common peroneal nerve (CPN) arises from the lateral portion of the sciatic nerve in the distal, posterior femur. In the thigh, the CPN innervates the short head of the biceps femoris and provides sensation to the proximal lateral leg.[15] The nerve travels inferolaterally in the popliteal fossa and descends obliquely toward the back of the head of the fibula. After winding around the lateral portion of the fibular head, the CPN trifurcates into the recurrent articular branch, superficial branch, and deep branch.[10,11,15] The CPN can be easily visualized on MR images, because it is surrounded by a significant amount of fat. Axial images through the distal thigh and into the knee joint reveal the CPN as it moves from the short head of the biceps femoris muscle to the lateral head of the gastrocnemius.[15] Even before physical bifurcation, the deep and superficial branches of the CPN can be visualized in the posterior distal thigh and knee joint.[15]

Deep peroneal nerve (fibular) nerve

The deep peroneal nerve (DPN) is first identified between the fibular neck and the peroneus longus muscle. Descending in the anterior compartment of the leg, the DPN travels on the anterior surface of the interosseous membrane, lateral to the tibialis anterior.[11] More distally, it runs between the extensor digitorum longus and the extensor hallucis longus tendons. In the leg, the DPN innervates the extensor muscles of the anterior compartment, including the tibialis anterior, extensor hallucis longus, extensor digitorum longus, and peroneus tertius muscles with little sensory innervation. At the ankle, the DPN passes under the hallucis longus tendon and the extensor retinaculum, entering the tarsal tunnel. In this region, branches of the nerve provide motor function to the extensor digitorum brevis and sensation to the first web space of the foot, ankle, and tarsal and metatarsophalangeal joints.[10,11,15]

On MR imaging, the distal portion of the DPN is easily visualized at the knee joint using axial images. To locate the nerve more proximally, the anterior tibial artery can be used as a guide, as it is often either medial or posterior to the DPN. In the foot, short-axis images of the midfoot are often used to evaluate the medial and lateral branches; however, given the medial branch's small size and proximity to other anatomic structures, it can be difficult to identify.[15]

Superficial peroneal (fibular) nerve

The superficial peroneal nerve (SPN) is a branch of the CPN, coursing anterior to the fibula in the lateral compartment of the leg and providing motor function to the peroneus longus and brevis as well as sensation to the anterolateral leg. More distally, the nerve becomes subcutaneous and pierces the deep fascia on the anterior surface of the lateral compartment.[15] The SPN then divides above the lateral malleolus into 2 distinct branches: the intermediate and medial dorsal cutaneous nerves.[10,11] On MR imaging, axial images are often best for tracing the course of the SPN. At the level of the knee, the SPN can be identified as the more posterior portion of the CPN. More distally, the nerve can be identified in a thin area of fat between the muscles of the anterior and lateral compartments of the leg.[15] The SPN is also well visualized through the ankle and foot as long as images are acquired perpendicular to the long axis of the nerve.

Sural nerve

The sural nerve is a sensory nerve formed from the medial sural cutaneous nerve (branch of the tibial nerve) and lateral sural cutaneous nerve (branch of the CPN). The sural nerve courses in the posterolateral leg, lateral to the Achilles tendon. More distally, the nerve travels superficial and posterior to the peroneal tendons, producing a branch to the heel and then terminating in the lateral foot.[10,15] The sural nerve provides sensation to the lateral foot and heel via the lateral calcaneal nerve and lateral dorsal cutaneous nerve branches.[10] On MR imaging, the sural nerve is best located at the lateral margin of the Achilles tendon and calcaneus, and courses adjacent to the often prominent lesser saphenous vein.

Medial plantar nerve

The medial plantar nerve is a terminal branch of the tibial nerve. Homologous to the median nerve in the hand, the medial plantar nerve courses medially in the foot with the medial plantar artery.[11] In the sole of the foot, the nerve can be found between the muscle of the abductor hallucis and the flexor digitorum brevis, traveling between the first and second layers of the plantar muscles.[11,15] The medial plantar nerve provides motor innervation to the abductor hallucis, flexor digitorum brevis, flexor hallucis brevis, and lumbricals.[10] On MR imaging, the medial plantar nerve is best visualized on thin axial images through the ankle and foot as well as far medial sagittal images through the foot.

Lateral plantar nerve

The lateral plantar nerve is the smaller of the 2 terminal branches of the tibial nerve. Homologous with the ulnar nerve in the hand and wrist, the lateral plantar nerve travels anterolaterally within the second plantar layer. Branches of the lateral plantar nerve innervate the abductor digiti minimi and flexor accessorius (quadratus plantae). The nerve also provides motor function to the 3 lateral-most lumbricals, as well as the dorsal and plantar interosseous muscles. It provides sensory innervation to the lateral aspect of the foot and toes.[10] At the medial portion of the base of the fifth metatarsal, the lateral plantar nerve divides into superficial and deep branches.[11] Similar to the medial plantar nerve, the lateral plantar nerve is best visualized on MR imaging using thin axial images through the area of clinical interest.

Medial and inferior calcaneal nerves

The medial calcaneal nerve arises from the posterior portion of the tibial nerve. The nerve pierces the flexor retinaculum and subsequent branches provide sensory innervation to the posteromedial heel as well as the medial side of the sole of the foot and the plantar fat pad.[16] The inferior calcaneal nerve, also known as the Baxter nerve, has been shown in cadaveric studies to originate from the lateral plantar nerve at the level of the medial malleolus.[17] The nerve travels between the abductor hallucis and the quadratus plantae along the medial aspect of the long plantar ligament.[16] In the hindfoot, the inferior calcaneal nerve makes a sharp 90° turn from vertical to horizontal as it travels laterally to supply the abductor digiti minimi.[15] The inferior calcaneal nerve provides motor function to the abductor digiti quinti muscle and the flexor digitorum brevis and provides sensation to the long plantar ligament and the heel of the foot.[16,18] On MR imaging, the inferior calcaneal nerve is most easily identified on coronal intermediate weighted or axial IR images through the area of clinical interest. This nerve can be traced as it branches off of the lateral plantar nerve and descends toward the abductor digiti minimi.[15]

IMAGING FINDINGS/PATHOLOGY

Pathologic conditions affecting the lower extremity nerves may be divided into a handful of general categories: these include traumatic and iatrogenic injury, entrapment, compression, inflammatory/infection, ischemic, toxic, metabolic, demyelinating/dysmyelinating, and radiation neuropathies. MR imaging is useful in discerning and differentiating neuropathy related to traumatic and iatrogenic injury, entrapment, extrinsic compression, and intrinsic lesions. Direct signs of nerve injury on imaging include alterations in normal signal and morphology (**Fig. 3**). Abnormal nerves appear to have one or a combination of these signs: fascicular thickening, focal or diffuse nerve enlargement when compared with adjacent arteries,

and effacement of the perineural fat planes. They classically appear hyperintense on STIR or T2-weighted images, with a fluidlike signal intensity comparable with adjacent vessels. This increase in signal intensity has been attributed to many factors, such as vascular congestion or the accumulation of endoneurial fluid.[3] Images parallel to the nerve can reveal changes in nerve contour, such as discontinuity or acute angulation, which is most commonly seen with traumatic injury. Secondary signs of nerve injury include denervation edema or fatty atrophy of muscles in a distribution characteristic to the affected nerve (**Fig. 4**); however, anatomic variation in muscle innervation may produce unexpected patterns of denervation.[1,15] These signal abnormalities can occur both acutely (within 24 hours of the nerve injury) or more chronically, showing fatty replacement and significant atrophy years after the initial injury.[3]

Nerve Entrapment

Predisposition to nerve entrapment is generally based on anatomic relationships. The close spatial relationship between the lower extremity nerves and certain anatomic structures predisposes them to entrapment at certain points along their respective courses. The term piriformis syndrome refers to a sciatic entrapment neuropathy based on the close anatomic relationship between the piriformis muscle and the sciatic nerve. Variant anatomy may be implicated in this syndrome; although the sciatic nerve typically exits the sciatic foramen anterior and inferior to the piriformis muscle, in some cases the nerve or a portion of the nerve may exit above the muscle or traverse the muscle belly itself, predisposing the variant portion of the nerve to entrapment (**Fig. 5**). In patients with a normal anatomic relationship between the piriformis muscle and sciatic nerve, piriformis syndrome may result from a variety of conditions affecting the piriformis muscle, including hypertrophy, inflammation, spasticity, trauma, and ischemia.[1,19,20]

Entrapment of the obturator nerve is rare, owing to the nerve's relatively deep, protected location; however, in athletes, particularly males, the nerve may become compressed by normal fascial structures anterior to the adductor brevis, where the nerve curves around the contour of the pelvis. Osteitis pubis may also secondarily affect the nerve.[1,19]

Mechanical compression of the lateral femoral cutaneous nerve at the level of the inguinal ligament may result in anterolateral sensory disturbances within the thigh, a condition termed meralgia paresthetica. Compression most commonly occurs as

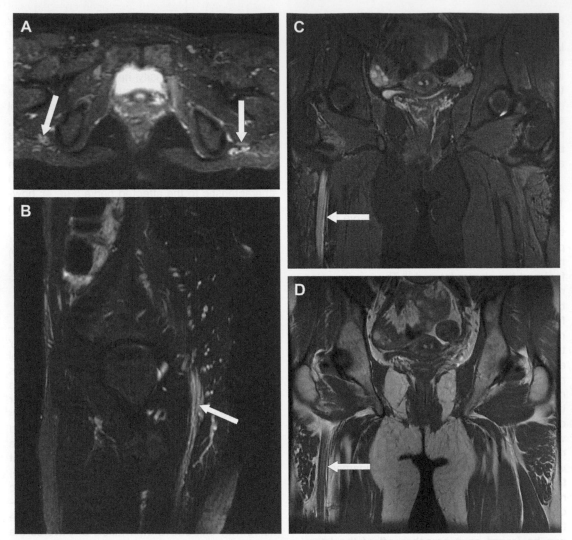

Fig. 3. Primary signs of nerve injury. (*A, B*) Axial (*A*) and sagittal (*B*) STIR images in a 38-year-old woman with lower extremity weakness following gynecologic surgery demonstrates hyperintensity of the bilateral sciatic nerves (*white arrows*). (*C, D*) Coronal STIR (*C*) and FSE (*D*) images in a 25-year-old woman following gynecologic surgery demonstrates hyperintensity and enlargement of the right sciatic nerve (*white arrows*). The findings indicate posttraumatic sciatic neuritis.

a result of tight-fitting clothing or belts, but may also derive from anatomic causes, such as abdominal pannus or a gravid uterus compressing the nerve against the inguinal ligament. Additionally, the sartorius muscle has been reported to compress the nerve in dancers when the leg is in the "turned out" position.[1,19]

Common peroneal neuropathy is the most common isolated neuropathy of the lower extremity. The CPN may rarely become entrapped proximally; however, entrapment at the level of the knee is much more common, occurring as the nerve crosses over the fibular neck, or as it passes beneath the origin of the peroneus longus.

Because of its superficial location at the level of the fibular neck, compression often occurs at this level, as has been reported in the setting of short leg casting and prolonged squatting (strawberry pickers' palsy).[15]

Impingement of the tibial nerve beneath the tendinous arch of the soleus muscle may result in an entrapment neuropathy termed "soleal sling syndrome." Although rare, this syndrome is an important differential diagnosis to popliteal artery entrapment syndrome, and responds similarly to surgical decompression.[21,22]

Entrapment of the tibial nerve at the level of the popliteal fossa and proximal leg is uncommon;

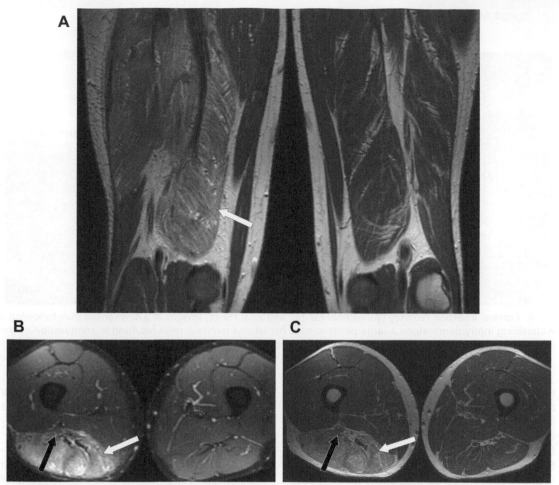

Fig. 4. Secondary signs of nerve injury. (*A–C*) Coronal FSE, axial STIR, and axial FSE images through the hamstrings demonstrates edema within the right hamstring muscle bellies (*white arrows*) in a 53-year-old man with right hamstring origin tear resulting in scar encasement of the sciatic nerve (*black arrows*).

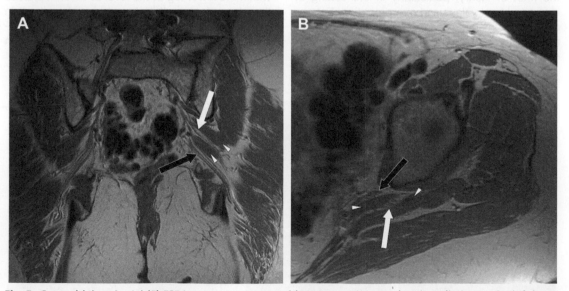

Fig. 5. Coronal (*A*) and axial (*B*) FSE images in a 70-year-old woman with buttock pain radiating to the left lower extremity demonstrates the common peroneal division (*white arrows*) of the left sciatic nerve traversing the muscle belly of the left piriformis (*white arrowheads*), whereas the tibial division (*black arrows*) maintains the typical anatomic relationship, an anatomic variant that may be implicated in piriformis syndrome.

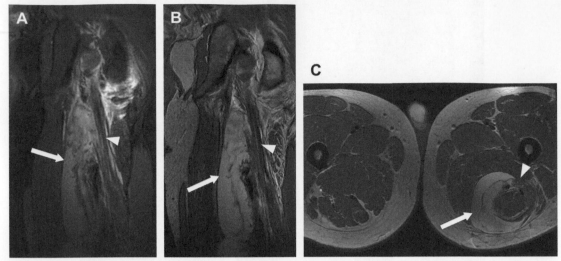

Fig. 6. Coronal inversion recovery (*A*), coronal FSE (*B*), and axial FSE (*C*) images in a 42-year-old man following a waterskiing injury demonstrate a large posttraumatic hematoma (*white arrow*) resulting in compression of the left sciatic nerve (*white arrowheads*), which is thickened and hyperintense.

more frequently, the nerve or its branches become compressed at the level of the ankle and foot. Tarsal tunnel syndrome is an entrapment neuropathy of the tibial nerve as it passes beneath the flexor retinaculum at the ankle. Pes planus, hindfoot valgus, and tarsal coalition may alter anatomic relationships in this area, predisposing the nerve to entrapment. Accessory muscles in the region may also predispose to entrapment. Jogger's foot refers to entrapment of the medial plantar nerve at the knot of Henry, particularly in the setting of increased heel valgus and overpronation. Entrapment of the inferior calcaneal nerve, termed Baxter neuropathy, typically occurs at 1 of 3 sites: adjacent to the fascial edge of the abductor hallucis,

at the medial edge of the quadratus plantae, or at the medial calcaneal tuberosity. Again, runners are at increased risk for this condition, particularly those who tend to overpronate.[15,19,23,24]

Anterior tarsal tunnel syndrome refers to entrapment of the DPN at the level of the inferior extensor retinaculum. Tight footwear, a high longitudinal arch, and the en pointe position in dancers may contribute to compression at this level.[15]

Finally, the SPN may become compressed within the lower leg at the level at which it pierces the deep fascia; this has been described in dancers, in whom repetitive inversion and/or plantarflexion results in stretching of the nerve with traction at this location.[15]

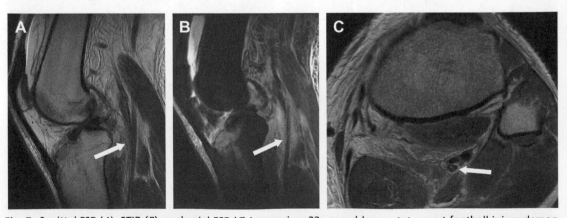

Fig. 7. Sagittal FSE (*A*), STIR (*B*), and axial FSE (*C*) images in a 23-year-old man status post football injury demonstrate hyperintensity and thickening of the tibial nerve (*white arrow*) with adjacent posttraumatic hemorrhage in the setting of a multiple ligament–injured knee.

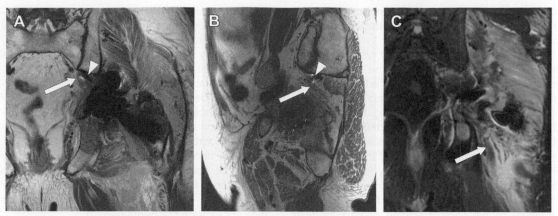

Fig. 8. Coronal FSE (*A*) and sagittal FSE (*B*) images in a 75-year-old man with foot drop following total hip arthroplasty 2 days prior demonstrates susceptibility related to an acetabular screw (*white arrowhead*) impinging the left sciatic nerve (*white arrow*), with associated hyperintensity and thickening of nerve fascicles (*white arrow*) demonstrated on coronal STIR (*C*).

Traumatic Injury

Trauma may result in neuropathy via direct nerve injury, or via injury to adjacent structures with secondary nerve involvement. Injury to certain structures is associated with a higher risk of concomitant neuropathy because of the close

anatomic relationships between these structures and the lower extremity nerves.

Within the pelvis and hip, severe injury, such as pelvic fracture, may result in direct nerve injury or compression by associated posttraumatic fluid collections. The vulnerability of a particular nerve depends on the location of the fracture and/or

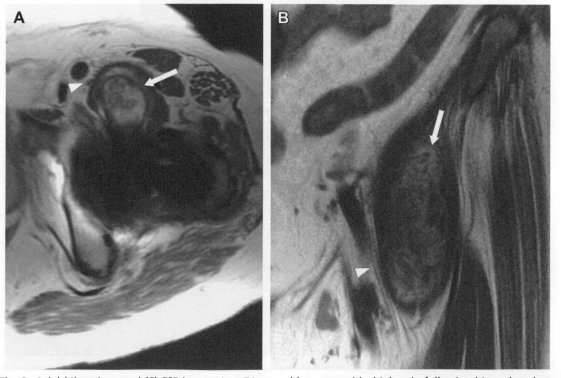

Fig. 9. Axial (*A*) and coronal (*B*) FSE images in a 74-year-old woman with thigh pain following hip arthroplasty 7 years prior demonstrates synovial expansion typical of wear induces synovitis decompressing anteriorly into the iliopsoas bursa (*white arrow*) and impinging on the left femoral nerve (*white arrowheads*).

collection; injury to the sciatic, femoral, and obturator nerves is not uncommon in the setting of pelvic trauma.[1,19]

Muscle and tendon injury may result in neuritis via secondary involvement of the nerve. In the acute setting, hemorrhage and edema from the injury may invest or frankly compress the nerve (**Fig. 6**). In a more chronic setting, the nerve may become encased in scar and/or tethered to adjacent structures. Hence, for example, a secondary sciatic neuritis may be observed in the setting of hamstring tear, and a secondary femoral neuritis in the setting of iliopsoas injury.[1,25,26]

At the level of the knee, trauma frequently results in injury to the CPN, because of its superficial location at this level. Fractures of the proximal fibula and ligamentous injury of the posterolateral corner structures are often associated with concurrent injury to the CPN. In a series of 21 patients with a clinical history of knee dislocation and resultant multiligament knee injury, Potter and colleagues[27] described MR imaging evidence of concomitant injury to the peroneal nerve in 10 patients, which was subsequently confirmed on surgical exploration. Because of its deeper location, the tibial nerve is less frequently injured in the setting of trauma; however, major trauma, such as posterior knee dislocation, may result in tibial nerve injury, and posttraumatic fluid collections may impinge on the nerve (**Fig. 7**).[15,19]

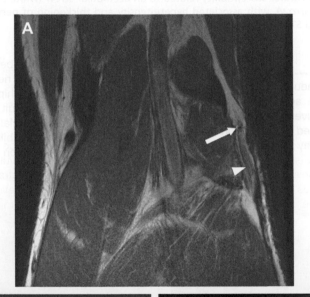

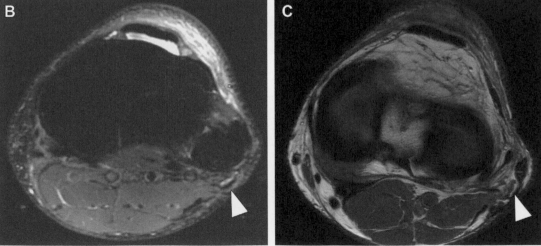

Fig. 10. Coronal FSE. (*A*) Image of the knee in a 45-year-old man with posterior knee pain and numbness radiating to the foot following proximal tibiofibular joint reconstruction demonstrates a focus of susceptibility artifact related to suture (*white arrow*) crossing the fascicles of the CPN (*white arrowhead*). Axial STIR (*B*) and FSE (*C*) images demonstrate associated hyperintensity and swelling of nerve fascicles (*white arrowheads*).

Within the foot and ankle, the nerves are particularly vulnerable to posttraumatic compression where they traverse the fibro-osseous tunnels formed by the retinacula; injury to adjacent bones, ligaments, or tendons can result in associated edema and/or hemorrhage, resulting in mass effect on the nerve. In the chronic setting, the nerves may become encased by scar or tethered to adjacent structures. Relatively superficial laceration to the dorsum of the foot may result in nerve injury, given the superficial position of the nerves in this area.[19] Although most traction injuries improve with conservative management, structural lesions, such as transection or neuroma, often require some type of intervention, such as neurolysis or repair/reconstruction; thus, the ability to differentiate the 2 injury types based on MR imaging findings is highly advantageous in terms of clinical decision making.[3,4]

Iatrogenic Injury

Iatrogenic injury is a relatively common cause of lower extremity neuropathy. Within the hip, arthroplasty is the most frequent cause of nerve injury, and the sciatic nerve is the most commonly involved, often manifesting as foot drop in the early postoperative period. In the acute setting, postoperative neuritis may be related to a variety of factors; commonly, postoperative edema and/or hemorrhage invest the sciatic nerve adjacent to the operative bed, resulting in a secondary neuritis. Less frequently, acute neuritis may be related to direct injury, traction, or impingement by hardware (**Fig. 8**); thus, although most acute postoperative sciatic neuritis will resolve given time, imaging is often warranted to exclude causes that may require intervention. In the subacute to chronic setting, neuropathy following hip arthroplasty may be related to a different subset of

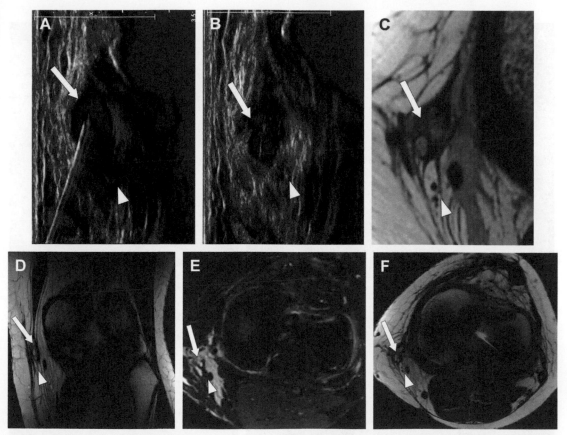

Fig. 11. Intraprocedural short-axis sonographic image of the medial knee (*A*) in a 20-year-old woman following multiple anterior cruciate ligament reconstructions demonstrates aspiration of a loculated fluid collection (*white arrow*) associated with the saphenous nerve (*white arrowhead*), consistent with saphenous nerve ganglion cyst. Postprocedural sonographic (*B*) and corresponding FSE image (*C*) demonstrate decrease in the size of the cyst, with small residual multilocular cystic structure (*white arrow*) along the course of the saphenous nerve (*white arrowhead*). Coronal FSE (*D*), axial STIR (*E*), and axial FSE (*F*) images demonstrate residual ganglion cyst (*white arrow*) along the course of the saphenous nerve (*white arrowhead*) following aspiration.

causes. Although hardware impingement missed in the early postoperative period may be a factor in the subacute/chronic setting, nerve impingement at this time point more frequently occurs because of synovial expansion, which may be secondary to a variety of etiologies, such as infection and adverse tissue reaction. Because of their close anatomic relationship to the hip joint, the sciatic and femoral nerves are most frequently affected; posterior decompression of synovitis often involves the sciatic nerve, whereas decompression of synovitis anteriorly into the iliopsoas bursa may impinge the femoral nerve (**Fig. 9**).[1,19,28]

A variety of other iatrogenic causes may result in nerve injury about the pelvis and hip. The femoral nerve is particularly vulnerable to injury during inguinal hernia repair, as well as during attempted vascular puncture.[1] Surgical positioning may also predispose to neuropathy; prolonged lithotomy position and the use of retractors during gynecologic surgery has been associated with secondary postoperative sciatic, femoral, and obturator neuritis.[1] Arthroscopic hip surgery has been associated with injury to the lateral femoral cutaneous nerve because of the proximity of the anterior arthroscopic portal to the nerve.[29] Radiation therapy may result in the formation of perineural scar tissue.[30]

Surgical intervention outside of the hip may also result in neuropathy. Impingement by hardware, entrapment by suture, and postoperative fluid collections may be implicated in the acute postoperative period (**Fig. 10**). Later, scar encasement, tethering, and ganglion formation may affect the nerves in the operative region (**Fig. 11**). Nerves in the path of desired arthroscopic portals are vulnerable to injury. Tunnel (retinacular) release may, paradoxically, result in the formation of hypertrophic scar tissue and neuroma, with worsening neuropathic symptoms (**Fig. 12**).[1,15,19,23]

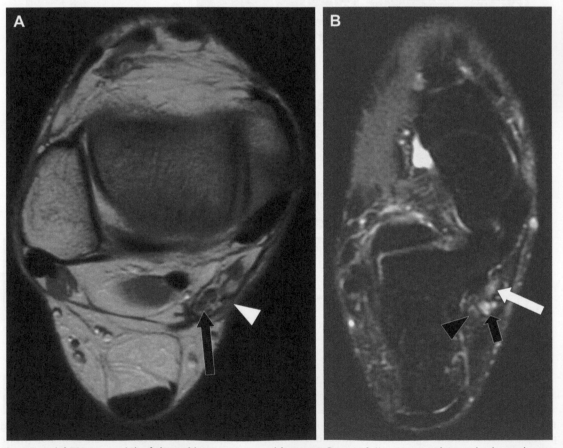

Fig. 12. Axial FSE image (*A*) of the ankle in a 38-year-old woman 2 years following tarsal tunnel release demonstrate scar reapproximation of the medial retinaculum (*white arrowhead*) at the level of the posterior tibial nerve (*black arrow*). Axial STIR image (*B*) demonstrates associated hyperintensity and swelling of the medial plantar nerve (*white arrow*), consistent with medial plantar neuritis; the lateral plantar nerve (*black arrowhead*) remains unaffected. Prominent veins (*short black arrow*) are noted coursing along with the nerves.

Extrinsic Mass Effect

Any extrinsic lesion along the course of a nerve may result in compression of that nerve and the development of secondary neuropathic symptoms. Osseous excrescences, such as poorly healed fractures, osteochondromas, and osteophytes, may result in impingement of adjacent nerves (**Fig. 13A, B**).[31] Abdominal and pelvic tumors may compress the sciatic, femoral, and obturator nerves intrapelvically.[1,19] Varices are not uncommon along the course of the sciatic nerve, and may result in impingement, the clinical symptoms of which can vary with patient position (see **Fig. 13C**). Soft tissue masses, vascular malformations, and ganglia may compress adjacent nerves,

which are particularly vulnerable at points of fixation, such as at fibro-osseous tunnels (**Fig. 14**).[32] Conditions causing soft tissue mineralization, such as tumoral calcinosis (see **Fig. 13D, E**), may encase and/or compress the nerves.[1,15,19]

Tumors and Tumorlike Lesions

Primary neurogenic lesions of the peripheral nerves may be benign or malignant, with benign nerve sheath tumors such as schwannomas and neurofibromas being more common (**Fig. 15**).[33,34] In general, nerve tumors are relatively rare within the peripheral nerves of the lower extremities, and are commonly seen in the setting of disorders, such as neurofibromatosis and schwannomatosis.

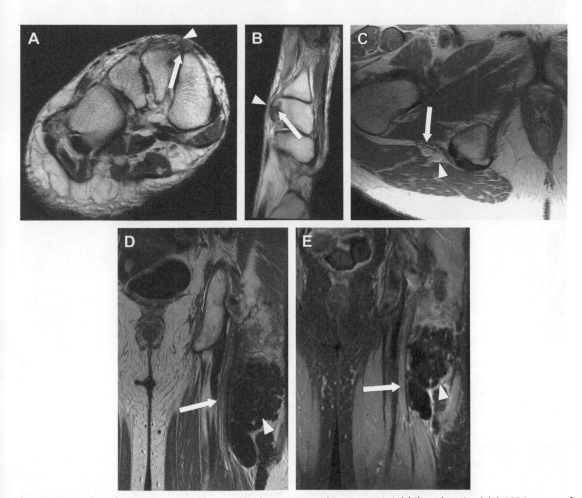

Fig. 13. Examples of extrinsic mass effect on the lower extremity nerves. Axial (*A*) and sagittal (*B*) FSE images of the midfoot in a 59-year-old woman with midfoot pain demonstrate osteophyte formation at the tarsometatarsal joint (*white arrows*) impinging the DPN (*white arrowheads*). Axial FSE (*C*) of the hip in a 64-year-old man with chronic buttock pain demonstrates varices (*white arrowhead*) abutting the sciatic nerve (*white arrow*). Coronal FSE (*D*) and STIR (*E*) images of the thigh in a 63-year-old woman with buttock and thigh pain radiating down the left leg demonstrate a large lobulated mineralized mass consistent with tumoral calcinosis (*white arrowhead*) impinging on the adjacent sciatic nerve (*white arrow*), with associated hyperintensity and thickening of nerve fascicles.

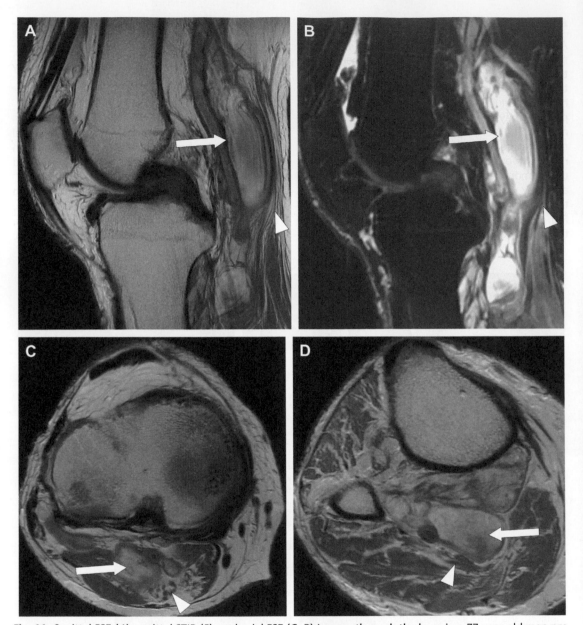

Fig. 14. Sagittal FSE (*A*), sagittal STIR (*B*), and axial FSE (*C, D*) Images through the knee in a 77-year-old man presenting with posterior knee and calf pain demonstrate a large posterior ganglion cyst (*white arrows*) impinging on the tibial nerve (*white arrowheads*), which is hyperintense and enlarged.

Neuromas, on the other hand, are extremely common, and are not true neurogenic tumors, but rather focal nodular areas of perineural fibrosis that form secondary to injury with subsequent scarring, axonal loss, and demyelination. Various types of injury may result in neuroma formation, including trauma, iatrogenic injury, and anatomic entrapment (**Fig. 16**). Neuroma formation is common following limb amputation. Interdigital (Morton) neuromas of the foot are extremely prevalent, and form secondary to chronic friction of the interdigital nerve against the adjacent transverse intermetatarsal ligament. These occur most commonly within the second and third web spaces, and appear as intermediate signal intensity nodules, often with an adjacent fluid-distended intermetatarsal bursa (**Fig. 17**). Joplin neuroma is a neuroma of the plantar proper digital nerve, which pierces the plantar aponeurosis to supply the flexor hallucis brevis muscle. Chronic pressure on the nerve as it crosses the plantar aspect of the first metatarsophalangeal joint may result in

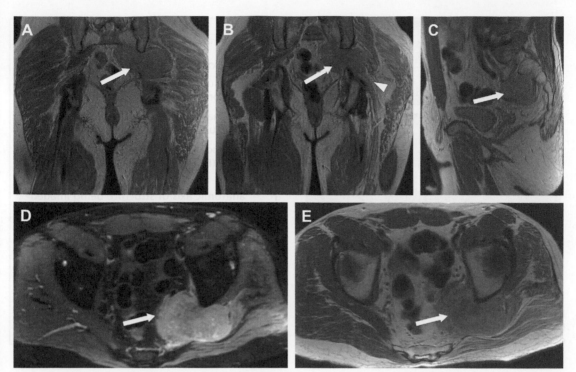

Fig. 15. Coronal FSE (*A, B*), sagittal FSE (*C*), axial STIR (*D*), and axial FSE (*E*) images of the pelvis in a 56-year-old man scheduled for spinal decompression for treatment of left sciatic symptoms demonstrates a large aggressive soft tissue sarcoma (*white arrows*) occupying the greater sciatic foramen, exerting mass effect on the sciatic nerve (*white arrowhead*).

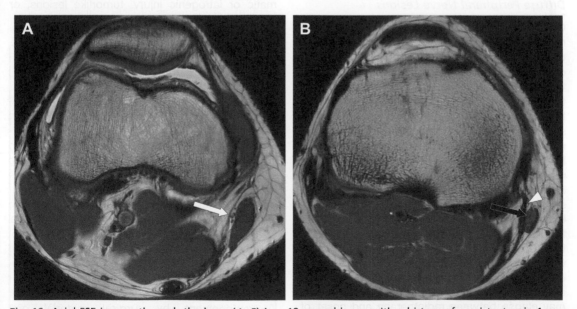

Fig. 16. Axial FSE images through the knee (*A, B*) in a 19-year-old man with a history of persistent pain 1 year following anterior cruciate ligament reconstruction using hamstring tendons demonstrates a normal appearing saphenous nerve at the level of the distal femur (*white arrow*), with frank neuroma formation (*black arrow*) distally at the level of the tibial plateau. Note the close proximity of the nerve to the stripped semitendinosus and gracilis tendon sheaths (*white arrowheads*).

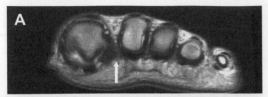

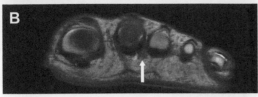

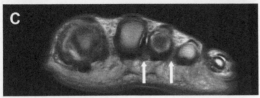

Fig. 17. Axial FSE images (*A–C*) through the forefoot in a 43-year-old woman with chronic plantar pain demonstrate intermetatarsal neuromas (*white arrows*) of the first, second, and third web spaces.

neuroma formation, particularly in ballet dancers and other athletes who commonly pivot on the ball of the foot.[15,35]

Diffuse Peripheral Nerve Lesions

Conditions that diffusely affect the peripheral nerves may be broadly categorized as inflammatory, infectious, hereditary, iatrogenic, metabolic, or neoplastic. These conditions may be difficult to differentiate based on imaging alone, and oftentimes detailed clinical history is necessary to reach the proper diagnosis. Inflammatory conditions, such as chronic inflammatory demyelinating polyneuropathy, the chronic counterpart of Guillain Barré Syndrome, may appear as diffuse asymmetric hyperintensity of nerves in the affected distribution. Charcot Marie Tooth, a hereditary sensorimotor neuropathy, manifests as fatty enlargement of the nerves with atrophy of the nerve fascicles, typically affecting all extremities. Leprosy commonly involves the peripheral nerves, with characteristic findings, such as nerve calcification, evident on imaging. The onset of severity and radiation neuritis is variable; weeks to years may elapse between radiotherapy and onset of neuritis, and the severity depends on radiation dose. Finally, conditions such as neurofibromatosis result in diffusely distributed neurogenic tumors.[34]

Box 1
General imaging protocol

General Extremity Imaging Protocol:

- Short Tau Inversion Recovery (STIR) or T2 with fat suppression

  ○ Coronal or sagittal plane, depending on structure being imaged

- High-resolution fast spin-echo (FSE) proton density (PD) weighted images

  ○ Axial, sagittal, and coronal oriented to anatomic axis of structure being imaged

Additional Sequences for the Evaluation of Nerves:

- Axial STIR images perpendicular to the long axis of the nerve in question

- Axial focused high resolution (512 × 384) thin FSE PD images

- Additional oblique coronal or sagittal FSE PD images depending on regional anatomy

---

SUMMARY

MRN is increasingly being used as a noninvasive means of evaluating patients with neurogenic symptoms. High-resolution imaging protocols aimed at imaging the nerves of the hip, thigh, knee, leg, ankle, and foot can demonstrate traumatic or iatrogenic injury, tumorlike lesions, or

---

Box 2
Diagnostic criteria

Primary Signs:

- Hyperintense on fluid-sensitive images (T2 weighted or STIR)

- Nerve enlargement

- Loss of normal fascicular architecture

- Discontinuity (partial or complete) or acute angulation

Secondary Signs:

- Edema or fatty muscle atrophy in a distribution characteristic to the affected nerve

Ancillary Findings:

- Entrapping or compressive lesions

- Impingement by surgical material or hardware

- Focal or abrupt alteration suggesting transition point

Box 3
Pearls, pitfalls, and variants

- When evaluating MR imaging in the setting of suspected neuropathy, direct and indirect signs of nerve injury should be interpreted in the context of ancillary imaging findings and clinical evaluation.
- The interpreting radiologist should remain cognizant of potential phenomena, such as magic angle, which may complicate the interpretation of potentially abnormal imaging findings.
- Edema or atrophy related to denervation may often be distinguished from that related to traumatic or infectious etiologies based on patterns of signal abnormality; however, variants in motor innervation may result in unexpected patterns of denervation.
- Variant anatomy, such as accessory musculature and variant spatial relationships between nerves and adjacent structures, may result in a predisposition to entrapment.
- Abundant fat within the sciatic nerve should not be mistaken for a lipomatous tumor.
- Imaging alone may not allow differentiation between regenerating and chronically degenerating nerves.

Box 4
What the referring physician needs to know

- MR imaging is useful postoperatively, even in the setting of metallic hardware.
- Although postoperative neuropathy commonly resolves over time, imaging is still recommended to exclude causes that require immediate intervention.
- Detailed clinical history is a useful to the radiologist when interpreting imaging findings
- Include in the MR imaging report:
  - The gross acuity versus chronicity of the finding
    - In the case of denervation, edema versus fatty atrophy
  - Partial versus complete disruption of nerve fascicles
  - Location and etiology of entrapment/ compression
  - Ancillary findings, such as concomitant osseous and soft tissue lesions

entrapment of the nerves, causing a potential loss of motor and sensory function in the affected area. Although dedicated MRN has evolved greatly in the past 2 decades, some still question its specificity for detecting neuropathies and differentiating between regenerating and chronically degenerating nerves.[3] Future research and developments in imaging techniques will hopefully make MRN more specific for detecting peripheral neuropathies, aiding in accurate diagnosis and helping to guide clinical management in years to come (Boxes 1–4).

REFERENCES

1. Petchprapa CN, Rosenberg ZS, Sconfienza LM, et al. MR imaging of entrapment neuropathies of the lower extremity. Part 1. The pelvis and hip. Radiographics 2010;30(4):983–1000.
2. Filler AG, Haynes J, Jordan SE, et al. Sciatica of non-disc origin and piriformis syndrome: diagnosis by magnetic resonance neurography and interventional magnetic resonance imaging with outcome study of resulting treatment. J Neurosurg Spine 2005;2(2): 99–115.
3. Chhabra A, Andreisek G, Soldatos T, et al. MR neurography: past, present, and future. AJR Am J Roentgenol 2011;197(3):583–91.
4. Chhabra A, Lee PP, Bizzell C, et al. 3 Tesla MR neurography—technique, interpretation, and pitfalls. Skeletal Radiol 2011;40(10):1249–60.
5. Chhabra A, Subhawong TK, Bizzell C, et al. 3T MR neurography using three-dimensional diffusion-weighted PSIF: technical issues and advantages. Skeletal Radiol 2011;40(10):1355–60.
6. Hagmann P, Jonasson L, Maeder P, et al. Understanding diffusion MR imaging techniques: from scalar diffusion-weighted imaging to diffusion tensor imaging and beyond. Radiographics 2006;26(Suppl 1): S205–23.
7. Oida T, Nagahara S, Kobayashi T. Acquisition parameters for diffusion tensor imaging to emphasize fractional anisotropy: phantom study. Magn Reson Med Sci 2011;10(2):121–8.
8. Kastel T, Heiland S, Baumer P, et al. Magic angle effect: a relevant artifact in MR neurography at 3T? AJNR Am J Neuroradiol 2011;32(5):821–7.
9. Chappell KE, Robson MD, Stonebridge-Foster A, et al. Magic angle effects in MR neurography. AJNR Am J Neuroradiol 2004;25(3):431–40.
10. Thompson JC, Netter FH. Netter's concise orthopaedic anatomy. 2nd edition. Philadelphia: Saunders Elsevier; 2010.
11. Cunningham DJ, Romanes GJ. Cunningham's Textbook of anatomy. 12th edition. London, New York: Oxford University Press; 1981.

12. Akkaya T, Comert A, Kendir S, et al. Detailed anatomy of accessory obturator nerve blockade. Minerva Anestesiol 2008;74(4):119–22.

13. Grothaus MC, Holt M, Mekhail AO, et al. Lateral femoral cutaneous nerve: an anatomic study. Clin Orthop Relat Res 2005;(437):164–8.

14. Chhabra A, Faridian-Aragh N. High-resolution 3-T MR neurography of femoral neuropathy. AJR Am J Roentgenol 2012;198(1):3–10.

15. Donovan A, Rosenberg ZS, Cavalcanti CF. MR imaging of entrapment neuropathies of the lower extremity. Part 2. The knee, leg, ankle, and foot. Radiographics 2010;30(4):1001–19.

16. Delfaut EM, Demondion X, Bieganski A, et al. Imaging of foot and ankle nerve entrapment syndromes: from well-demonstrated to unfamiliar sites. Radiographics 2003;23(3):613–23.

17. Louisia S, Masquelet AC. The medial and inferior calcaneal nerves: an anatomic study. Surg Radiol Anat 1999;21(3):169–73.

18. Recht MP, Grooff P, Ilaslan H, et al. Selective atrophy of the abductor digiti quinti: an MRI study. AJR Am J Roentgenol 2007;189(3):W123–7.

19. Beltran LS, Bencardino J, Ghazikhanian V, et al. Entrapment neuropathies III: lower limb. Semin Musculoskelet Radiol 2010;14(5):501–11.

20. Jawish RM, Assoum HA, Khamis CF. Anatomical, clinical and electrical observations in piriformis syndrome. J Orthop Surg Res 2010;5:3.

21. Chhabra A, Williams EH, Subhawong TK, et al. MR neurography findings of soleal sling entrapment. AJR Am J Roentgenol 2011;196(3):W290–7.

22. Williams EH, Rosson GD, Hagan RR, et al. Soleal sling syndrome (proximal tibial nerve compression): results of surgical decompression. Plast Reconstr Surg 2012;129(2):454–62.

23. Chhabra A, Subhawong TK, Williams EH, et al. High-resolution MR neurography: evaluation before repeat tarsal tunnel surgery. AJR Am J Roentgenol 2011;197(1):175–83.

24. Gould JS. Tarsal tunnel syndrome. Foot Ankle Clin 2011;16(2):275–86.

25. Puranen J, Orava S. The hamstring syndrome. A new diagnosis of gluteal sciatic pain. Am J Sports Med 1988;16(5):517–21.

26. Young IJ, van Riet RP, Bell SN. Surgical release for proximal hamstring syndrome. Am J Sports Med 2008;36(12):2372–8.

27. Potter HG, Weinstein M, Allen AA, et al. Magnetic resonance imaging of the multiple-ligament injured knee. J Orthop Trauma 2002;16(5):330–9.

28. Bader R, Mittelmeier W, Zeiler G, et al. Pitfalls in the use of acetabular reinforcement rings in total hip revision. Arch Orthop Trauma Surg 2005;125(8):558–63.

29. Robertson WJ, Kelly BT. The safe zone for hip arthroscopy: a cadaveric assessment of central, peripheral, and lateral compartment portal placement. Arthroscopy 2008;24(9):1019–26.

30. Moore KR, Tsuruda JS, Dailey AT. The value of MR neurography for evaluating extraspinal neuropathic leg pain: a pictorial essay. AJNR Am J Neuroradiol 2001;22(4):786–94.

31. Paik NJ, Han TR, Lim SJ. Multiple peripheral nerve compressions related to malignantly transformed hereditary multiple exostoses. Muscle Nerve 2000;23(8):1290–4.

32. Van Gompel JJ, Griessenauer CJ, Scheithauer BW, et al. Vascular malformations, rare causes of sciatic neuropathy: a case series. Neurosurgery 2010;67(4):1133–42 [discussion: 1142].

33. Kuntz CT, Blake L, Britz G, et al. Magnetic resonance neurography of peripheral nerve lesions in the lower extremity. Neurosurgery 1996;39(4):750–6 [discussion: 756–7].

34. Thawait SK, Chaudhry V, Thawait GK, et al. High-resolution MR neurography of diffuse peripheral nerve lesions. AJNR Am J Neuroradiol 2011;32(8):1365–72.

35. Chhabra A, Williams EH, Wang KC, et al. MR neurography of neuromas related to nerve injury and entrapment with surgical correlation. AJNR Am J Neuroradiol 2010;31(8):1363–8.

Magnetic Resonance Neurography of Peripheral Nerve Tumors and Tumorlike Conditions

Shivani Ahlawat, MD[a], Avneesh Chhabra, MD[b], Jaishri Blakely, MD[c],*

KEYWORDS

- Peripheral nerve tumors • Schwannoma • Neurofibroma • Perineurioma
- Peripheral nerve tumor mimics • Neurolymphoma • Malignant peripheral nerve sheath tumor • MR

KEY POINTS

- MR imaging characteristics of many lesions in and around the peripheral nerves are unique and a confident diagnosis of such lesions including lipoma, fibrolipoma, ganglion cyst and perineurioma can be prospectively suggested.
- Multiple MR imaging findings can suggest the possibility of a neurogenic tumor but do not reliably distinguish between schwannoma and neurofibroma.
- Although there are certain MR features that increase the likelihood of MPNST, biopsy is still necessary to confirm the diagnosis.
- Understanding of the clinical features of a broad range of neuropathy conditions and a multidisciplinary approach is essential for proper and timely patient management.

INTRODUCTION

Patients with signs and symptoms of focal neuropathy are often referred for nerve imaging, which may consist of regional magnetic resonance (MR) imaging of different areas of the body. The imaging may be designed to provide an overview of tumor burden (whole-body MR [WBMR] imaging) or detailed anatomy of a specific nerve (MR neurography [MRN]). When peripheral nerve enlargement is seen, there is a common differential that includes benign peripheral nerve sheath tumors (PNSTs), malignant PNSTs (MPNSTs), hereditary

or inflammatory neuropathy, posttraumatic neuroma, intraneural ganglion or other secondary nonneurogenic malignancies such as neurolymphoma and other intraneural epithelial or mesenchymal tumors (Table 1).

Neurofibromas account for 5% of all benign soft tissue tumors with 95% occurring sporadically.[1] Schwannomas also account for 5% of all benign soft tissue tumors and 95% also occur sporadically.[1] The remainder of neurofibromas and schwannomas are related to genetic neurocutaneous syndromes, including neurofibromatosis

Disclosure: A. Chhabra, research grants from GE-AUR, Siemens, Integra Life Sciences; Gatewood fellowship, MSK CAD; consultant, Siemens.
a The Russell H. Morgan Department of Radiology and Radiological Science, The Johns Hopkins Hospital, 601 N. Caroline Street, Baltimore, MD 21287, USA; b University of Texas Southwestern, 5323 Harry Hines Blvd, Dallas, TX 75390, USA; c Department of Neurology, The Johns Hopkins Hospital Comprehensive Neurofibromatosis Center, The Johns Hopkins Hospital, CRB II, Suite 1M16, 1550 Orleans Street, Baltimore, MD 21231, USA
* Corresponding author.
E-mail address: jblakel3@jhmi.edu

Neuroimag Clin N Am 24 (2014) 171–192
http://dx.doi.org/10.1016/j.nic.2013.03.035
1052-5149/14/$ – see front matter © 2014 Elsevier Inc. All rights reserved.

Table 1
Differential diagnosis of peripheral nerve mass–like enlargement on MR imaging

	Clinical Features	Imaging Features
Neurogenic Lesions		
Benign PNST		
Neurofibroma	Young to middle age Solitary slow-growing lesion Incidental discovery Mild to moderate sensory or motor symptoms and signs Isolated or associated with neurocutaneous syndromes (can occur at early age)	Continuity with nerve (tail sign) and/or multiple fascicles, can be centrally located Target sign Split fat sign Fascicular sign Unencapsulated Homogeneous or targetoid enhancement High ADC (min) on DTI >1.1–1.2 × 10^{-3} mm/s^2 Low SUV$_{max}$ (<2–3) on early and delayed F^{18} FDG-PET scan
Schwannoma	Young to middle age Solitary slow-growing lesion Incidental discovery or painful lesion Mild to moderate sensory or motor symptoms and signs Isolated or associated with neurocutaneous syndromes (can occur at early age)	Continuity with nerve (tail sign) and/or 1 or 2 fascicles, can be eccentrically located Target sign Split fat sign Fascicular sign Encapsulated Cystic changes, hemorrhage, calcification (10%–20%) Homogeneous or targetoid or heterogeneous enhancement High ADC (min) on DTI >1.1–1.2 × 10^{-3} mm/s^2 Low SUV$_{max}$ (<2–3) on early and delayed F^{18} FDG-PET scan
Perineurioma	Young to middle age Isolated Slowly progressive mononeuropathy with few or no sensory symptoms or signs	Continuity with nerve (tail sign) and/or multiple fascicles Most commonly in lower limbs, and in sciatic or femoral distributions Uniform homogeneous fascicular enlargement and hyperintensity (Honeycomb pattern) High ADC (min) on DTI >1.1–1.2 × 10^{-3} mm/s^2 Low SUV$_{max}$ (<2–3) on early and delayed F^{18} FDG-PET scan
Malignant PNST	New-onset sensory and/or motor deficit New or intensified pain Rapid enlargement of a known PNST	Irregular or round shape Usually larger than 5 cm Perilesional edema Intratumoral nodularity, necrosis/cystic change or hemorrhage T1 heterogeneity and lack of targetoid appearance Heterogeneous enhancement Restricted diffusion: low ADC (min) on DTI <1.1 × 10^{-3} mm/s^2 Increased SUV$_{max}$ (>3–4) on early and delayed F^{18} FDG-PET scan
Neurocutaneous syndromes	Younger age of presentation and family history	—
NF1	Cutaneous lesions Skeletal deformities Glioma Lisch nodule First-degree relative	Plexiform neurofibroma or multiple PNSTs (usually NF) Multifocal diffuse nerve thickening(s) and nodularity Malignant PNST

(continued on next page)

Table 1
(continued)

	Clinical Features	Imaging Features
NF2	Vestibular tumors Ependymomas with other schwannomas or multiple meningiomas First-degree relative	Multiple benign PNST (usually SW) Malignant PNST (very rare)
Schwannomatosis	No vestibular tumors (rare reports of unilateral vestibular schwannoma) Possible meningioma Multiple PNST	Multiple benign PNST
Tumor Mimics		
Neuroma	Prior trauma or surgery	Fusiform shape Spindle (neuroma in continuity) or end-bulb neuroma (complete nerve transection) Heterogeneous T1 and T2 signal alterations with loss of fascicular continuity Lack of significant enhancement Perineural scarring
Lipoma	Mononeuropathy with gradual-onset motor and/or sensory symptoms Most commonly in median nerve distribution Macrodactyly and/or association with macrodystrophia lipomatosa	Shape: fusiform or rounded. Diffuse long segment or, less commonly, focal nerve enlargement Fatty and fibrous infiltration with typical MR signal characteristics Spaghetti appearance on long-axis images and coaxial-cable appearance on short-axis images
Hereditary neuropathy	Positive family history Hyporeflexia, high arches Foot deformities Two-thirds CMT 1A Two-thirds with positive PMP22 gene	Symmetric and bilateral nerve enlargement Peripheral appendicular and axial pan plexus involvement Most enlargement with CMT 1A Uniform fascicular enlargement Variable to no enhancement Multiple nerve entrapments may be identified, especially with HNPP variant
Inflammatory neuropathy: AIDP/CIDP/MMN	AIDP/CIDP: albuminocytologic dissociation. Increased CSF protein Prognosis: good in AIDP, poor in CIDP. In MMN, prognosis is variable	Diffuse (often asymmetrical) > fusiform enlargement of cauda equina, nerve roots/plexus and peripheral nerves MMN common in upper limbs. CIDP common in lower limbs Mild to moderate enhancement. No focal masses as with neurocutaneous syndromes Skeletal survey and cross-sectional examinations may show underlying malignancy, particularly myeloma association with CIDP
Infectious neuropathy: leprosy	Endemic area Neuropathic ankles and wrists Neuropathic acro-osteolysis	Ulnar or peroneal involvement Peripheral nerve enlargement with hyperintensity Abscess formation

(continued on next page)

Table 1
(continued)

	Clinical Features	Imaging Features
Nonneurogenic Lesions		
Tumor Mimics		
Intraneural ganglion	With internal joint derangement Slow or fluctuating functional motor loss Prognosis: good with surgical resection of the intra-articular feeding nerve	In close proximity to a joint with evidence of internal joint derangement, such as Baker cyst, paralabral cyst, ganglion cyst Elongated shape Cystic intraepineural mass. Mutiloculated Nerve hyperintensity ± peripheral enhancement
Amyloidosis	Pertinent long-standing clinical history of chronic kidney disease, myeloma, chronic infection, and so forth Bilateral sensorimotor symptoms. Gradual deterioration Negative birefringent deposits in the epineurium and other layers of the nerve on Congo red staining	Lower extremity more commonly involved, particularly LS plexus and sciatic nerves Diffuse or, less commonly, focal nerve enlargement with nodularity similar to neurocutaneous syndromes, but less pronounced Variable enhancement
Tumors		
Lymphoma	Known hematologic malignancy Painful sensorimotor neuropathy	Can present as adjoining adenopathy with compression or infiltration of the nerves or, less commonly, with primary enlargement of the peripheral nerve with multifocal nodularity and areas of T2 hypointensity Intense enhancement on contrast
Intraneural epithelial or mesenchymal tumors	Known malignancy in cases of metastasis In primary epithelioid or mesenchymal sarcoma, gradual mononeuropathy symptoms and/or signs	Evidence of direct invasion but local metastasis or sarcoma Evidence of other metastases Heterogeneous fusiform enlargement of the nerve with intraneural primary sarcoma or granular cell tumor Heterogeneous enhancement with tumors. No significant enhancement with lipoma along with its fatty tissue characteristics

Abbreviations: ADC, apparent diffusion coefficient; AIDP, acute inflammatory demyelination polyneuropathy; CIDP, chronic inflammatory demyelinating polyneuropathy; CMT, Charcot-Marie-Tooth; CSF, cerebrospinal fluid; DTI, diffusion tensor imaging; FDG-PET, fluorodeoxyglucose positron emission tomography; HNPP, hereditary neuropathy with liability to pressure palsies; LS, lumbosacral; MMN, multifocal mononeuropathy; NF1, neurofibromatosis type 1; SUV$_{max}$, maximal standardized uptake value; SW, Schwannomatosis.

type 1 (NF1), neurofibromatosis type 2 (NF2), and schwannomatosis (SW).

NF1 is one of the most common autosomal dominant neurogenetic syndromes with well-established clinical criteria (**Box 1**). Benign PNSTs called neurofibromas are the hallmark of NF1. There are 3 main types of neurofibromas: localized, diffuse, and plexiform, and all can be present in patients with NF1. Plexiform neurofibromas are benign but complex tumors that cause diffuse enlargement of deep nerves such as the plexuses or may present as diffuse cutaneous and nerve thickening. These lesions are classic for NF1. They are difficult to manage clinically because they can cause pain, disfigurement, and neurologic dysfunction and can progress to malignant sarcomas.

NF2 is also an autosomal dominant inherited syndrome that predisposes individuals to multiple tumors of the nervous system. Although intracranial

Box 1
Diagnostic criteria for NF1, NF2, and schwannomatosis

NF1:

At least 2 of the following:

- More than 6 café au lait macules (>1.5 cm in adults and >0.5 cm in prepubertal individuals)
- More than 2 neurofibromas of any type or 1 plexiform neurofibroma
- Axillary or inguinal freckling
- Optic pathway glioma
- Two or more Lisch nodules
- An osseous lesion specific for NF1, including sphenoid dysplasia or thinning or pseudoarthrosis
- A first-degree relative with NF1 by the criteria listed earlier

NF2:

At least 1 of the following scenarios:

1. Bilateral masses of the eighth cranial nerve consistent with vestibular schwannoma
2. First-degree relative, and:
   a. Unilateral lesion consistent with vestibular schwannoma in someone <30 years old

   Or:

   b. At least 2 of the following:
      - Meningioma
      - Glioma
      - Schwannoma
      - Juvenile cortical cataract
3. Unilateral lesion consistent with vestibular schwannoma in someone <30 years old

   And:

   a. At least 2 of the following:
      - Meningioma
      - Glioma
      - Schwannoma
      - Juvenile cortical cataract
4. More than 2 meningiomas and:
   a. Unilateral lesion consistent with vestibular schwannoma in someone <30 years old

   Or:

   b. At least 2 of the following:
      - Meningioma
      - Glioma
      - Schwannoma
      - Juvenile cortical cataract

schwannomatosis:

1. More than 30 years old and all of the following:
   a. More than 2 schwannomas (1 with pathologic confirmation)
   b. No vestibular schwannoma by MR imaging with thin cuts through the internal auditory canals
   c. No NF2 gene mutation

   Or:

2. More than 1 nonvestibular schwannoma (with pathologic confirmation) and a first-degree relative

schwannomas, such as vestibular schwannomas, are pathognomonic for NF2, patients with NF2 often have peripheral schwannomas. In contrast, patients with schwannomatosis generally have no intracranial lesions but a preponderance of peripheral schwannomas. Familial schwannomatosis is also thought to be caused by autosomal dominant inheritance, although most patients with schwannomatosis have no known familial occurrence. Patients with schwannomatosis develop peripheral schwannomas involving spinal roots, plexuses, and peripheral nerves. The major clinical manifestation of schwannomatosis is pain, often requiring multiple surgical procedures.

Because these syndromes account for a great number of the lesions detected on peripheral nerve imaging and can be difficult to distinguish from either nontumor causes or nonsyndromic causes, this article reviews the typical imaging appearance of PNST and tumorlike conditions with an emphasis on MRN features that distinguish benign tumors from malignant tumors and from conditions that mimic tumors.

Neurogenic Lesions

Benign peripheral nerve tumors
Neurogenic tumors represent 10% to 12% of all benign soft tissue neoplasms.[1,2] Benign PNSTs often have distinctive features including location in relation to the neurovascular bundle, clinical history, and intrinsic imaging features. The common neurogenic tumors include neurofibroma, schwannoma, and, rarely, perineurioma. Although neurogenic tumors can be diagnosed on MR imaging, it is difficult to differentiate between the schwannomas and neurofibromas. Perineuriomas are

less likely to represent a diagnostic dilemma because of their rarer occurrence, location, and more typical clinical and imaging presentation. Jee and colleagues[3] reported that MR imaging findings can aid in differentiating schwannomas and neurofibromas; however, no single imaging finding or combination allows definitive diagnosis, which is not surprising because they share several features and can be difficult to distinguish pathologically.[4]

Neurofibroma Neurofibromas are benign PNSTs that arise from Schwann cells, but have multiple additional cell types making up the tumor mass, including neuronal axons, fibroblasts, mast cells, macrophages, perineural cells, and extracellular matrix materials such as collagen.[5] These tumors are inseparable from the normal nerve, and therefore complete surgical excision must include the functional nerve.[6] Neurofibromas can occur both in the context of NF1 and sporadically. They also come in several forms including a localized or solitary form, a diffuse form, and plexiform neurofibroma. One of the complexities is that there is not uniform agreement about the definition of neurofibromas across or even within medical subspecialties. However, using the terms most commonly encountered in radiology, the solitary neurofibroma is the most common type encountered clinically overall. These neurofibromas are also termed nodular neurofibromas and are the variety that is most commonly encountered in patients who do not have NF1. These neurofibromas typically present in young to middle-aged adults with a slow-growing mass. They can be incidentally discovered or patients may present with mild to moderate sensorimotor symptoms.

The diffuse, superficial form involves the subcutaneous tissues and is often seen in the region of the head and neck, but can be anywhere in the body (**Fig. 1**).[6] Plexiform neurofibromas grow along the nerve sheath spreading the axons as the abnormal cells proliferate and increased extracellular matrix is deposited. They may involve multiple fascicles and branches of nerve and can involve nerves in any region of the body. The most common location for plexiform neurofibromas in patients with NF1 is the trunk including the paraspinal region (41%), followed by the neck/upper trunk (24%) and the extremities (17%). Between 15% and 30% of plexiform neurofibromas are isolated to the head and neck region.[6–8] Diffuse and plexiform neurofibromas are more likely to be found in the setting of NF1.

Localized or solitary neurofibromas are often indistinguishable from schwannomas based on imaging features. They are usually well-defined,

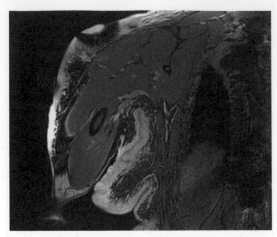

Fig. 1. Benign PNST: diffuse superficial neurofibroma. Coronal T2 spectral adiabatic inversion recovery (SPAIR) image on a patient with large diffuse superficial neurofibroma shows marked hyperintensity and skin thickening circumferentially extending from the axilla into the chest wall and proximal arm.

unencapsulated, fusiform or round soft tissue masses typically less than 5 cm in diameter. The fusiform shape and continuity with the nerve (tail sign) is useful in establishing a neurogenic origin because it reflects the nerve entering and exiting the mass. This morphology is better seen when a large and deep nerve is involved as opposed to small superficial nerve.[9] On T1-weighted (T1W) images, they are usually isointense to muscle.[9–12] On T2-weighted (T2W) images, they show heterogeneous high signal intensity. The presence of target sign, fascicular sign, split fat sign, and continuity with a peripheral nerve points to a neurogenic origin.[9–11] These lesions show variable enhancement with gadolinium contrast agent.[10,12] The target sign refers to high peripheral signal and low to intermediate central signal on fluid-sensitive sequences. The intralesional architecture with more myxoid material peripherally and fibrous tissue centrally accounts for this appearance.[9] Although the target sign was initially thought to be pathognomonic of neurofibroma, it has been observed in both neurofibromas and schwannomas and has even been reported in MPNSTs.[9] The fascicular sign describes multiple ringlike prominent structures within the lesion, possibly reflecting the enlarged fascicular bundles seen histologically. A thin, hypointense capsule might be identified on T2W images, particularly if the tumor is surrounded by fat. This finding is slightly more common in schwannomas than in neurofibromas. On contrast-enhanced images, small nerve sheath tumors often show intense and homogeneous or targetoid enhancement. Large lesions may show predominantly peripheral, central, or heterogeneous nodular enhancement. Specific evaluation for edemalike signal on T2W images, fatty infiltration, and atrophy of innervated muscles is recommended to strengthen the diagnosis of a neurogenic tumor. On advanced diffusion tensor imaging (DTI), these lesions are associated with high apparent diffusion coefficient (ADC) values ($>1.1–1.2 \times 10^{-3}$ mm/s^2).

MR imaging of plexiform neurofibromas shows a tortuous mass of thickened nerve branches that can invade surrounding tissues (**Fig. 2**). In general, plexiform neurofibromas share the same signal characteristics and enhancement pattern as a solitary lesion.[9] Developing in childhood, plexiform neurofibromas can precede cutaneous neurofibromas. Depending on their location, plexiform neurofibromas can be deep, superficial, or a combination of both. Deep plexiform neurofibromas do not involve the skin or subcutaneous tissues. The superficial plexiform neurofibromas can be asymmetric in distribution, with a diffuse or infiltrative morphology, extend to the skin surface in an arborizing pattern, with smaller fascicles or nodules, and lack a target sign.[13] Superficial neurofibromas can mimic venous malformations on MR imaging, and MR angiography or Doppler ultrasound evaluation may be needed for further differentiation.

Schwannoma Schwannoma (neurilemoma or neurinoma) is also a tumor of Schwann cells.[9] Schwannomas, unlike neurofibromas, are typically encapsulated and do not have multiple cell types inherent to the tumor. They can be seen at any age but are more commonly diagnosed in patients 20 to 30 years of age.[9] They are usually solitary, slow-growing small lesions (<5 cm) that are incidentally discovered or present with mild to moderate sensorimotor symptoms. They can be found in the cranial, spinal, and sympathetic nerve roots as well as the peripheral nerves of the flexor surfaces of the extremities.[9,11]

Schwannomas are fusiform masses, eccentric to and separate from the adjacent nerve but encapsulated within the perineurium (**Fig. 3**). When they arise from cutaneous or other small nerves, the nerve may be obliterated by the mass on MR imaging. They have 2 components: a hypercellular Antoni A region and a loosely organized, hypocellular Antoni B region.[9,11] Surgical excision of schwannomas, unlike neurofibroma, can spare the affected peripheral nerve.[9] This eccentric and separate relationship of the schwannoma relative to the involved peripheral nerve is not confidently shown on MR imaging to distinguish between neurofibroma and schwannoma. However, dedicated MRN can show the 1 or 2 prominent fascicles individually affected by the tumor, similar to surgical findings. Large tumors may exhibit cystic degeneration, calcification, hemorrhage, and fibrosis, and are described as ancient schwannomas.[9,14] They only rarely undergo malignant transformation.

Schwannomas share MR imaging features with other neurogenic tumors, especially nodular neurofibromas. A hypointense capsule representing the epineurium is more commonly seen with

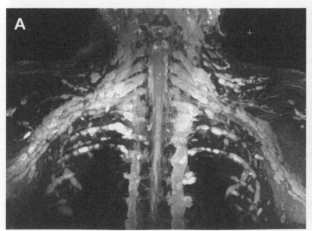
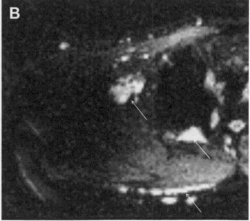

Fig. 2. Benign PNST: plexiform neurofibromas in the setting of NF1. A 21-year-old man with known clinical history of NF1. Coronal maximal intensity projection (MIP) three-dimensional (3D) short tau inversion recovery (STIR) sampling perfection with application optimized contrasts by using different flip angle evolutions (SPACE) image (*A*) shows innumerable neurofibromas with plexiform neurofibromas involving the bilateral brachial plexuses, intercostal nerves, and paraspinal nerves. The ADC map (*B*) shows no restricted diffusion in any of these lesions (*arrows*) (minimal ADC value of 1.8×10^{-3} mm/s^2 and average ADC value of 2.4×10^{-3} mm/s^2).

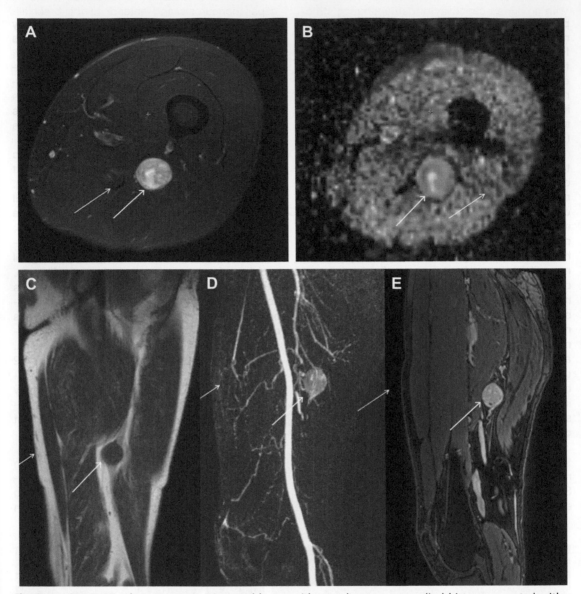

Fig. 3. Benign PNST: schwannoma. A 59-year-old man with no relevant past medical history presented with a palpable mass in the posterior left thigh for 2 years with pain radiating to the great toe. Physical examination showed mild weakness in the foot flexor muscles. Axial T2 SPAIR (*A*) shows a heterogeneous, hyperintense mass (*arrow*) associated with the left sciatic nerve without perilesional edema. The ADC map (*B*) revealed no restricted diffusion with an average ADC value of 1.5×10^{-3} mm/s^2 (range 1.1–2.1 mm/s^2). The mass was surgically confirmed as schwannoma. The coronal T1W (*C*) image better showed the fusiform shape with continuity with the left sciatic nerve depicting the tail and split far signs (*arrow*); these findings suggest a neurogenic origin. The time-resolved dynamic MR angiogram (*D*) reveals early arterial enhancement (*arrow*). The delayed postcontrast image (*E*) shows homogeneous enhancement (*arrow*).

schwannomas than with neurofibromas. On MR imaging, schwannomas are isointense to skeletal muscle on T1W-images and heterogeneously hyperintense on T2W-images and variable contrast enhancement. Similar to neurofibromas, they can show target sign, fascicular sign, and split fat sign. The target pattern is usually absent in large masses and in tumors with cystic,

hemorrhagic, or necrotic degeneration.[11] On advanced DTI, these lesions also show high ADC values or lack of restricted diffusion similar to neurofibromas. Just as neurofibromas can be plexiform, schwannomas can also be plexiform.[15,16] In general, when evaluating for possible malignant potential in a PNST, heterogeneity in a schwannoma is less concerning than in a neurofibroma, because the latter are generally more homogeneous or simply targetoid.

Perineurioma Perineurioma are categorized into 2 main types based on location: intraneural or extraneural. Intraneural perineuriomas are benign neoplasms composed of whorls of perineural cells surrounding the peripheral nerves. Because of their histologic origin, they are located in the periphery of the nerves. Cross-sectional histologic examination reveals irregularly enlarged, hypercellular nerve fascicles composed of spindled perineural cells arranged in pseudo-onion bulblike whorls. The mitotic rate is low, accounting for the slowly progressive or static symptoms. The nature of intraneural perineurioma has been debated in the literature, with some investigators speculating a reactive posttraumatic cause.[17] The recent evidence has confirmed its neoplastic nature.[18] These benign tumors are typically seen in teenagers with progressive muscle weakness. Pain and sensory disturbances are less common. As opposed to neurofibroma and schwannoma, which are both

associated with good prognosis, perineurioma have poor prognosis with slow functional loss over time.

On MR imaging, the affected peripheral nerve is enlarged, T1 hypointense, T2 hyperintense, with associated avid enhancement on postcontrast imaging (**Fig. 4**). There is gradual increase of the nerve caliber followed by gradual taper.[19] Fat-saturated postcontrast T1W images are most helpful to show the extent of the lesions. Separating the lesions from adjacent vessels can be difficult and the lesion can be mistakenly characterized as a vascular malformation on imaging.[20] The sciatic nerve or common peroneal nerves are most commonly affected. The fascicular architecture is maintained on axial and longitudinal MRN images. The individual fascicles are uniformly enlarged, resulting in a honeycomb appearance.[21] Although the imaging appearance can mimic other neurogenic benign neoplasms, the clinical history of slowly progressive mononeuropathy, the patient's young age, and lack of known tumor syndrome makes the diagnosis likely.[22] Because these

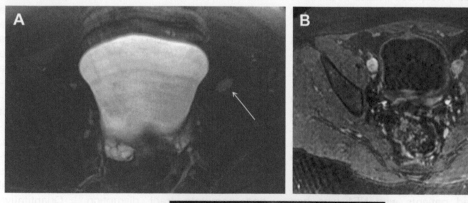

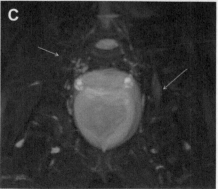

Fig. 4. Benign PNST: perineurioma. An 11-year-old girl with no past medical history presented with left lower extremity weakness, difficulty climbing stairs, and dysesthesia for 1 year duration. The patient was noted to have atrophy in the left quadriceps muscle group with associated lower extremity weakness on physical examination. Axial T2 SPAIR image (*A*) shows hyperintense enlargement of the left femoral nerve (*arrow*). Mild associated enhancement (*arrow*) is noted on the postcontrast images (*B*). Coronal 3D MIP STIR SPACE (*C*) image shows asymmetric fusiform mass associated with left femoral nerve (*large arrow*). Note normal right femoral nerve (*small arrow*). Surgical pathology confirmed the diagnosis of perineurioma.

tumors are static or slowly progressive, they can be followed clinically and with imaging as indicated. Treatment of choice is resection of the lesion with end-to-end nerve grafting. However, few patients do well, despite extensive surgery.[22]

Malignant peripheral nerve tumors

Malignant peripheral nerve tumor (malignant schwannoma, neurofibrosarcoma, malignant neurolemmimas, and neurogenic sarcoma) is a spindle cell sarcoma arising from a peripheral nerve or neurofibroma or showing nerve tissue differentiation. MPNSTs account for 3% to 10% of all soft tissue sarcomas with 15% to 70% occurring in patients with NF1.[9,23] This sarcoma is a high-grade malignancy with an overall poor prognosis. MPNST more commonly occurs in young persons between 20 and 50 years of age without gender predilection.[9,23] Patients with NF1 with MPNST present at a younger age and are mostly male.[9] MPNSTs most commonly involve large peripheral nerves including sciatic nerve, brachial plexus, and lumbosacral plexus.[24] Malignant PNST can also be a secondary neoplasm related to previous radiation therapy. Such tumors develop after a long latent period (10–20 years) and account for 11% of malignant PNSTs.[2,23] Clinical signs and symptoms suggesting an MPNST include new-onset pain, the intensification of existing pain, and the rapid enlargement of a peripheral tumor. Anatomic and metabolic imaging is used in an attempt to distinguish benign neurofibromas in a growth phase from an MPNST.

Using F[18] fluorodeoxyglucose positron emission tomography (FDG-PET), multiple studies have shown usefulness in differentiation between benign tumours and MPNSTs. In 2008, Ferner and colleagues[25] studied patients with NF1 who had symptomatic neoplasms, using early (60–90 minutes) and delayed (240 minutes) FDG-PET acquisitions, and reported a sensitivity and specificity of 89% and 95% respectively for diagnosing an NF1-associated MPNST. Warbey and colleagues[26] subsequently showed the reproducibility of the early and delayed PET/computed tomography (CT) technique with sensitivity and specificity of 97% and of 87% respectively. Benz and colleagues[27] examined the usefulness of FDG-PET/CT to distinguish histologically proven MPNSTs from benign PNSTs. The difference in standardized uptake values (SUVs) observed in MPNSTs compared with those of schwannomas was not as striking as the difference between SUVs of MPNSTs and neurofibromas, with 3 of 14 schwannomas exhibiting maximal SUV (SUV_{max}) greater than 5. Such investigations suggest that, although PET is useful for differentiating an MPNST from a neurofibroma, PET is less specific for distinguishing an MPNST from a schwannoma. This limitation is similar to that of anatomic MR imaging, in which imaging features that suggest malignancy, such as large size, necrosis, hemorrhage, and heterogeneity, are similarly observed in schwannomas and MPNSTs.

Using anatomic MR imaging, a few studies have described some distinguishing characteristics for benign and malignant PNSTs.[28–30] Matsumine and colleagues[30] assessed MR imaging features of neurofibromas and MPNSTs in patients with NF1 and showed that, although irregular tumor shape, indistinct margins, and heterogeneous enhancement were important factors, only intratumoral lobulation and the presence of T1-hyperintense areas were considered diagnostic indicators of malignancy. Four specific MR imaging features were recently reported that can be used to distinguish MPNSTs from neurofibromas with a sensitivity and specificity of 61% and 90% respectively (when 2 or more of the following features were observed: large size, peripheral enhancement pattern, perilesional edema, and intratumoral cystic changes).[30]

Functional and metabolic MR sequences have also been described for the assessment of nerve sheath tumors. Preliminary functional DTI studies in assessing nerve tract integrity in the presence of various peripheral nerve sheath lesions have been performed. Benign PNSTs show near-normal appearance or partial nerve tract disruption in benign tumors, with the exception of degenerated schwannoma and plexiform neurofibroma; however, neurolymphoma, perineurioma, and hereditary neuropathy also showed near-normal appearance of the tracts.[31] Two MPNSTs were also studied using DTI and showed partial and complete tract disruption.[31] Quantitative diffusion-weighted imaging has been reported to be of questionable value for distinguishing benign and malignant soft tissue tumors including PNSTs.[32–37] In addition, metabolic MR imaging with MR spectroscopy has been studied for the characterization of musculoskeletal lesions for malignancy, and can aid in distinguishing between these two lesions.[38–41]

Malignant triton tumor (MTT) is a rare subtype of MPNST, histologically defined as a MPNST with additional rhabdomyoblastic differentiation (Fig. 5). The mean age of patients with MTT has been estimated to be 31.7 years.[42,43] There seems to be an equal sex distribution in those affected, and the tumor coexists with NF1 in 44% to 69% of cases. When associated with NF1, MTT tends to present at a younger age, and in men, than has been observed in sporadic cases. MTT is a highly aggressive tumor with low overall survival

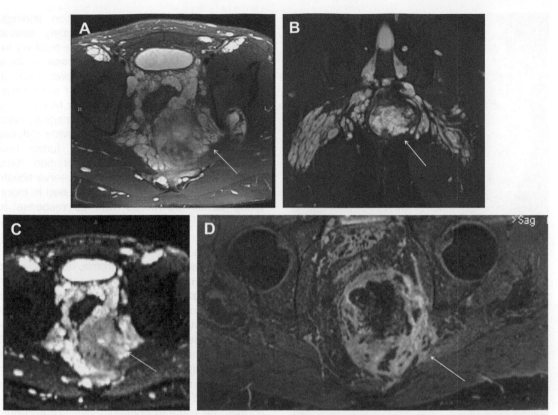

Fig. 5. MPNST. A 21-year-old man with known history of NF1 presented with severe left scrotal pain to the emergency room and was found to have a pelvic mass on CT imaging. Axial T2 SPAIR imaging (*A*) reveals plexiform and innumerable neurofibromas in the pelvis. There is a large left hemipelvic mass (*arrow*) with heterogeneous internal signal. Coronal 3D STIR SPACE sequence (*B*) also shows innumerable plexiform neurofibromas (note the target signs) with a dominant pelvic mass (*arrow*). Axial ADC map (*C*) shows restricted diffusion with a minimal ADC value of 0.4×10^{-3} mm/s^2 and an average ADC value of 0.8×10^{-3} mm/s^2 (*arrow*). Contrast-enhanced examination (*D*) shows heterogeneous peripheral enhancement with internal necrosis (*arrow*). Percutaneous biopsy revealed MPNST with skeletal muscle components consistent with triton tumor.

rates (estimated 5-year survival rates are 26%),[43] high rates of metastasis (48%), and local recurrence (43%).[42–46]

Tumor syndromes

The neurofibromatoses are hereditary syndromes caused by genetic mutations in the *NF1*, *NF2*, and *SMARCB1* tumor-suppressor genes, respectively.[47–50] NF1, NF2, and schwannomatosis increase the likelihood to develop Schwann cell tumors. These related syndromes have overlapping clinical features making clinical and imaging differentiation difficult in some cases; however, there are established diagnostic criteria that assist in reliable clinical differentiation (see **Box 1**).[50–52]

Despite the benign histology of neurofibromas and schwannomas, they can cause significant morbidity and even mortality. Patients with NF1 have increased mortality caused by MPNSTs, central nervous system gliomas, cardiovascular disease, and organ compression by neurofibromas.[53,54] Even the benign tumors of NF1 (neurofibromas and optic pathway gliomas), NF2 (schwannoma, ependymoma, and meningioma), and schwannomatosis (schwannoma) increase morbidity because of continuous tumor growth and frequent surgical inaccessibility. Pain is a debilitating consequence of schwannomatosis.[55] Patients suffering from schwannomatosis tend to be younger than those presenting with solitary schwannomas. Therefore, schwannomatosis should be suspected in young individuals presenting with multiple schwannomas but not meeting the criteria for NF2. Increased growth and new pain in a known benign PNST in the context of tumor syndrome should raise suspicion of malignant transformation.[55]

NF1 and NF2 as well as schwannomatosis occur in mosaic forms caused by somatic mutations (**Fig. 6**). Early somatic mutations cause generalized disease, clinically identical to nonmosaic forms. Later somatic mutations cause localized

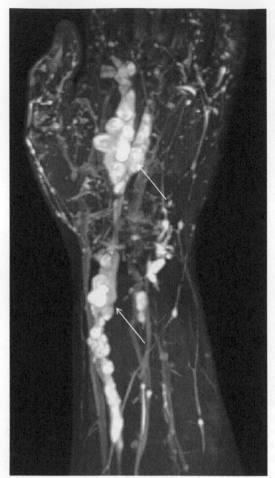

Fig. 6. Neurocutaneous syndrome: segmental schwannomatosis. A 36-year-old woman with no past medical or family history presented with multiple palpable masses in the right upper extremity. She did not meet the criteria for NF1 and had no vestibular schwannomas based on prior brain imaging. The patient was clinically diagnosed with segmental or mosaic form of schwannomatosis. Coronal MIP 3D STIR SPACE image shows multiple lobulated masses along the median nerve distribution (*arrows*).

symptoms and physical examination findings. However, these studies inadequately assess whole-body tumor burden and make tracking tumor behavior for tumors that cross multiple anatomic regions more difficult over time. In large centers managing these tumor syndromes, there is a move toward whole-body MR imaging with fluid-sensitive and anatomic imaging. Such a whole-body examination can provide detailed information regarding whole-body tumor burden including the number, distribution, type (localized or plexiform), and size of nerve sheath tumors in a patient. It can also be used in monitoring tumor growth as well as response to treatment.[57–60]

PNST mimics

Neuroma Posttraumatic neuroma, also known as neuroma, is related to disorganized proliferation of axonal tissue as a response to injury such as chronic friction or transection. Pain is the most common clinical symptom and can be reproduced with tapping on the lesion (Tinel sign). A soft tissue mass that is firm at a focal pressure site may be apparent. The most common location for traumatic neuroma is the lower extremity after amputation. They can be divided into 2 major categories: neuroma in continuity (NIC) or end-bulb neuroma. NIC is a localized, fusiform enlargement caused by a fibroinflammatory response to chronic friction or irritation.[61] NIC is subdivided into 2 pathologic types: spindle neuromas with intact perineurium or lateral neuromas with partially disrupted perineurium. End-bulb neuromas result from entangled regenerating axons attempting to reestablish continuity after an injury or surgery (amputation). They can develop within 1 to 12 months of the traumatic event and can present as a painful mass.[4]

MR images show fusiform (NIC) or bulbous (end-bulb neuroma) masses in continuity with the injured or transected nerves, respectively. Most traumatic neuromas are of intermediate signal intensity on T1W images and of intermediate to heterogeneously high signal intensity on T2W images with loss of fascicular continuity (**Fig. 7**). Contrast enhancement is variable.[4] NIC has a similar fusiform morphology to previously described PNST; however, presence of perineural scarring, lack of split fat or target sign, and usually lack of significant enhancement aids in distinguishing the two entities.[62]

Initial nonoperative treatment has been successful in up to 50% of patients. Failure of nonoperative therapy may require surgical resection.[62–64] Prognosis can be variable depending on the extent of nerve circumference involvement.

or segmental. In individuals with mosaic or localized manifestations of NF1, disease manifestations are limited to the affected area. Distribution is usually unilateral but can be bilateral, either in a symmetric or asymmetrical arrangement. Individuals with the mosaic form, even with a generalized phenotype, typically have milder disease and decreased risk for transmission of the gene to their children than individuals with the nonmosaic form, although the risk cannot be accurately quantified.[56]

At present, localized MRN examinations are performed on these patients based on concerning

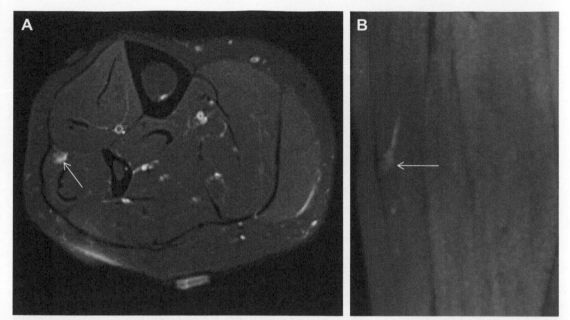

Fig. 7. Neurogenic tumor mimics: end-bulb neuroma. A 21-year-old man sustained a penetrating injury to the lower leg and presented with sensory loss along the superficial peroneal nerve distribution. Axial T2 SPAIR (*A*) shows fusiform enlargement of the superficial peroneal nerve (*arrow*) with internal heterogeneity and loss of the normal fascicular pattern. The coronal MIP 3D diffusion-weighted (DW) reversed fast imaging with steady state precession (PSIF) image (*B*) shows an end-bulb neuroma from Sunderland grade V injury (*arrow*).

LIPOMA/neural fibrolipoma Lipoma can involve the nerve intraneurally or perineurally. Neural fibrolipoma (lipomatosis or nerve or fibrolipomatous hamartoma) refers to a tumorlike process with intraepineural as well as perineural infiltration of fatty and fibrous tissue. It presents before the age of 30 years, and most commonly affects the median or ulnar nerve in the wrist.[4] The lesions can be associated with macrodactyly in the hand or foot. The slow-growing mass can cause increased pain, paresthesia, and weakness.

MR imaging is pathognomonic in lipoma with simple fatty component in close proximity to the nerve. Neural fibrolipoma shows diffuse enlargement of the affected nerve (**Fig. 8**). The fatty and fibrous infiltration causes a cablelike appearance of the thickened fascicles (**Fig. 9**). There is a typical spaghetti appearance on the long-axis images and a coaxial-cable appearance on the axial images.[65] The signal intensity of the tissue surrounding the nerves is variable, related to the relative amounts of fat and fibrous tissue encompassing the lesion.[66]

Hereditary neuropathy Charcot-Marie-Tooth (CMT) syndrome is a rare hereditary motor and sensory neuropathy that can have a confounding MR appearance imitating tumor syndromes such as neurofibromatosis. A positive family history is present in 80% of patients.[67] The typical clinical presentation includes chronic degeneration of peripheral nerves and nerve roots with predominantly distal muscle atrophy and sensory impairment, hyporeflexia, and foot deformities such as high arch and pes cavus. Two-thirds of these lesions are CMT type 1A (demyelinating type) and two-thirds are positive for PMP22 gene.

Bilateral peripheral nerve and lumbosacral plexus involvement are typically present.[67,68] Typical MRN findings include fusiform T1 hypointense and T2 hyperintense masslike symmetric enlargement of the peripheral nerves and/or cauda equina (**Fig. 10**).[69,70] Type II (axonal variety) shows minimal nerve enlargement but abnormal hyperintensity is also observed. Some of the hereditary neuropathy can show abnormal contrast enhancement.[69] Multiple nerve entrapments can be identified, especially with the type III (hereditary neuropathy with liability to pressure palsies [HNPP]) variant.

Treatment is usually conservative with surgery reserved for orthopedic deformity correction or release of disabling or painful nerve entrapments. Prognosis is poor with slow progression over time.

Inflammatory neuropathy Chronic inflammatory demyelinating polyneuropathy (CIDP) is a chronic (greater than 8 weeks) analog to Guillain-Barré syndrome. The patients present with muscle weakness, sensory involvement, and areflexia. Lumbar puncture reveals albuminocytologic

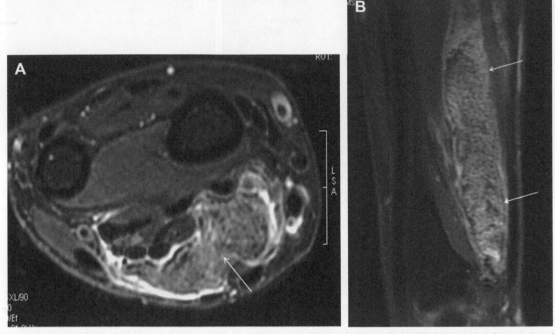

Fig. 8. Neurogenic tumor mimics: fibrolipoma. A 56-year-old man presented with palpable mass in the wrist with thenar muscle weakness. Axial and coronal fat-saturated T2W (*A, B*) images show markedly enlarged median nerve replaced by fibrofatty proliferative tissue (*arrows*) in keeping with fibrolipoma.

dissociation with high cerebrospinal fluid protein. Acute inflammatory demyelination polyneuropathy (AIDP) or Guillain-Barré is the acute form with a better long-term prognosis. AIDP is usually diagnosed clinically with history of prior infection, typical physical examination findings, and lumbar puncture. Multifocal mononeuropathy (MMN) is an additional inflammatory condition with a variable prognosis. CIDP is more common in the lower extremity, whereas MMN is more common in the upper extremity.

MRN findings include focal or diffuse, asymmetric fusiform enlargement of cauda equina, nerve roots/plexus, and peripheral nerves **(Fig. 11)**.[71] The affected nerves are T1 isointense, T2 hyperintense with mild to moderate contrast enhancement.[71] Although the diagnosis is typically made on clinical grounds, many patients have atypical presentation

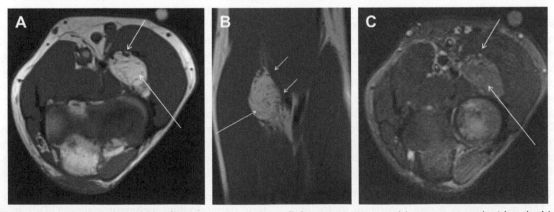

Fig. 9. Neurogenic tumor mimics: lipoma encasing the radial nerve. A 56-year-old man presented with palpable mass in the forearm with radial-sided forearm pain. Axial T1W image (*A*) and coronal T1W image (*B*) shows a hyperintense fat signal mass (*large arrows*) enveloping the radial nerve (*small arrows*). Axial fat-saturated T2W image (*C*) shows fat signal suppression (*large arrow*) and mild hyperintensity of the radial nerve (*small arrow*) in keeping with compressive neuropathy.

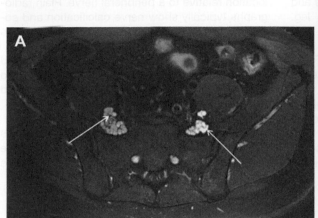
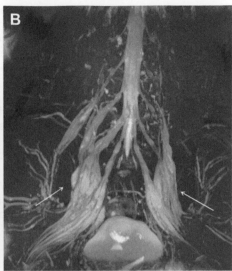

Fig. 10. Neurogenic tumor mimics: hereditary neuropathy. A 51-year-old man presenting with right lower extremity weakness had peripheral nerve root enlargement of bilateral lumbar plexuses. Axial T2 SPAIR (A) image shows bilateral peripheral nerve root enlargement with maintenance of the fascicular pattern (*arrows*). Coronal MIP 3D STIR SPACE image (B) shows diffuse, nearly symmetric peripheral nerve enlargement (*arrows*). There was no associated contrast enhancement. The patient had a strong family history of neuropathy and the constellation of findings are consistent with hereditary neuropathy.

requiring imaging and nerve biopsy for confirmation. Skeletal survey and cross-sectional studies can aid in detection of underlying malignancy, particularly myeloma, which can be seen in association with CIDP.

Infectious neuropathy Although infection can affect the peripheral nervous system, it is rare and does not usually produce masslike enlargement of the affected nerve. However, leprosy is an exception. Leprosy is caused by *Mycobacterium*

leprae with a predilection for dermal and neural cells. In most cases, the neural lesion remains as a granuloma; however, in some cases an abscess can be identified. There are 3 types of leprosy: tuberculoid, lepromatous, and borderline. Abscess formation is most often seen in the tuberculoid form. Differentiation between the three forms of leprosy is based on the clinical picture, bacterial load, and the individual's immune response. Tuberculoid leprosy primarily affects pressure-dependent nerves. Lepromatous leprosy causes

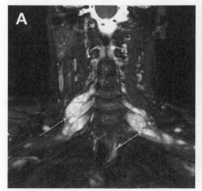
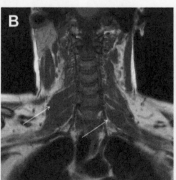
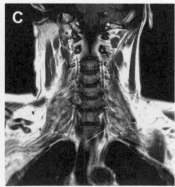

Fig. 11. Neurogenic tumor mimics: inflammatory neuropathy. CIDP. A 48-year-old woman with a history of thyroid carcinoma presented with sensory neuropathy. Coronal STIR (A) image shows bilateral brachial plexus enlargement (*arrows*). Coronal T1W image (B) shows homogeneous nerve enlargement bilaterally (*arrows*). Coronal postcontrast T1W image (C) shows homogeneous mild to moderate enhancement (*arrows*). The patient underwent biopsy confirmation of chronic inflammatory demyelinating polyneuropathy. The patient also improved with plasmapheresis.

widespread symmetric nerve damage with extensive intracutaneous nerve involvement, resembling symmetric polyneuropathy. Sensory loss occurs in the coolest areas of body, such as the hands and feet, ears, and anterolateral parts of the leg. Borderline leprosy has characteristics of both tuberculoid and lepromatous types.

MR imaging has limited role in leprosy. MR imaging shows diffuse enlargement and hypersensitivity of the peripheral nerve.[72,73] Ulnar and peroneal nerves are most commonly involved, but this is nonspecific and can be seen in other conditions such as hereditary or inflammatory neuropathy. The presence of granuloma or abscess formation suggests leprosy. Leprosy-associated nerve abscess follows the same signal characteristics as abscess in remainder of the body with peripheral enhancement.[73] The key to diagnosis is location relative to a peripheral nerve. Plain radiographs typically show nerve calcification and so-called licked-candy-stick stigmata in small bones of hands.

Treatment includes steroid treatment followed by epineurotomy and external decompression to decrease the pressure throughout the involved nerve segment.

Intraneural ganglion Intraneural ganglion cysts are mucinous cysts arising from neural connective tissue. However, many of the lesions classified as

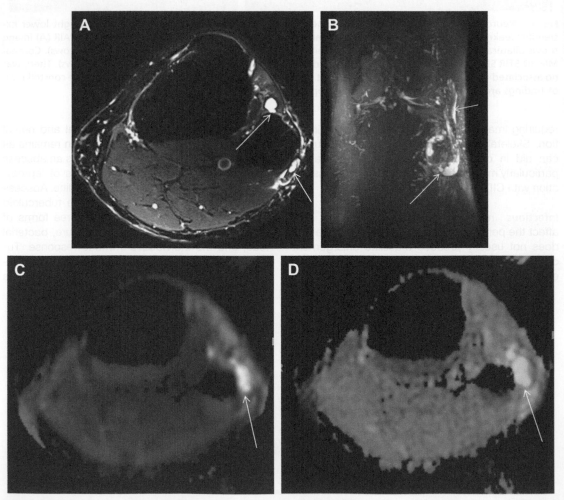

Fig. 12. Nonneurogenic tumor mimics: common peroneal nerve ganglion. A 59-year-old man presented with foot drop. Axial T2 SPAIR images (*A*) and coronal MIP 3D DW PSIF image (*B*) show a multilocular complex cyst (*large arrows*) arising from the proximal tibial fibular joint, extending retrograde along the intra-articular branch of the common peroneal nerve (CPN) and enveloping the CPN (*small arrows*). DTI (*C*) and apparent diffusion map (*D*) show T2 shine-through artifact with lack of restriction in the lesion in keeping with a cyst (*arrow*). The findings were confirmed surgically and the ganglion as well as the intra-articular branch was resected.

intraneural ganglion are extraneural ganglion cysts originating from adjacent joint capsules and tendon sheaths with extension into the epineurium. Approximately three-quarters of reported intraneural ganglion are associated with the common peroneal nerve arising from the proximal tibiofibular joint.[66,74] The adjacent joint shows evidence of internal derangement. The clinical presentation includes slow or fluctuating motor loss.

On MR imaging, the lesion is a unilocular or multilocular cystic mass that is T1 hypointense, T2 hyperintense, with thin peripheral enhancement in close proximity to a joint with internal derangement such as a Baker cyst, paralabral cyst, or ganglion cyst (**Fig. 12**). MRN imaging can show the relationship of the cyst with the affected nerve and its various branches.

Amyloidosis Primary systemic amyloidosis is related to deposition of insoluble, monoclonal immunoglobulin light changes in various tissues with hepatic, cutaneous, cardiac, renal, and, less commonly, peripheral nervous system manifestations. Amyloidosis can be primary or secondary related to chronic kidney disease, multiple myeloma, chronic infections such as tuberculosis, or osteomyelitis. The patients present with severe progressive mixed neuropathy and autonomic dysfunction. The diagnosis is confirmed with apple-green birefringence on Congo red stain.

On MRN imaging, there can be focal amyloidoma or diffuse bilateral multifocal nerve enlargement with variable enhancement and occasional T2-hypointense foci (**Fig. 13**).[75-77] The lower extremity is more commonly involved, particularly the lumbosacral plexus and sciatic nerves. The prognosis is variable but generally poor with a slow progressive deterioration.

Lymphoma Neurolymphoma or lymphomatous infiltration of the peripheral nerves has been

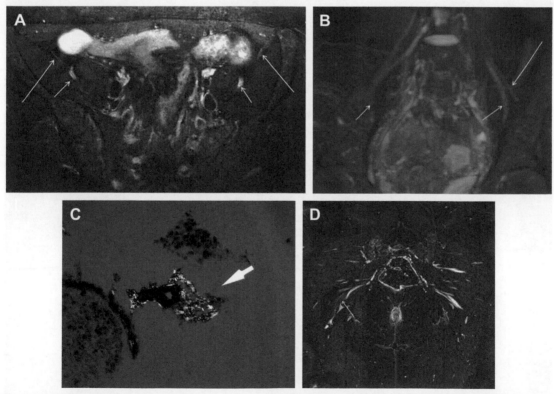

Fig. 13. Nonneurogenic tumor mimics: amyloidosis. A 37-year-old woman with known history of multiple myeloma presented with progressive, chronic right-sided foot drop. Axial T2 SPAIR image (*A*) shows abnormally hyperintense and mildly enlarged bilateral femoral nerves (*small arrows*) and lateral femoral cutaneous nerves (*large arrows*), left worse than right. There was also sciatic neuropathy (not shown). Coronal MIP 3D STIR SPACE image (*B*) shows thickened femoral nerves (*small arrows*) and left lateral femoral cutaneous nerve (*large arrow*) suggesting the diagnosis of amyloidosis in view of the history of myeloma. The patient underwent sural nerve biopsy, which showed apple-green birefringence (*arrow*) on Congo red stain (*C*), confirming the diagnosis. Coronal postcontrast Volume Interpolated Breath-hold Examination (VIBE) subtraction image (*D*) shows minimal asymmetric hyperintensity of the right sciatic nerve (*arrow*).

reported in less than 40% of patients dying with lymphoma. It is seen in the setting of known hematologic malignancy. It is related to non-Hodgkin lymphoma in 90% and leukemia or chloroma in 10%.[77–81] It presents with progressive painful sensorimotor neuropathy. Most commonly, enlarged lymph nodes compress or infiltrate the affected peripheral nerve. Primary neurolymphomatosis, which is extremely rare, involves the peripheral nerves without systemic hematologic malignancy. The diagnosis is confirmed with nerve biopsy or autopsy.

MR findings of enhancing mass within a peripheral nerve in a patient with known leukemia or lymphoma or immunocompromised status should raise concern for neurolymphoma (Fig. 14).[66] MRN imaging typically shows diffuse enlargement of the nerves and/or multifocal nodularity with intense enhancement.[79]

Intraneural epithelial or mesenchymal tumor Intraneural metastasis from carcinoma is extremely rare. Nerve involvement occurs because of direct extension of disease rather than intraneural development or hematogenous spread. Kim and colleagues[64] reported the brachial plexus as the most common site of neural metastases, typically by breast or lung primary cancer. It is most commonly seen in head and neck neoplasms, especially adenoid cystic carcinoma with cranial

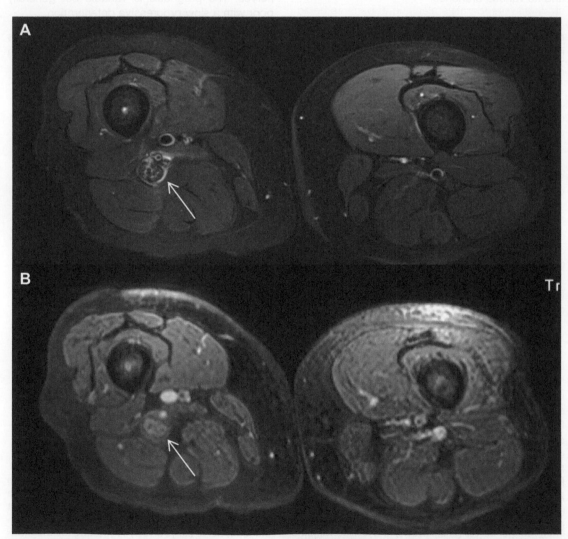

Fig. 14. Nonneurogenic tumors: neurolymphoma. A 68-year-old woman with known history of lymphoma presented with right lower extremity weakness. Axial T2 SPAIR image (A) shows asymmetric enlargement of the right sciatic nerve with internal heterogeneity and enlarged as well as disrupted fascicles (arrow). Postcontrast VIBE image (B) shows enhancement of the abnormal region (arrow).

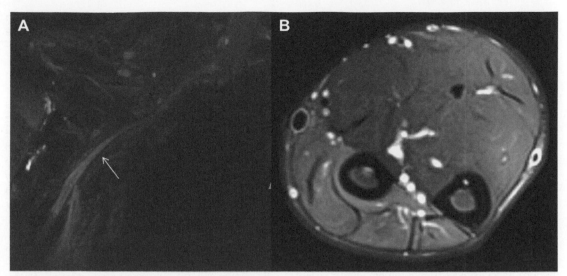

Fig. 15. Nonneurogenic tumors: intraneural epithelial sarcoma. A 24-year-old man presented with right arm weakness. Coronal 3D MIP image (*A*) shows peripheral nerve enlargement (*arrow*) and abnormal signal with associated enhancement on postcontrast images. Axial T2 SPAIR image (*B*) shows denervation edema in the posterior compartment as well as enlargement of the radial nerve.

nerve involvement. In primary epithelioid or mesenchymal sarcoma, patients present with gradual mononeuropathy symptoms.

MR findings that may aid in differentiating metastatic from primary lesions include multiplicity, evidence of direct invasion, and evidence of other metastases such as nodal or osseous disease.[82] Evidence of direct invasion but local metastasis or sarcoma can help as well. With primary sarcoma or granulosa cell tumor, there is heterogeneous fusiform enlargement of the nerve with heterogeneous enhancement with tumors (**Fig. 15**). Prognosis is typically poor with malignant lesions and better with benign lesions.

SUMMARY

Peripheral nerve enlargement is associated with a large range of diagnoses (see **Table 1**). There are multiple MR imaging findings that invoke the possibility of a neurogenic tumor. These imaging features do not reliably distinguish between schwannoma and neurofibroma. The various differentiating features between benign PNSTs and MPNSTs are discussed because of the higher likelihood of MPNST in patients with tumor syndromes. Although there are multiple MR features that increase the likelihood of MPNST, the difference between the benign tumor and malignancy cannot be confidently made with anatomic imaging alone. The sensitivity and specificity is increased with metabolic PET imaging and in the future possibly with functional MR spectroscopy and DTI. The addition

of functional diffusion tractography imaging can provide vital information about neural integrity in benign and malignant peripheral nerve lesions. Future directions will include combinations of metabolic, functional, and anatomic imaging to differentiate these clinical entities. A close working relationship with the clinician is necessary, especially for relevant past medical and family histories in the setting of inflammatory or hereditary neuropathy. Although MRN imaging can show peripheral nerve enlargement as the cause of the patient's symptoms, a definitive diagnosis sometimes may not be reached and a biopsy may be necessary. It is essential for the radiologist to provide a relevant differential diagnosis and obtain advanced imaging in appropriate cases because it directly influences patient care paradigms.

REFERENCES

1. Kransdorf MJ. Benign soft-tissue tumors in a large referral population: distribution of specific diagnoses by age, sex, and location. AJR Am J Roentgenol 1995;164:395–402.
2. Enzinger FM, Weiss SW. Benign tumors of peripheral nerves. Soft tissue tumors. 3rd edition. St Louis (MO): Mosby; 1995. p. 821–88.
3. Jee WH, Oh SN, McCauley T, et al. Extraaxial neurofibromas versus neurilemmomas: discrimination with MRI. AJR Am J Roentgenol 2004; 183:629–33.
4. Harder A, Wesemann M, Hagel C, et al. Hybrid neurofibroma/schwannoma is overrepresented

among schwannomatosis and neurofibromatosis patients. Am J Surg Pathol 2012;36(5):702–9.

5. Le LQ, Liu C, Shipman T, et al. Susceptible stages in Schwann cells for NF1-associated plexiform neurofibroma development. Cancer Res 2011; 71(13):4686–95.

6. Waggoner DJ, Towbin J, Gottesman G, et al. Clinic-based study of plexiform neurofibromas in neurofibromatosis 1. Am J Med Genet 2000; 92(2):132–5.

7. Tonsgard JH, Kwak SM, Short MP, et al. CT imaging in adults with neurofibromatosis-1: frequent asymptomatic plexiform lesions. Neurology 1998; 50(6):1755–60.

8. Prada CE, Rangwala FA, Martin LJ, et al. Pediatric plexiform neurofibromas: impact on morbidity and mortality in neurofibromatosis type 1. J Pediatr 2012;160(3):461–7.

9. Murphey MD, Smith WS, Smith SE, et al. From the archives of the AFIP. Imaging of musculoskeletal neurogenic tumors: radiologic-pathologic correlation. Radiographics 1999;19:1253–80.

10. Banks KP. Signs in imaging. The target sign: extremity. Radiology 2005;234(3):899–900.

11. Varma DG, Moulopoulos A, Sara AS, et al. MR imaging of extracranial nerve sheath tumors. J Comput Assist Tomogr 1992;16:448–53.

12. Bhargava R, Parham DM, Lassater OE, et al. MR imaging differentiation of benign and malignant peripheral nerve sheath tumors: use of the target sign. Pediatr Radiol 1997;27:124–9.

13. Lim R, Jaramillo D, Poussaint TY, et al. Superficial neurofibroma: a lesion with unique MRI characteristics in patients with neurofibromatosis type I. AJR Am J Roentgenol 2005;184:962–8.

14. Isobe K, Shimizu T, Akahane T, et al. Imaging of ancient schwannoma. AJR Am J Roentgenol 2004;183(2):331–6.

15. Capone F, Pravatà E, Novello M, et al. A rare case of life-threatening giant plexiform schwannoma. Spine J 2012;12(1):83.

16. Rodriguez FJ, Folpe AL, Giannini C, et al. Pathology of peripheral nerve sheath tumors: diagnostic overview and update on selected diagnostic problems. Acta Neuropathol 2012;123(3):295–319. http://dx.doi.org/10.1007/s00401-012-0954-z.

17. Heibrun ME, Tsurda JS, Townsend JJ, et al. Intraneural perineurioma of the common peroneal nerve: case report and review of the literature. J Neurosurg 2001;94:811–5.

18. Emory TS, Scheitbauer BW, Hirose T, et al. Intraneural perineurioma: a clonal neoplasm associated with abnormalities of the chromosome 22. Am J Clin Pathol 1995;103:696–704.

19. Wadhwa V, Thakkar R, Maragakis N, et al. Sciatic nerve tumors and tumor like lesions – uncommon pathologies. Skeletal Radiol 2012;41:763–74.

20. Merlini L, Viallon M, De Caoulon G, et al. MRI neurography and diffusion tensor imaging of sciatic perineurioma in a child. Pediatr Radiol 2008;38: 1009–12.

21. Lacour-Petit MC, Lozeron P, Ducreux D. MRI of peripheral nerve lesions of the lower limbs. Neuroradiology 2003;45(3):166–70.

22. Mauremann ML, Armrami KK, Kuntx NL, et al. Longitudinal study of intraneural perineurioma – a benign focal hypertrophic neuropathy of the youth. Brain 2009;132(8):2265–76.

23. Ducatman DB, Scheithauer BW, Piepgras DG, et al. Malignant peripheral nerve sheath tumors: a clinicopathologic study of 120 cases. Cancer 1986;57:2006–21.

24. Mautner VF, Friedrich RE, von Deimling A, et al. Malignant peripheral nerve sheath tumours in neurofibromatosis type 1: MRI supports the diagnosis of malignant plexiform neurofibroma. Neuroradiology 2003;45:618–25.

25. Ferner RE, Golding JF, Smith M, et al. [18F]2-fluoro-2-deoxy-D-glucose positron emission tomography (FDG PET) as a diagnostic tool for neurofibromatosis 1 (NF1) associated malignant peripheral nerve sheath tumours (MPNSTs): a long-term clinical study. Ann Oncol 2008;19(2): 390–4.

26. Warbey VS, Ferner RE, Dunn JT, et al. FDG PET/CT in the diagnosis of malignant peripheral nerve sheath tumours in neurofibromatosis type-1. Eur J Nucl Med Mol Imaging 2009;36(5):754–7.

27. Benz MR, Czernin J, Dry SM, et al. Quantitative F18-fluorodeoxyglucose positron emission tomography accurately characterizes peripheral nerve sheath tumors as malignant or benign. Cancer 2010;116(2):451–8.

28. Wasa J, Nishida Y, Tsukushi S, et al. MRI Features in the differentiation of malignant peripheral nerve sheath tumors and neurofibromas. AJR Am J Roentgenol 2010;194(6):1568–74.

29. Chhabra A, Soldatos T, Durand DJ, et al. The role of magnetic resonance imaging in the diagnostic evaluation of malignant peripheral nerve sheath tumors. Indian J Cancer 2011;48(3):328–34.

30. Matsumine A, Kusuzaki K, Nakamura T, et al. Differentiation between neurofibromas and malignant peripheral nerve sheath tumors in neurofibromatosis 1 evaluated by MRI. J Cancer Res Clin Oncol 2009;135(7):891–900.

31. Chhabra A, Thakkar RS, Andresiek G, et al. Anatomic MR imaging and functional diffusion tensor imaging of peripheral nerve tumors and tumor like conditions. AJNR Am J Neuroradiol 2013;34(4):802–7.

32. Oka K, Yakushiji T, Sato H, et al. Ability of diffusion-weighted imaging for the differential diagnosis between chronic expanding hematomas and

malignant soft tissue tumors. J Magn Reson Imaging 2008;28(5):1195–200.

33. Tamai K, Koyama T, Saga T, et al. The utility of diffusion-weighted MR imaging for differentiating uterine sarcomas from benign leiomyomas. Eur Radiol 2008;18:723–30.

34. van Rijswijk CS, Kunz P, Hogendoorn PC, et al. Diffusion-weighted MRI in the characterization of soft-tissue tumors. J Magn Reson Imaging 2002; 15(3):302–7.

35. Nagata S, Nishimura H, Uchida M, et al. Diffusion-weighted imaging of soft tissue tumors: usefulness of the apparent diffusion coefficient for differential diagnosis. Radiat Med 2008;26:287–95.

36. Einarsdottir H, Karlsson M, Wejde J, et al. Diffusion-weighted MRI of soft tissue tumours. Eur Radiol 2004;14(6):959–63.

37. Genovese E, Cani A, Rizzo S, et al. Comparison between MRI with spin-echo echo-planar diffusion-weighted sequence (DWI) and histology in the diagnosis of soft-tissue tumours. Radiol Med 2011;116(4):644–56.

38. Wang CK, Li CW, Hsieh TJ, et al. Characterization of bone and soft tissue tumors with in vivo 1H MR spectroscopy: initial results. Radiology 2004; 232(2):599–605.

39. Fayad LM, Salibi N, Wang X, et al. Quantification of muscle choline concentrations by proton MR Spectroscopy at 3 T: technical feasibility. AJR Am J Roentgenol 2010;194(1):73–9.

40. Fayad LM, Wang X, Salibi N, et al. A feasibility study of quantitative molecular characterization of musculoskeletal lesions by proton MR spectroscopy at 3 T. AJR Am J Roentgenol 2010;195(1):69–75.

41. Lee CW, Lee JH, Kim DH, et al. Proton magnetic resonance spectroscopy of musculoskeletal lesions at 3 T with metabolite quantification. Clin Imaging 2010;34(1):47–52.

42. Brooks JS, Freeman M, Enterline HT. Malignant "Triton" tumors. Natural history and immunohistochemistry of nine new cases with literature review. Cancer 1985;55:2543–9.

43. Yakulis R, Manack L, Murphy AI. Postradiation malignant triton tumor. A case report and review of the literature. Arch Pathol Lab Med 1996;120:541–8.

44. Woodruff JM, Chernik NL, Smith MC, et al. Peripheral nerve tumors with rhabdomyosarcomatous differentiation (malignant "Triton" tumors). Cancer 1973;32:426–39.

45. Stasik CJ, Tawfik O. Malignant peripheral nerve sheath tumor with rhabdomyosarcomatous differentiation (malignant triton tumor). Arch Pathol Lab Med 2006;130:1878–81.

46. Terzic A, Bode B, Gratz KW, et al. Prognostic factors for the malignant triton tumor of the head and neck. Head Neck 2009;31:679–88. http://dx.doi.org/10.1002/hed.21051.

47. Cawthon RM, Weiss R, Xu GF, et al. A major segment of the neurofibromatosis type 1 gene: cDNA sequence, genomic structure, and point mutations. Cell 1990;62:193–201.

48. Trofatter JA, MacCollin MM, Rutter JL, et al. A novel moesin-, ezrin-, radixin-like gene is a candidate for the neurofibromatosis 2 tumor suppressor. Cell 1993;75:826.

49. Rouleau GA, Merel P, Lutchman M, et al. Alteration in a new gene encoding a putative membrane-organizing protein causes neuro-fibromatosis type 2. Nature 1993;363:515–21.

50. Hulsebos TJ, Plomp AS, Wolterman RA, et al. Germline mutation of INI1/SMARCB1 in familial schwannomatosis. Am J Hum Genet 2007;80: 805–10.

51. MacCollin M, Chiocca EA, Evans DG, et al. Diagnostic criteria for schwannomatosis. Neurology 2005;64:1838–45.

52. NIH Consensus Conference. Neurofibromatosis. Conference statement. National Institutes of Health Consensus Development Conference. Arch Neurol 1988;45:575–8.

53. Duong TA, Sbidian E, Valeyrie-Allanore L, et al. Mortality associated with neurofibromatosis 1: a cohort study of 1895 patients in 1980-2006 in France. Orphanet J Rare Dis 2011;6:18.

54. Evans DG, O'Hara C, Wilding A, et al. Mortality in neurofibromatosis 1: in North West England: an assessment of actuarial survival in a region of the UK since 1989. Eur J Hum Genet 2011;19(11): 1187–91. http://dx.doi.org/10.1038/ejhg.2011.113.

55. Gonzalvo A, Fowler A, Cook RJ, et al. Schwannomatosis, sporadic schwannomatosis, and familial schwannomatosis: a surgical series with long-term follow-up. Clinical article. J Neurosurg 2011; 114(3):756–62.

56. Ruggieri M, Huson SM. The clinical and diagnostic implications of mosaicism in the neurofibromatoses. Neurology 2001;56(11):1433–43.

57. Plotkin SR, Bredella MA, Cai W, et al. Quantitative assessment of whole-body tumor burden in adult patients with neurofibromatosis. PLoS One 2012;7(4): e35711. http://dx.doi.org/10.1371/journal.pone. 0035711.

58. Chhabra A, Blakely J. Whole-body imaging in schwannomatosis. Neurology 2011;76:2035.

59. Cai W, Kassarjian A, Bredella MA, et al. Tumor burden in patients with neurofibromatosis types 1 and 2 and schwannomatosis: determination on whole-body MR images. Radiology 2009;250:665–73.

60. Bhattacharyya AK, Perrin R, Guha A. Peripheral nerve tumors: management strategies and molecular insights. J Neurooncol 2004;69:335–49.

61. Boutin RD, Pathria MN, Resnick D. Disorders in the stumps of amputee patients: MR imaging. AJR Am J Roentgenol 1998;171(2):259–62.

62. Chhabra A, Williams EH, Wang KC, et al. MR neurography of neuromas related to nerve injury and
entrapment with surgical correlation. AJNR Am J
Neuroradiol 2010;31:1363–8.

63. Burchiel KJ, Johans TJ, Ochoa J. The surgical
treatment of painful amputation neuromas.
J Neurosurg 1993;78:714–9.

64. Kim DH, Murovic JA, Tiel RL, et al. A series of
146 peripheral non-neural sheath nerve tumors:
30 year experience at Louisiana State University
Health Sciences Center. J Neurosurg 2005;102(2):
256–66.

65. Marom EM, Helms CA. Fibrolipomatous hamartoma: pathognomonic on MR imaging. Skeletal Radiol 1999;28(5):260–4.

66. Van Breuseghem I, Sicot R, Pans S, et al. Fibrolipomatous hamartoma in the foot: atypical MR imaging
findings. Skeletal Radiol 2003;32(11):651–5.

67. Berciano J, Combarros O. Hereditary neuropathies. Curr Opin Neurol 2003;16(5):613–22.

68. Choi SK, Bowers RP, Buckthal PE. MR imaging in
hypertrophic neuropathy: a case of hereditary motor and sensory neuropathy, type I (Charcot-Marie-
Tooth). Clin Imaging 1990;14(3):204–7.

69. Chung KW, Suh BC, Shy ME, et al. Different clinical
and magnetic resonance imaging features between Charcot-Marie-Tooth disease type 1A and
2A. Neuromuscul Disord 2008;18(8):610–8.

70. Aho TR, Wallace RC, Pitt AM, et al. Charcot-Marie-
Tooth Disease: extensive cranial nerve involvement
on CT and MR imaging. AJNR Am J Neuroradiol
2004;25(3):494–7.

71. Rowin J. MR imaging of demyelinating hypertrophic polyneuropathy. Neurology 2010;74(14):1155.
http://dx.doi.org/10.1212/WNL.0b013e3181d7d8f3.

72. Sethi S, Solanki RS, Mehandiratta V. Leprotic nerve
abscess. Appl Radiol 2006;35:44–7.

73. Kulkarni M, Chauhan V, Bharucha M. MR imaging
of ulnar leprosy abscess. J Assoc Physicians India
2009;57:175–6.

74. Moore KR, Tsuruda JS, Dailey AT, et al. The value
of MR neurography for evaluating extraspinal
neuropathic leg pain: pictorial essay. AJNR Am J
Neuroradiol 2001;22(4):786–94.

75. Metzler JP, Fleckenstein JL, White CL 3rd, et al.
MRI evaluation of amyloid myopathy. Skeletal Radiol 1992;21:463–5.

76. Thawait SK, Chaudhry V, Thawak GK, et al. High
resolution MR neurography of diffuse peripheral
nerve lesions. AJNR Am J Neuroradiol 2011;32:
1365–72.

77. Misdraji J, Ino Y, Louis DN, et al. Primary lymphoma
of peripheral nerve: report of four cases. Am J Surg
Pathol 2000;24(9):1257–65.

78. Quiñones-Hinojosa A, Friedlander RM, Boyer PJ,
et al. Solitary sciatic nerve lymphoma as an initial
manifestation of diffuse neurolymphomatosis.
Case report and review of the literature.
J Neurosurg 2000;92(1):165–9.

79. Descamps MJ, Barrett L, Groves M, et al. Primary
sciatic nerve lymphoma: a case report and review
of the literature. J Neurol Neurosurg Psychiatry
2006;77(9):1087–9.

80. Baehring JM, Batchelor TT. Diagnosis and management of neurolymphomatosis. Cancer J 2012;
18(5):463–8.

81. Wadhwa V, Salaria S, Thakkar RS, et al. Epithelioid
sarcoma presenting as radial mononeuropathy-
Anatomic magnetic resonance neurography and
diffusion tensor imaging appearances. Skeletal
Radiol 2013. [Epub ahead of print].

82. Woertler K. Tumors and tumor-like lesions of peripheral nerves. Semin Musculoskelet Radiol
2010;14(5):547–58.

Peripheral Nerve Surgery
Primer for the Imagers

Jonathan Pindrik, MD[a], Allan J. Belzberg, MD[b],*

KEYWORDS

- Peripheral nerve trauma • Nerve sheath tumor • Entrapment • Nerve repair • Neurotization

KEY POINTS

- Peripheral nerves may be affected individually or in concert by various pathologic conditions, including trauma, entrapment, tumor, or iatrogenic injury.
- After Wallerian (anterograde) and retrograde degeneration, peripheral nerves may undergo physiologic regeneration, aided by Schwann cells and nerve growth factors.
- Peripheral nerve sheath tumors include more common benign and infrequent malignant pathologic-conditions. The operative approach varies depending on tumor pathology.
- Numerous operative techniques foster peripheral nerve regeneration, including nerve repair with coaptation, nerve grafting with autologous or synthetic grafts, and nerve transfers (neurotization).
- Goals of nerve transfer in brachial plexus injuries include elbow flexion, shoulder stability, and arm abduction. Numerous intraplexal and extraplexal donor nerves exist for neurotization.

INTRODUCTION

The peripheral nervous system represents a complex, organized network of nerves providing sensory, motor, and autonomic control of various end organs within the human body. Because of the anatomy and potential mechanisms of injury, multiple specialties collaborate in the care of patients with peripheral nerve pathologic conditions. The patient population represents a similarly wide spectrum, including neonates with birth-related brachial plexus injuries (BRBPI) to young adults sustaining brachial plexus trauma, and to older adults with nerve entrapments, tumors, or iatrogenic causes of peripheral nerve injury. The variety of pathologic conditions and anatomic regions invites a broad array of surgical techniques used within peripheral nerve surgery. Clear understanding of nerve structure and the peripheral nervous system aids diagnostic and therapeutic approaches to patients with peripheral nerve pathologic conditions.

SURGICAL ANATOMY
Components of a Peripheral Nerve

Peripheral nerves possess a hierarchical internal configuration composed of neural and connective tissue elements[1] surrounded by endoneurium, and multiple myelinated axons join in parallel to form a fascicle. Perineurium envelopes each fascicle and contributes paramount strength to nerve structure.[2–4] The perineurium also represents the blood nerve barrier. Multiple fascicles travel in parallel, surrounded by internal epineurium and an external layer of epineurium. Connective tissue and vasa nervorum reinforce the external layer of epineurium, providing extra support and blood supply. Several nerves within the human body coalesce

Disclosures: None.
[a] Department of Neurosurgery, The Johns Hopkins Hospital, 1800 Orleans Street, Zayed Tower 6-007, Baltimore, MD 21287, USA; [b] Department of Neurosurgery, Johns Hopkins University School of Medicine, 600 North Wolfe Street, Meyer 5-181, Baltimore, MD 21287, USA
* Corresponding author.
E-mail address: abelzbe1@jhmi.edu

Neuroimag Clin N Am 24 (2014) 193–210
http://dx.doi.org/10.1016/j.nic.2013.03.034
1052-5149/14/$ – see front matter © 2014 Elsevier Inc. All rights reserved.

into networks, including the cervical, brachial, and lumbosacral plexuses.

Cervical Plexus

The cervical plexus originates deep to the sternocleidomastoid and emerges anterolateral to the middle scalene muscle. Organized into multiple loops, the cervical plexus controls sensory and motor functions within the neck, posterolateral scalp, and superolateral thorax. Ventral rami from C1-C5 contribute to the cervical plexus and split (except C1) into ascending and descending divisions that join segments from adjacent levels. The ansa cervicalis represents a prominent loop of nerves originating from C1 (superior root) and C2-C3 (inferior root) serving primarily motor functions.

Posterior branches from the cervical plexus provide sensory innervation to the anterolateral neck, scalp between the pinna and external occipital protuberance, and superolateral thorax (**Table 1**).[5] Anterior motor branches from the cervical plexus control suprahyoid and infrahyoid muscles and the diaphragm (see **Table 1**). The ansa cervicalis sends motor branches to infrahyoid muscles, including the sternohyoid, sternothyroid, and omohyoid muscles. Arising mainly from the C4 ventral ramus with contributions from C3 and C5, the phrenic nerve provides the sole motor control of the diaphragm along with innervating the mediastinal pleura and pericardium.[5]

Brachial Plexus

The brachial plexus usually originates from the cervicothoracic spinal roots of C5-T1. As anatomic variants, a prefixed plexus spans the cervical roots C4-C8, whereas a postfixed plexus encompasses roots C6-T2, with negligible contributions from T1 and C5, respectively. Plexus elements are organized in the following sequence:

Roots → Trunks → Divisions → Cords → Branches.

The brachial plexus runs inferolaterally from the vertebral foramina, between the anterior and middle scalene muscles, to below the clavicle and above the first thoracic rib. Plexus elements continue through the axilla, neighboring the axillary artery, to the ipsilateral upper extremity. The C5 and C6 roots join to form the upper trunk, whereas roots C8 and T1 combine to form the lower trunk. The middle trunk arises from the spinal root of C7 alone. The subclavian artery lies deep to the upper and middle trunks and ventral to the lower trunk.[6]

Excluding the anterior and posterior divisions, each segment of the plexus contains peripheral nerve branches. Representing one of the first major branches, the long thoracic nerve emanates from roots C5-C7 to provide motor control of the serratus anterior muscle. Deficits of this nerve result in the familiar examination finding of scapular winging. Important in brachial plexus repair surgery, the suprascapular nerve originates from the upper trunk, traveling posteriorly through the suprascapular notch to innervate the supraspinatus and infraspinatus muscles.

Each trunk divides into anterior and posterior divisions just proximal to the upper margin of the clavicle. Running below and distal to the clavicle, the divisions coalesce into cords, labeled anatomically:

Table 1
Sensory and motor branches of the cervical plexus

Nerve Branch	Origin	Function	Distribution or Target
Lesser occipital n.	C2-C3	Sensory	Posterolateral scalp behind auricle, superolateral neck
Greater auricular n.	C2-C3	Sensory	Skin superficial to parotid gland and around ear; posterior portion of auricle
Transverse cervical n.	C2-C3	Sensory	Anterior neck
Supraclavicular n.	C3-C4	Sensory	Lower neck, superolateral thorax, skin over shoulder
Branch traveling with hypoglossal n.	C1	Motor	Geniohyoid and thyrohyoid mm.
Ansa cervicalis	C1-C3	Motor	Infrahyoid mm.: sternohyoid, sternothyroid, omohyoid mm.
C1-C2 branches	C1-C2	Motor	Rectus capitis anterioris and lateralis mm., longus capitis mm.
C2-C4 branches	C2-C4	Motor	Longus colli and capitis mm.
C3-C4 branches	C3-C4	Motor	Levator scapulae and scalene mm.
Phrenic n.	C3-C5	Motor	Diaphragm

Abbreviations: mm., muscle(s); n., nerve.

- The lateral cord (from anterior divisions of the upper and middle trunk) resides lateral and superficial to the axillary artery.
- The medial cord forms solely from the anterior division of the lower trunk, traveling medial and deep to the axillary artery.
- The 3 posterior divisions combine to form the posterior cord, located dorsal to the axillary artery.

Several terminal branches originate from the cords of the plexus to innervate distal targets (**Table 2**). Between the clavicle and axilla, these cords separate into their respective terminal branches. The lateral cord splits into the musculocutaneous nerve and lateral contribution to the median nerve. The medial cord ultimately forms the ulnar nerve and medial contribution to the median nerve. After sending off the axillary nerve, the posterior cord continues distally as the radial nerve.

The peripheral nerve branches of the brachial plexus provide motor and sensory control of the upper extremities (see **Table 2**). The anatomic location of the divisions implies the functionality of their distal branches:

- The anterior divisions ultimately provide motor control of flexors.[6]
- The posterior divisions ultimately control upper extremity extensors.[6]

Lumbosacral Plexus

Serving sensory, motor, and autonomic functions of the lower half of the body, the lumbosacral plexus arises from lumbar roots L1-L5 and sacral roots S1-S4. Although not organized into divisions or cords, the lumbosacral plexus sends off various branches to the lower trunk, reproductive organs, and lower extremities (**Table 3**). Major proximal branches include the femoral and obturator nerves, both originating from roots L2-L4. The sciatic nerve (L4-S3) traverses the greater sciatic foramen and travels down the dorsal aspect of the thigh, splitting into the tibial and common peroneal nerves proximal to the knee. The common peroneal nerve splits proximally in the upper leg into the deep (L4-L5) and superficial (L5-S1) peroneal nerves. Serving important autonomic functions in the reproductive organs, bowel, and bladder, the pudendal and pelvic nerves originate from roots S2-S4.

PATHOLOGY
Peripheral Nerve Injury

Injuries to peripheral nerves occur through various mechanisms including penetrating or blunt trauma, compression, crush, stretch or traction,

and iatrogenic injury. Civilian nerve trauma most commonly involves stretch or crush injury due to motor vehicle accidents, whereas military nerve trauma frequently involves blast injuries.[7] Nearly 5% of all soft tissue injuries involve damage to nearby peripheral nerves.[8] Peripheral nerve trauma affects the upper extremities in greater than 70% of cases.[7] For instance, the brachial plexus frequently sustains injury in high-velocity motorcycle accidents and BRBPI.[9] The mechanism of injury often predicts the type of peripheral nerve damage:

- Motorcycle accidents frequently involve nerve root avulsions.[9]
- Car collisions typically cause peripheral nerve crush injuries.[9]
- BRBPI can cause transient deficits due to stretch injury or more serious deficits due to nerve root avulsion.

Regardless of the injury mechanism, damage to axonal integrity initiates Wallerian degeneration. This process represents the degeneration of axon segments distal to the site of injury in anterograde fashion.[8] Wallerian degeneration begins soon after axonal injury and results in axonal and myelin disintegration. Macrophages responsible for debris removal can be seen along injured peripheral nerves as early as 3 days following trauma.[8] Endoneurial tubes remain intact and devoid of neural components after phagocytic clearance of axonal and myelin debris.[1]

Neuronal damage proximal to the site of injury also occurs because of axonal dysfunction. The decline in retrograde transport of nutrients along the axon toward the neuronal cell body ultimately leads to a breakdown of cell constituents.[1,8] Microscopy of degenerating neurons reveals chromatolysis, or the destruction of Nissel substance in the nerve cell body. Distal muscle fibers also undergo degeneration and fibrosis when lacking peripheral nerve innervation. Fibrotic change initiates 3 weeks after axonal damage and completes within 18 months of denervation.[1,7] The timeline of muscle atrophy, Wallerian degeneration, and loss of Schwann cells in the distal nerve carries significant implications for nerve grafting and repair.

Sunderland Classification of Peripheral Nerve Injury

Despite their higher resistance to mechanical deformation than central nerves, peripheral nerves undergo reproducible phases of injury.[8] The Sunderland classification represents the most commonly used system of grading peripheral nerve

Table 2
Peripheral nerve branches of the brachial plexus

Peripheral Nerve	Nerve Roots	Site of Origin	Innervated Target	Function
Dorsal scapular n.	C5	C5 root	Levator scapulae and rhomboid mm.	Elevate and adduct scapula
Suprascapular n.	C5, C6	Upper trunk	Supraspinatus, infraspinatus mm.	Arm abduction (<90°), external rotation
Long thoracic n.	C5-C7	Roots	Serratus anterior mm.	Stabilizes scapula to chest wall
Lateral pectoral n.	C5-C7	Lateral cord	Pectoralis major/minor mm.	Arm adduction, internal rotation
Medial pectoral n.	C8, T1	Medial cord	Pectoralis major/minor mm.	Arm adduction, internal rotation
Thoracodorsal n.	C6-C8	Posterior cord	Latissimus dorsi mm.	Arm adduction
Axillary n.	C5, C6	Posterior cord	Deltoid, teres minor mm.	Arm abduction (>90°), external rotation
Radial n.	C5-C8	Posterior cord	Triceps, supinator, brachioradialis mm., extensor carpi radialis longus/brevis	Forearm and radial hand extension; forearm supination
Posterior interosseous n.	C7, C8	Radial n.	Extensor carpi ulnaris, extensor digitorum, extensor pollicis longus/brevis, abductor pollicis longus, extensor indicis and digiti minimi	Hand and finger extension, thumb abduction and extension
Musculocutaneous n.	C5-C7	Lateral cord	Biceps, brachialis, and coracobrachialis mm.; forearm radial skin	Forearm flexion and supination; cutaneous sensation to radial aspect of forearm
Medial brachial cutaneous n.	T1	Medial cord	Arm ulnar skin	Cutaneous sensation to ulnar aspect of arm
Medial antebrachial cutaneous n.	C8, T1	Medial cord	Forearm ulnar skin	Cutaneous sensation to ulnar aspect of forearm
Ulnar n.	C8, T1	Medial cord	Flexor carpi ulnaris, lumbricals 3–4, flexor digitorum profundus 3–4, hand interossei, adductor pollicis mm.; abductor, opponens, and flexor digiti minimi mm.	Ulnar hand and finger (digits 4–5) flexion; finger abduction and adduction; thumb adduction; little finger abduction, opposition, and flexion
Median n.	C6-T1	Lateral and Medial cords	Palmaris longus, flexor carpi radialis, pronator teres, flexor digitorum superficialis; lumbricals 1–2, opponens pollicis, abductor and flexor pollicis brevi mm.	Hand and finger flexion; forearm pronation; thumb opposition, abduction, and flexion
Anterior interosseous n.	C7-T1	Median n.	Flexor digitorum profundus 1–2, flexor pollicis longus, pronator quadratus mm.	Finger (digits 2–3) and thumb flexion

Abbreviations: mm., muscle(s); n., nerve.

Table 3
Peripheral nerve branches of the lumbosacral plexus

Peripheral Nerve	Origin	Sensory Distribution	Motor Function	Additional Comments
Iliohypogastric n.	L1	Inferior trunk/abdomen	—	
Ilio-inguinal n.	L1	Inguinal region	—	
Genitofemoral n.	L1-L2	Genital region, groin	—	
Lateral femoral cutaneous n.	L2-L3	Lateral thigh	—	Entrapment causes meralgia paresthetica
Femoral n.	L2-L4	Anterior thigh to knee (anterior femoral cutaneous n.); medial leg from knee to foot (saphenous n.)	Hip flexion via iliopsoas and sartorius mm.; knee extension via quadriceps femoris mm.	
Obturator n.	L2-L4	—	Thigh adduction via adductor longus, magnus, and brevis mm., gracilis mm.	
Superior gluteal n.	L4-S1	—	Thigh abduction via gluteus medius and minimus mm.; thigh flexion via tensor fascia lata mm.	
Inferior gluteal n.	L5-S2	—	Thigh abduction via gluteus maximus mm.	Tested with patient prone
Sciatic n.	L4-S3	Posterior thigh (posterior femoral cutaneous n.); lower leg, sole of foot (tibial n.); sural n.	Knee flexion via biceps femoris, semitendinosus, and semimembranosis mm.; adductor magnus mm.	Semimembranosus, semitendinosus, and biceps femoris mm. commonly referred to as hamstrings
Tibial n.	L4-L5	—	Plantarflexion via soleus, plantaris, gastrocnemius mm.; foot inversion via tibialis posterior mm.; toe flexion via flexor hallucis longus/brevis, flexor digitorum longus/brevis mm.	Tibial n. splits into medial and lateral plantar n. that supply mm. in foot
Deep peroneal n.	L4-L5	—	Foot dorsiflexion via tibialis anterior mm.; toe extension via extensor digitorum longus/brevis, extensor hallucis longus mm.	Extensor hallucis longus mm. represents best test for L5 function
Superficial peroneal n.	L5-S1	—	Foot eversion, plantarflexion of pronated foot via peroneus longus/brevis mm.	Common peroneal n. splits into superficial and deep peroneal n.
Pudendal n.	S2-S4	Perineum and external genitalia	Urethral and external anal sphincters; contraction of pelvic floor	Sympathetic branches regulate ejaculation
Pelvic n.	S2-S4	—	Parasympathetic branches control bowel, bladder, and sexual function	Parasympathetic branches regulate erection

Abbreviations: mm., muscle(s); n., nerve(s).

damage. Divided into 5 ascending degrees of severity, the Sunderland classification stratifies nerve injury based on damage to neural anatomic components (Table 4).

Grade I injuries spare the continuity of the axon, but result in electrical conduction loss. Negligible structural damage with loss of nerve function describes a neurapraxia. The conduction deficit typically resolves, leading to complete recovery.[10] A Sunderland degree II injury involves severing the axon and subsequent Wallerian degeneration distal to the injury. All structural components beyond the axonal level are preserved. Grade III classification indicates damage or disorganization to axons and endoneurium within the fascicles. In addition to Wallerian degeneration, retrograde injury is more pronounced than seen in grade II injuries.[10] Sunderland degree IV injuries involve structural disruption to axons, fascicles, and perineurium with a loss of fascicular anatomy. The most severe class of peripheral nerve injury, Sunderland grade V, involves complete nerve discontinuity. With structural damage to all peripheral nerve anatomic components, nerve regeneration without intervention does not typically occur.[10]

Peripheral Nerve Regeneration and Neuroma Formation

Distal targets of peripheral nerves release trophic factors to promote growth and survival of axons and neuronal cell bodies. Following axonal damage, proximal axonal sprouts grow distally, seeking these trophic factors. Chemotactic factors released by distal targets also help guide sprouting axons to the appropriate destination. Peripheral nerve regeneration occurs at an approximate rate of 1 mm/d or 1 inch/mo.[1] After extending beyond a discontinuity, growing axons may enter endoneurial tubes previously vacated by Wallerian degeneration. The endoneurial tubes, along with trophic and chemotactic factors, act as guides to direct axonal regeneration toward the proper distal target. The entrance of Schwann cells into the endoneurial tubes further supports peripheral nerve reconstitution via myelin formation around budding axons.

The misdirection of axonal sprouting results in neuroma formation. Budding axons that do not properly cannulate an endoneurial tube grow astray, creating a focal tangle of regenerating axons, Schwann cells, and fibrotic tissue. Scarring of endoneurial tubes exacerbates this process as sprouting axons lack proper channels to enter. Intrafascicular hemorrhage and edema in significant nerve injury also contribute to the process of scarring in neuroma formation.[1,10]

Multiple factors influence the success of peripheral nerve regeneration following injury. In general, younger patients show better rates of recovery and functional improvement than older patients.[9] The location of the lesion also bears considerable weight on the success of peripheral nerve regeneration. Proximal lesions, including nerve root avulsions, exhibit poor rates of recovery.[9] Similarly, proximal injuries require prolonged regeneration times to reach their targets, increasing the risk of muscle atrophy before reinnervation.

Schwann Cells and Nerve Growth Factors

Schwann cells and nerve growth factors (NGFs) play critical roles in the development, maintenance, and regeneration of peripheral nerves. Beyond providing myelin sheaths to enhance action potential conduction, Schwann cells aid peripheral nerve regeneration along with NGFs:

Table 4
Sunderland classification of peripheral nerve injury

Sunderland Degree	Components Damaged	Clinical Outcome Expected	Additional Comments
I	No structural damage; only conduction loss	Complete recovery	Consistent with neurapraxia
II	Axon, myelin	Complete recovery	Longer recovery period than degree I injuries
III	Axon, endoneurium, fascicle	Incomplete recovery with residual deficit	Intrafascicular hemorrhage and fibrosis complicate recovery
IV	Axon, endoneurium, fascicle, perineurium, internal epineurium	Partial spontaneous recovery; limited function of involved distal targets	Typically requires surgical repair
V	Entire nerve structure	Negligible recovery	Typically requires surgical repair

Data from Sunderland S. A classification of peripheral nerve injuries producing loss of function. Brain 1951;74:491–516.

- Schwann cells contribute to the formation of longitudinal Hanken-Bungner's cell cords that guide sprouting axons toward the appropriate target.[8]
- Schwann cells secrete NGFs and neurotrophins to provide sustenance for regenerating axons.
- Schwann cells also produce collagen and laminin, integral components of peripheral nerve basal laminae.[8]
- Acting as positive chemotactic agents, NGFs help guide sprouting axons to their destination.
- Neurotrophic factors stunt retrograde degeneration from the proximal nerve stump.[8]

CLINICAL EVALUATION

Peripheral nerve injury may lead to motor or sensory deficits, hyperalgesia, or neuropathic pain. Sensory deficits include those of touch, pain, proprioception, or joint sensation, whereas motor deficits range from minor weakness to complete plegia of an affected extremity.[7,10] The clinical evaluation of a patient with suspected nerve pathologic condition broadly includes history, physical examination, and ancillary studies including imaging findings.

Elements of the medical history may provide clues or lead directly to the diagnosis in peripheral nerve disorders. For instance, history of trauma or surgical procedures often suggests the mechanism of peripheral nerve injury. In addition, certain diseases like diabetes mellitus cause higher susceptibility to entrapment or peripheral neuropathy.[1] Physical examination techniques isolate the peripheral nerves involved by assessing sensory and motor function and evaluating palpable masses. Several examination maneuvers (Tinel sign, Froment sign, scapular winging) highlight peripheral nerve deficits.

Imaging modalities and ancillary studies provide valuable information in peripheral nerve disorders. Plain films or computed tomography (CT) may depict a cervical rib in thoracic outlet syndrome (Fig. 1), whereas magnetic resonance (MR) imaging, especially MR neurography, may display a peripheral nerve tumor or pseudomeningocele in the context of nerve root avulsion (Fig. 2). Additional diagnostic tests, including electromyography (EMG) and nerve conduction study (NCS), evaluate neuromuscular function to assess denervation, preservation of motor units, or conduction loss.

TIMING OF SURGICAL INTERVENTION

Timing of surgical intervention depends on several factors including suspected peripheral nerve

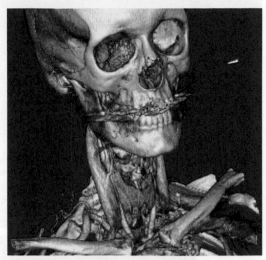

Fig. 1. CT reconstruction of a right cervical rib. Note how it articulates with the first rib.

pathologic conditon, mechanism of injury, neurologic findings, and the presence of physiologic regeneration. Masses along peripheral nerves causing intractable pain or neurologic deficit may warrant early surgical intervention for diagnosis and debulking. Asymptomatic lesions stable in size with a presumed diagnosis (neurofibromatosis or schwannomatosis) may be followed nonoperatively. In traumatic lesions, shorter durations of time between nerve injury and repair offer better chances for regeneration.[9] Prolonged delay between the inciting event and surgical intervention may result in muscle atrophy and loss of support cells in the distal nerve, preventing functional recovery despite adequate nerve regeneration.[9]

Timing in Peripheral Nerve Trauma

The mechanism of peripheral nerve trauma dictates the timing of diagnostic and/or surgical intervention (Table 5). Penetrating injuries causing nerve transection or laceration warrant early surgical exploration. Such lesions can be repaired in the acute setting after stabilization of other traumatic injuries.[1,7] Nerve deficits due to blunt or stretch injury can be evaluated 2 weeks following trauma with NCS and EMG.[1] Abnormal results should prompt clinical follow-up with repeat EMG and NCS at 3 months after injury. Improvement in neuromuscular function warrants nonoperative management with serial examinations and EMG/NCS.[1] However, persistent deficits favor surgical exploration 3 to 6 months after injury.[7] Nerve transfers should be attempted within 6 months after injury to offer the best chance of successful reinnervation.[11] Muscle fibers atrophy and scar

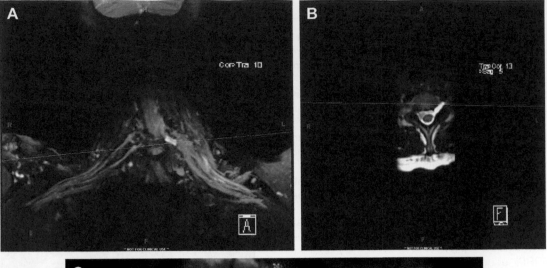

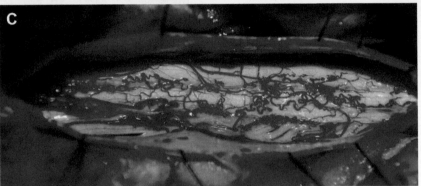

Fig. 2. Nerve root avulsions extending from C6 through T1 on the left with prominent pseudomeningocele formation involving the C8 and T1 nerve root sleeves (*A, B*). An intraoperative image (*C*) follows that shows the avulsion of dorsal nerve rootlets on the left side with preservation on the right side.

Table 5
Timing of diagnostic evaluation and surgical intervention in peripheral nerve injury

Type of Nerve Injury	Acute Setting	Medium Term Follow-Up	Longer Term Follow-Up
Nerve laceration	Early surgical intervention after stabilization of other traumatic injuries	Postoperative clinical examination	Adjuvant surgery as required (tendon or muscle transfers)
Progressive loss of function over 12–24 h	Urgent diagnostic evaluation, surgery for compressive hematoma, pseudo-aneurysm, etc	Postoperative clinical examination	Clinical follow-up to assess recovery
Blunt or stretch injury	Initial clinical examination, stabilization of other traumatic injuries	EMG and NCS at 2 wk following injury	Clinical examinations and repeat EMG/NCS at 3-mo intervals; surgery as needed
Obstetric brachial plexus injury	Initial clinical examination	Repeat clinical assessment at age 3 mo; consider surgical intervention at age 3–6 mo	Delayed repair as needed (tendon or muscle transfers)
Entrapment neuropathy	Clinical history and examination; EMG and NCS	Conservative management, physical therapy, analgesic medications	Surgical considerations if conservative management ineffective

by 12 to 18 months following denervation, whereas vacant endoneurial tubes degenerate 18 to 24 months after Wallerian degeneration, complicating repair.[7] Innervation of free muscle transfers can be performed in delayed fashion after peripheral nerve injury.

Timing in Special Circumstances

Certain clinical contexts require unique consideration regarding timing of intervention (see **Table 5**). Motor deficits progressing over 12 to 24 hours after trauma warrant urgent diagnostic evaluation. Lesions such as a compressive hematoma, pseudoaneurysm, or compartment syndrome may be amenable to operative correction.[1] In contrast, BRBPI undergo evaluation over a longer time course to monitor physiologic recovery. At the age of 3 months, infants with severe BRBPI lacking signs of reinnervation may become surgical candidates. The lack of external shoulder rotation, biceps muscle contraction, or meaningful hand movements indicate severe BRBPI, warranting surgical intervention within the 3- to 6-month age range.[12,13] However, the ideal timing for surgical intervention in BRBPI remains controversial.[13]

DEFINING LESION LOCATION

Clinical history, physical examination, and imaging findings usually predict the location of a peripheral nerve injury or lesion. Blunt trauma or stretch injuries to the brachial plexus rely heavily on examination findings and EMG/NCS to locate the region of damage. The presence of pseudomeningocele on MR imaging or CT myelography suggests nerve root avulsion, consistent with preganglionic injury. The distinction between preganglionic and postganglionic nerve injury significantly impacts surgical decision-making.[11]

Intraoperative Exploration

Intraoperative exploration helps define the precise location of a peripheral nerve lesion. Visual inspection and palpation may reveal the site of injury in cases of peripheral nerve transection, neuroma formation, entrapment, intraneural cyst, or tumor. Blunt or stretch injuries may require more sophisticated techniques including intraoperative nerve stimulation and recordings. Nerve stimulation helps confirm axonal preservation or regeneration by producing observable contractions within distal muscle targets. Intraoperative NCS also helps define the location of injury by confirming the presence or absence of action potential conduction along peripheral nerve segments. Lack of conduction between stimulating

and recording electrodes indicates the absence of functioning axons between electrodes.

Precise localization of injury significantly impacts surgical planning in peripheral nerve repair. Several different methods (neurolysis, direct coaptation, nerve graft, nerve transfer) may be used depending on the current level of neuromuscular function, length of defect, and anticipated rate of regeneration. Determining the specific location of nerve dysfunction helps minimize gap distances when planning for direct repair, grafting, or transfer. NCS and intraoperative nerve stimulation also help determine the extent of surgical intervention. The presence of muscular contraction on nerve stimulation warrants less aggressive measures due to the presence of physiologic regeneration.

PERIPHERAL NERVE ENTRAPMENT

Entrapment neuropathies occur at various locations in the body, often near joints or rigid structures. Peripheral nerves affected by entrapment include the suprascapular, ulnar, median, lateral femoral cutaneous, and common peroneal nerves (**Table 6**). Some peripheral nerve entrapments cause familiar syndromes, including carpel tunnel syndrome and meralgia paresthetica. Peripheral nerve compression typically causes pain, sensory abnormalities, or weakness and muscular wasting in advanced stages.

Pathophysiology of Entrapment

Sites of entrapment occur most frequently near joints, including the wrist, elbow, and knee. Neighboring structures along the nerve, including bone, muscle, tendon, or fibrous tissue, may create an anatomically confined region.[14] Compression of peripheral nerves causes structural and functional damage through multiple mechanisms:

- A fibro-osseous tunnel may cause static compression of a peripheral nerve, especially when tendons or joint capsules become inflamed or edematous.[14]
- A fibrotendinous arcade causes dynamic compression of a peripheral nerve on muscular contraction and narrowing of the arcade.[14]
- Sustained compressive forces cause structural damage and axonolysis, leading to Wallerian degeneration.
- Interruption of microvascular blood flow to peripheral nerves causes ischemia and edema, further compounding entrapment.[14]
- Mechanical compressive forces cause cessation of retrograde and anterograde transport, further aggravating nerve dysfunction.[14]

Table 6
Examples of peripheral nerve entrapment

Peripheral Nerve	Anatomic Region	Compressive Structures and Mechanism	Additional Comments
Brachial plexus lower trunk	Superolateral thorax, supraclavicular region	Cervical rib, elongated C7 TP, or fibrous band between C7 TP and 1st thoracic rib; static compression	Thoracic outlet syndrome; surgical correction places subclavian vessels at risk
Suprascapular n.	Scapula, shoulder	Ligamentous roof of suprascapular notch (transverse scapular ligament)	
Ulnar n.	Medial elbow, cubital tunnel	Osborne's band between 2 heads of flexor carpi ulnaris mm.; dynamic compression	Cubital tunnel syndrome
	Wrist	Guyon's canal; static compression	
Median n.	Wrist, carpal tunnel	Flexor retinaculum or transverse carpal ligament; static compression	Carpal tunnel syndrome; most common entrapment
	Elbow, distal humerus	Ligament of Struthers or supracondylar bony process; static compression	Relatively uncommon
	Upper forearm	Pronator teres mm.; dynamic compression	
Lateral femoral cutaneous n.	Hip, near anterior superior iliac spine	Inguinal ligament; static compression	Meralgia paresthetica; surgical correction risks hernia formation
Common peroneal n.	Knee, proximal fibula	Fibular neck, peroneus longus muscle; static or dynamic compression	
Posterior tibial n.	Foot, tarsal tunnel	Flexor retinaculum between medial malleolus and calcaneus; static or dynamic compression	Tarsal tunnel syndrome

Abbreviations: mm., muscle; n., nerve; TP, transverse process.

Anatomic location of peripheral nerves often dictates the mechanism of entrapment. Median nerve compression in carpal tunnel syndrome occurs via static compression, whereas ulnar nerve entrapment between the 2 heads of the flexor carpi ulnaris occurs via dynamic compression. NCS typically show slowed conduction across a region of entrapment.[14]

Surgical Treatment of Nerve Entrapment

Nerve entrapments refractory to nonoperative measures may be treated surgically with various approaches. Thoracic outlet syndrome due to a cervical rib or elongated C7 transverse process typically requires brachial plexus exploration, definition of the compressed lower trunk, and removal of the aberrant bone or fibrous band. To

decompress the median nerve in the carpal tunnel, the flexor retinaculum of the distal wrist is divided superficial to the nerve. In the case of ulnar entrapment neuropathy, several methods accomplish decompression near the elbow. Dissection along the ulnar nerve with division of Osborne's band between the 2 heads of the flexor carpi ulnaris may suffice. More aggressive measures include a submuscular transposition of the ulnar nerve or medial epicondylectomy. Treatment of meralgia paresthetica typically involves dissection along the lateral femoral cutaneous nerve of the thigh, with division of the compressive inguinal ligament.

PERIPHERAL NERVE TUMORS

Accounting for less than 5% of upper extremity oncologic lesions, peripheral nerve tumors occur infrequently in the lower extremities as well.[6,15] Anatomically, nerve tumors may arise from the nerve sheath, nerve cell, or nonneural precursors (Table 7). Benign nerve sheath tumors occur most commonly, whereas malignant peripheral nerve sheath tumors (MPNSTs) carry the worst prognosis. Peripheral nerve tumors may cause pain, sensory and motor deficits, or cosmetic deformity. Nonneoplastic lesions like intraneural cysts may mimic peripheral nerve tumors; MR neurography aids in their characterization (Fig. 3). Diagnosis of peripheral nerve tumors may be suggested by imaging and examination findings, but are confirmed by surgical sampling and pathologic evaluation.

Schwannoma

The 3 types of nerve sheath tumors, schwannoma, neurofibroma, and MPNST, differ with respect to nerve fascicle involvement, histopathology, and patient presentation (Table 8). Schwannomas occur anywhere along the length of nerve encapsulated by a myelin sheath. In rare instances, multiple schwannomas occur throughout the body in the absence of vestibular tumors (Schwannomatosis). Schwannomas typically displace, rather than encase, neighboring fascicles.[15] Although usually asymptomatic, patients may note cosmetic deformity or a palpable mass. On clinical examination, these lesions can be mobilized orthogonal to the longitudinal axis of the nerve.[15] On microscopic analysis, schwannomas appear solid or cystic and exhibit specific patterns:

- The Antoni A type has a spindle-cell array with collagen matrix arranged into palisading Verocay bodies.[15]
- The Antoni B pattern exhibits a looser structure of mucinous matrix with fewer interspersed spindle cells.[15]
- Cellular schwannomas display high cellular density and nuclear atypia, but contain fewer mitotic figures than malignant schwannomas.[15]

Schwannoma Resection

As schwannomas displace nerve fascicles, careful dissection from peripheral nerves can spare damage to nerve structure and function. The appropriate surgical plane must be found between the tumor capsule and nerve fascicles to accomplish safe and complete resection. Schwannomas carry a low risk of malignant degeneration and rarely recur following excision.[15] The rare disease Schawannomatosis defies these rules however, showing elevated rates of fascicular involvement.

Neurofibroma and Neurofibromatosis

Neurofibromas represent benign nerve sheath tumors and occur within the skin and subcutaneous tissue, or along major peripheral nerves. Nerve fascicles typically traverse the tumor, leading to pain or neurologic deficits in addition to cosmetic deformity. Histologically, neurofibromas appear mucinous with interspersed fusiform tumor cells, collagen matrix, and traversing nerve fascicles.[15] Neurofibromas arise solitarily or as part of neurofibromatosis type I (NF1). The presence of a plexiform neurofibroma suggests NF1 and warrants a search for other stigmata. Neurofibromatosis (NF1 and NF2) represents an autosomal-dominant disorder of neural crest cells with variable phenotype and high proclivity for neoplasia. NF1 exhibits a high rate of malignant transformation, with up to 10% of plexiform neurofibromas converting to malignancy.[15]

Neurofibroma Resection or Biopsy

Neurofibromas offer more challenging surgical resection due to the intimate relationship between nerve fascicles and tumor. Although dermal or subcutaneous neurofibromas can be resected without significant neural impairment, neurofibromas along major peripheral nerves carry higher risks of sensory or motor deficits following resection. Biopsy or cautious debulking may avoid

---

Table 7
Peripheral nerve tumor types

Nerve Sheath Tumors	Nerve Cell Tumors	Nonneural Tumors
Benign nerve sheath tumors	Ganglioneuroma	Metastases
Schwannoma	Neuroblastoma	Lipofibromatosis of the
Neurofibroma	Pheochromocytoma	median nerve
Malignant peripheral nerve sheath tumors		Intraneural lipoma
Malignant scwhannoma		Hemangioma
Fibrosarcoma		Ganglioma

Data from Mackinnon SE, Dellon AL. Surgery of the peripheral nerve. New York: Thieme; 1988.

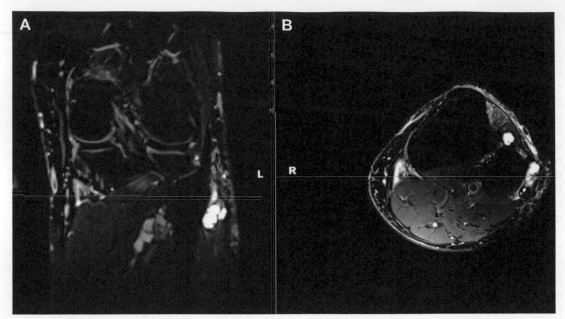

Fig. 3. MR imaging appearance of an intraneural ganglion cyst extending from the tibiofibular joint along the articular branch of the common peroneal nerve (*A, B*).

functional impairment.[15] More aggressive neurofibroma resection may cause peripheral nerve damage or discontinuity, requiring nerve repair or grafting.

Malignant Peripheral Nerve Sheath Tumor

Occurring less commonly than benign nerve sheath tumors, MPNSTs include malignant schwannomas and fibrosarcomas. These tumors often develop from malignant degeneration of neurofibromas in NF1. Patients may present with pain or sensory or motor deficit. Histologically, MPNSTs exhibit hypercellularity, frequent mitoses, and necrosis.[15]

These tumors exhibit high rates of metastatic spread and local recurrence following resection. Identifying neurofibromas with malignant degeneration in patients with NF1 represents a clinical challenge; positron emission tomography and sampling are useful in such contexts.

MPNST Resection

MPNSTs require more aggressive surgical approaches than benign nerve sheath tumors because of their high metastatic potential and local recurrence rates. The greatest chances for prolonged survival often necessitate amputation of

Table 8
Common peripheral nerve sheath tumors

Nerve Sheath Tumor	Histopathology	Nerve Fascicle Involvement	Additional Comments
Schwannoma	Antoni A type: spindle cells and collagen matrix in palisading Verocay bodies	Fascicles displaced	Mostly benign tumor pathologic conditions; malignancy uncommmon
	Antoni B type: loose structure of mucinous matrix with interspersed spindle cells	Fascicles displaced	Mostly benign tumor pathologic conditions; malignancy uncommmon
Cellular Schwannoma	Hypercellularity, nuclear atypia	Fascicles displaced	Fewer mitoses than malignant schwannoma
Neurofibroma	Mucinous matrix of collagen fibers and fusiform tumor cells	Fascicles within tumor	May be solitary or part of neurofibromatosis
MPNST	Hypercellularity, high mitotic activity, necrosis	Fascicles within tumor	High rate of metastatic spread and local recurrence

Data from Mackinnon SE, Dellon AL. Surgery of the peripheral nerve. New York: Thieme; 1988.

the involved extremity or wide local excision with negative margins.[15] In the context of wide local excision, nerve discontinuity can be corrected through a variety of techniques, including nerve repair, grafting, or nerve transfers.

NEUROLYSIS AND NEUROMA RESECTION

Scarring or fibrosis may occur diffusely or focally along the course of traumatized peripheral nerves. Focal neuromas may form at the site of nerve transection or incomplete injury. In the context of neuroma-in-continuity, the involved peripheral nerve may still conduct action potentials along some preserved axons and produce minimal muscular contractions on stimulation. In this context, traumatized peripheral nerves may be treated with neurolysis. Internal neurolysis involves careful dissection along the longitudinal plane of a nerve to expose functioning fascicles. Definition of healthy fascicles and release of scar tissue may enhance nerve regeneration; however, this may also lead to further scarring.

The absence of nerve conduction across a neuroma requires other methods of repair. Neuroma resection and grafting across the nerve defect offer acceptable chances of functional recovery. The proximal and distal nerve stumps should be trimmed back sequentially until the healthy appearance of fascicles. When excessive length of the nerve gap and timing of regeneration preclude grafting, nerve transfers may be used to optimize recovery.

NERVE REPAIR

Nerve repair encompasses different techniques of reapproximating transected nerves. Primary repair with end-to-end coaptation fosters efficient reapproximation with limited morbidity. Coaptation allows sprouting axons from the proximal stump to course along the distal nerve toward the appropriate target, promoting reinnervation and functional recovery. With inconsistent rates of success, end-to-side coaptation may be performed when end-to-end approximation cannot be achieved.[7] Proximal and distal nerve stumps may be realigned using epineurial or perineurial sutures, with fibrin glue reinforcement. Perineurial sutures offer better results for reinnervation if similarly functioning fascicles are lined up appropriately.[7,8] This technique is usually reserved for very distal repairs.

During nerve repair, proximal and distal nerve stumps should be sequentially trimmed back to yield healthy-appearing nerve. The nerve cross-sections should exhibit minimal scarring and normal-appearing fascicles. This process maximizes chances for axonal regeneration but may complicate attempts at nerve coaptation by increasing the gap. Coaptation under tension should be avoided by using other methods of surgical repair.[7]

NERVE GRAFTING
Autologous Nerve Grafting

Nerve grafts or guides may be harvested from multiple sites or created in various ways (**Table 9**). Representing the standard therapy for bridging gaps, autogenous nerve grafts are harvested directly from the patient at the time of exploration and repair.[7] Sural and MABCN represent frequent examples of autografts. The graft ends may be aligned with proximal and distal nerve stumps using small-caliber nylon suture or fibrin glue. Similar to direct coaptation, grafting must be achieved without tension across the nerve construct. Advantages of autografting include the following:

- Presence of Schwann cells that help create an ideal environment for nerve regeneration[8]
- Lack of immunogenicity
- Longitudinal structure of the nerve graft
- Presence of Bungner's bands that help mechanically direct sprouting axons toward the distal target[8]

Disadvantages of autogenous nerve grafts include the following:

- Additional operative time for harvesting grafts
- Limited sources of autologous nerve
- Donor site morbidity
- Potential recipient site reactions (scarring, neuroma formation)[8]

Because of drawbacks of donor site morbidity, limited autograft sources, and prolonged operative times, alternatives to autologous nerve grafting have been explored.

Biologic Nerve Guides

Other anatomic structures may be used as biologic nerve guides to bridge peripheral nerve gaps. Several clinical studies have shown similar results between vein and autologous nerve grafts for gaps up to 30 mm.[8] In addition to their abundant supply, veins offer benefits of no immunogenicity, minimal donor site morbidity, and the presence of collagen and laminin to help foster nerve regeneration.[7,8] The potential drawbacks of using venous nerve guides include compressibility of the venous wall potentially obstructing axonal growth and limited applicability beyond gaps of 30 mm.[8] To

Table 9
Different types of nerve grafts or guides

Type of Nerve Graft or Guide	Examples	Applications	Advantages	Disadvantages
Autologous nerve graft	• Sural nerve • MABCN	• Long nerve gaps • Multiple cable graft repairs	• Superior to coaptation under tension • Presence of Schwann cells • Lack of immunoreaction • Longitudinal structure guides axonal sprouting	• Prolonged operative time for harvesting • Donor site morbidity • Limited graft sources • Complete recovery rare
Biologic nerve graft	• Vein graft • Vein filled with muscle • Vein filled with nerve	• Nerve gaps ≤30 mm • Nerve gaps ≤45 mm	• Lack of immunoreaction • Minimal donor site morbidity • Many harvesting sources • Collagen and laminin content, favorable matrix • Longitudinal structure	• Compressible venous wall • Inconsistent clinical and experimental results • Lack of clinical data for gaps >20–30 mm
Nerve allograft	• Cadaveric donor nerve	• Large nerve gaps	• No donor site morbidity • Shorter operative times • Unlimited graft supply	• Nerve graft rejection • Complications of immunosuppression
Synthetic nerve graft	• Silicon tubes • Collagen • Polyglycolic acid conduits	• Nerve gaps ≤30 mm	• No donor site morbidity • Shorter operative times • Avoids axonal mismatch • Prevents errant axonal outgrowth • Limited neuroma formation • Absorbable materials limit scar formation	• Rigid structure may lead to nerve compression • Inflexible material risks damage and foreign body reaction • Nonpermeable material limits exchange of nerve growth factors

Abbreviation: MABCN, medial antebrachial cutaneous nerve.
   Data from Dornseifer U, Matiasek K, Fichter MA, et al. Surgical therapy of peripheral nerve lesions: current status and new perspectives. Zentralbl Neurochir 2007;68:101–10.

enhance the firmness of venous guides, both denatured muscle and nerve tissue have been infused inside the graft with successful results up to 20-mm and 45-mm gaps, respectively.[8]

Nerve Allografts

Cadaveric nerve grafts represent attractive options for bridging large nerve gaps that exceed the length of available autografts. Furthermore,

this technique avoids donor site morbidity and prolonged operative times of harvesting. However, allografting carries significant risks of nerve graft rejection and complications associated with immunosuppression.[7] Freeze-drying and irradiation techniques have been applied to decrease the immunogenicity of nerve allografts with some success. Nevertheless, nerve allografting has achieved limited clinical exposure since its reintroduction in 2001.[7] Recently, the use of detergent-washed cadaveric nerve grafts has been introduced. These grafts lack cells including Schwann cells, but do retain laminin. They do not require immunosuppression and have been approved for gaps less than 30 mm.

Synthetic Nerve Guides

Artificial nerve guides offer several benefits over using autologous grafts. Without the need for harvesting, synthetic nerve grafts avoid donor site morbidity and prolonged operative times. Furthermore, the firm structure of neural tubes constricts axonal growth in a longitudinal direction, guarding against errant axonal sprouting and neuroma formation.[8] As opposed to autologous nerve grafts, artificial grafts avoid problems of axonal mismatch between sensory and motor fascicles.[8]

Drawbacks of synthetic nerve guides include their rigid structure, risking destruction, or nerve compression in the setting of foreign body reactions.[8] Furthermore, impermeable nerve conduits prevent the exchange of neurotrophic factors with the neighboring environment. Absorbable and permeable artificial nerve guides help reduce these problems and limit scar tissue formation. Despite these advancements, synthetic nerve grafts lack encouraging results for repairs greater than 30 mm in length.[7,8] Based on their limited success in experimental and clinical trials, artificial nerve guides are currently approved only for short peripheral nerve gap repair (≤30 mm).[7]

NERVE TRANSFER

Neurotization, or nerve transfer, involves the redistribution of function from intact to nonfunctioning nerves. A working peripheral nerve or subset of fascicles can be realigned with the distal stump of a nonfunctional nerve to promote peripheral nerve regeneration and reinnervation of selected distal targets, which occurs at the expense of eliciting motor deficits in muscles innervated by the donor nerves. Neurotization promotes meaningful functional recovery by preferentially targeting muscle groups serving basic, evolutionary roles.

Goals, Donors, and Targets in Nerve Transfer

In brachial plexus injuries involving upper trunk deficits, the ultimate goals of nerve transfer include the following:

- Elbow flexion
- Shoulder stability
- Arm abduction

Neurotization represents the preferred approach in preganglionic injuries (nerve root avulsion), as the absence of proximal nerve precludes grafting.[11] In postganglionic injuries, nerve transfers can supplant or accompany nerve grafting or allow innervation of a free muscle flap.

Several donor nerve options exist within and outside of the brachial plexus. Regarding upper trunk injuries, intraplexal donor nerves include the ulnar, median, medial pectoral, and radial nerves. In the same clinical setting, extraplexal donor nerves include the spinal accessory, intercostal, and phrenic nerves. In the context of complete plexus avulsion, the contralateral C7 nerve root may serve as a contributing element in neurotization.[11]

The type of nerve transfer used must be selected based on the specific injury and donor nerve function. Despite various mechanisms and types of injury, brachial plexus lesions can be approached similarly with the common objective of achieving meaningful functional recovery. To recover elbow flexion, shoulder stability, and/or shoulder abduction, the primary distal nerve targets include the following:

- Musculocutaneous nerve motor branches innervating the biceps and brachialis muscles
- Suprascapular nerve innervating the supraspinatus and infraspinatus muscles
- Axillary nerve innervating the deltoid muscle

Examples of Nerve Transfer: Extraplexal Donors

Donor nerves outside of the injured plexus include the spinal accessory nerve, intercostal nerves, and contralateral C7 root. The ipsilateral spinal accessory nerve may be neurotized to the suprascapular, musculocutaneous, or axillary nerves. Transfer to the musculocutaneous or axillary nerves requires a bridging nerve graft due to the length of separation. Frequently used in preganglionic injuries, intercostal nerve transfer represents an alternative method of neurotizing the musculocutaneous nerve. In complete plexus injuries or avulsions, the contralateral C7 root represents a potential donor to the median nerve via a bridging, vascularized ulnar nerve graft.[11] In select cases, the phrenic nerve also may be used for contribution in neurotization; however, the risk of pulmonary compromise typically precludes its usage.

The spinal accessory and intercostal nerves or a fascicle from an ulnar nerve can be used as donors to a free gracilis muscle transfer. Gracilis muscle transfers allow recapitulation of elbow flexion and potentially wrist extension beyond the acute or subacute setting.[11] During gracilis muscle transfer, the obturator nerve will represent the recipient in neurotization.

Examples of Nerve Transfer: Intraplexal Donors

Intraplexal nerve donors receive frequent attention in the context of upper trunk deficits. The classic Oberlin technique involves neurotization between a functioning ulnar nerve and nonfunctioning musculocutaneous nerve. As a modification, the median nerve represents a potential donor to biceps or brachialis branches of the musculocutaneous nerve. Neurotization of a free muscle transfer may also use the ulnar and median nerves as donors.[11] To help preserve shoulder stability and recover arm abduction, a radial (triceps branch)

Table 10
Examples of nerve transfer in brachial plexus injury

Brachial Plexus Components Injured	Donor Nerve	Recipient Nerve	Desired Functional Recovery	Additional Comments
Upper trunk, C5 root	Spinal accessory n.	Suprascapular n.	Shoulder stability, abduction	
Upper trunk	Spinal accessory n.	Musculocutaneous n. Axillary n.	Elbow flexion Shoulder abduction	Requires bridging sural n. graft
Upper trunk	Spinal accessory n.	Obturator n., gracilis muscle transfer	Elbow flexion, wrist extension	May be performed in acute or late setting
Upper trunk, C5-C6 avulsion	Intercostal n.	Musculocutaneous n.	Elbow flexion	Requires 2–3 intercostal n. fibers per transfer Contraindications include major anterior chest trauma
Upper trunk, C5-C6 avulsion	Intercostal n.	Obturator n., gracilis muscle transfer	Elbow flexion	Requires 2–3 intercostal n. fibers per transfer
Complete plexus avulsion	Intercostal n.	Obturator n., gracilis muscle transfer	Finger flexion, elbow extension	Requires 2–3 intercostal n. fibers per transfer
Complete plexus injury	Contralateral C7 nerve root	Median n. Axillary or Suprascapular n.	Hand function Shoulder stability	Requires bridging ulnar n. graft
Complete plexus avulsion	Phrenic n.	Suprascapular n.	Shoulder stability, abduction	Risk of pulmonary compromise; contraindicated in children
Complete plexus avulsion	Phrenic n.	Axillary n. Musculocutaneous n.	Shoulder stability Elbow flexion	Requires bridging n. graft Same risks as above
Upper trunk, C5-C6 roots	Ulnar n. Median n.	Musculocutaneous n.	Elbow flexion	Classic Oberlin technique Modified Oberlin technique
Upper trunk, C5-C6 roots	Ulnar n.	Obturator n., gracilis muscle transfer	Elbow flexion	
C5-C6 avulsion	Radial n.	Axillary n.	Shoulder stability	Short distance of reinnervation through quadrangular space

Abbreviation: n., nerve(s).

Data from Shin AY, Spinner RJ, Bishop AT. Nerve transfers for brachial plexus injuries. Oper Tech Orthop 2004;14:199–212.

to axillary nerve transfer provides reasonable benefit due to the short reinnervation distance through the quadrangular space.[11]

The different types of neurotization may be used individually or in concert. Furthermore, these techniques may be combined with other methods of peripheral nerve repair, including grafting. The various techniques of neurotization used in brachial plexus injuries are summarized in **Table 10**.

FUTURE DIRECTIONS: NERVE GROWTH FACTORS, SCHWANN CELL TRANSPLANTATION, NERVE ALLOGRAFTS

Due to their supportive roles in nerve growth and regeneration, NGFs and Schwann cells represent attractive targets in peripheral nerve research.[7] Multiple experimental studies have shown positive effects of transplanted Schwann cells on nerve regeneration across gaps up to 40 to 60 mm in length.[8] Continued advancement in stem cell biology may offer novel techniques to harvest and cultivate autologous Schwann cells for autotransplantation. Despite experimental success with NGFs and Schwann cells, no major clinical success has been reported. Future testing in animals, including primates, and clinical research efforts may help exhibit the beneficial roles of NGFs and Schwann cells in peripheral nerve repair. Nerve allografting also represents an important area for further research and development to overcome issues related to immunogenicity and immunosuppression.[7]

SUMMARY POINTS

- Peripheral nerves maintain a hierarchical structure composed of axons (surrounded by endoneurium) running in parallel to form groups of fascicles sequentially enveloped by perineurium and epineurium.
- Several peripheral nerves coalesce into networks, forming the cervical, brachial, and lumbosacral plexuses.
- Peripheral nerves may be affected individually or in concert by various pathologic conditions, including trauma, entrapment, tumor, or iatrogenic damage.
- The Sunderland classification grades traumatic peripheral nerve injury based on structural damage with ascending levels of severity. Grade I injuries (neurapraxia) typically recover completely, whereas grade V lesions do not exhibit regeneration without intervention.
- Following Wallerian (anterograde) and retrograde degeneration, peripheral nerves may undergo physiologic regeneration, aided by Schwann cells and NGFs.
- Neuroma formation occurs because of misdirection of sprouting axons from a proximal nerve stump. Compounded by intraneural hemorrhage and edema, fibrosis results in a tangle of axons and scar tissue.[1]
- Neuromas can be treated surgically with neurolysis or resection and grafting depending on the presence of nerve conduction across the lesion.
- Suggested by patient symptomatology, examination findings, and EMG/NCS, entrapment neuropathies occur near joints or rigid structures and can be treated with different methods of nerve decompression.
- Peripheral nerve sheath tumors include more common benign (schwannoma, neurofibroma) and infrequent malignant (MPNST) pathologic conditions. The operative approach varies depending on tumor pathology.
- Timing of surgical intervention in peripheral nerve trauma depends on the mechanism of injury. Nerve transection or laceration warrants early repair following stabilization of other traumatic injuries.
- Nerve deficits due to blunt or stretch injury warrant initial EMG/NCS at 2 weeks following injury. Lack of improvement at 3 months, based on clinical follow-up and repeat EMG/NCS, favors surgical intervention.
- Numerous operative techniques foster peripheral nerve regeneration, including nerve repair with coaptation, nerve grafting with autologous or synthetic grafts, and nerve transfers.
- Neurotization involves the redistribution of function from intact to nonfunctioning nerves to promote peripheral nerve regeneration and reinnervate selected targets.
- The ultimate goals of nerve transfer in the setting of brachial plexus injury include elbow flexion, shoulder stability, and arm abduction. Numerous intraplexal and extraplexal donor nerves exist for neurotization.
- Research efforts target Schwann cells, NGFs, and allografting to enhance peripheral nerve regeneration.

REFERENCES

1. Belzberg AJ. Acute nerve injuries. In: Rengachary SS, Ellenbogen RG, editors. Principles of neurosurgery. 2nd edition. Philadelphia: Elsevier Mosby; 2005. p. 387–95.
2. Kwan MK, Wall EJ, Massie J, et al. Strain, stress and stretch of peripheral nerve: rabbit experiments

in vitro and in vivo. Acta Orthop Scand 1992;63(3): 267–72.

3. Rickett T, Connell S, Bastijanic J, et al. Functional and mechanical evaluation of nerve stretch injury. J Med Syst 2010;35(5):787–93.

4. Sunderland S, Bradley KC. Stress-strain phenomena in human peripheral nerve trunks. Brain 1961;84: 125–7.

5. Moore KL, Dalley AF. Clinically oriented anatomy. 4th edition. Baltimore (MD): Lippincott Williams & Wilkins; 1999. p. 1004–12.

6. Huang JH, Zaghloul K, Zager EL. Surgical management of brachial plexus region tumors. Surg Neurol 2004;61:372–8.

7. Siemionow M, Brzezicki G. Current techniques and concepts in peripheral nerve repair. Int Rev Neurobiol 2009;87:141–71.

8. Dornseifer U, Matiasek K, Fichter MA, et al. Surgical therapy of peripheral nerve lesions: current status and new perspectives. Zentralbl Neurochir 2007; 68:101–10.

9. Lanaras TI, Schaller HE, Sinis N. Brachial plexus lesions: 10 years of experience in a center for microsurgery in Germany. Microsurgery 2009;29: 87–94.

10. Sunderland S. A classification of peripheral nerve injuries producing loss of function. Brain 1951;74: 491–516.

11. Shin AY, Spinner RJ, Bishop AT. Nerve transfers for brachial plexus injuries. Oper Tech Orthop 2004; 14:199–212.

12. Malessy MJ, Pondaag W. Obstetric brachial plexus injuries. Neurosurg Clin N Am 2009;20:1–14.

13. Hale HB, Bae DS, Waters PM. Current concepts in the management of brachial plexus birth palsy. J Hand Surg Am 2010;35:322–31.

14. Belzberg AJ. Entrapment neuropathies. In: Rengachary SS, Ellenbogen RG, editors. Principles of neurosurgery. 2nd edition. Philadelphia: Elsevier Mosby; 2005. p. 397–405.

15. Mackinnon SE, Dellon AL. Surgery of the peripheral nerve. New York: Thieme; 1988.

Magnetic Resonance Neurography–Guided Nerve Blocks for the Diagnosis and Treatment of Chronic Pelvic Pain Syndrome

Jan Fritz, MD[a],*, Avneesh Chhabra, MD[b],
Kenneth C. Wang, MD, PhD[a], John A. Carrino, MD[a]

KEYWORDS

- MR neurography (MRN) - Pudenda nervel block - Posterior femoral cutaneous nerve block
- MR guidance - Pain injection - Nerve block - Piriformis syndrome

KEY POINTS

- Magnetic resonance neurography (MRN)–guided interventional magnetic resonance imaging (MRI) describes a technique for selective nerve blocks, in which limited MRN and interventional MRI are used in combination.
- MRN-guided nerve pelvic blocks favorably combine the benefits of direct visualization of the nerve targets, objective assessment of the distribution of the injectant, and absence of ionizing radiation.
- MRN-guided nerve pelvic blocks achieve high face validity by directly visualizing the target, needle tip, injectant surrounding the nerve, and detection of spread to confounding structures.
- Selective MRN-guided nerve blocks are especially suited for deeply situated and small nerves, which are difficult to visualize and target with other imaging modalities.
- Selective MRN-guided nerve blocks can help diagnose and treat pelvic neuropathies causing chronic pelvic pain syndrome.

INTRODUCTION

Chronic pelvic pain is a multifactorial condition with a high prevalence in the general population and a substantial socioeconomic impact. The estimated prevalence of chronic pelvic pain in women is 3.8%, which is very similar to the prevalence of back pain.[1] An estimated 15% to 20% of women between 18 and 50 years of age experience chronic pelvic pain, which accounts for up to 40% of patients visiting gynecologic outpatient clinics and $881.5 million dollars spent each year on outpatient management in the United States alone.[1–4] The diagnostic workup and management frequently represent a major challenge to health care providers because of multiple possible causes and often poor response to treatment. Patients with chronic pelvic pain use 3 times more medication, have 4 times more nongynecologic surgeries, and are 5 times more likely to have hysterectomy.[5] Chronic pelvic pain syndrome represents a subdivision of chronic pelvic

[a] Musculoskeletal Radiology, The Russell H. Morgan Department of Radiology and Radiological Science, The Johns Hopkins Hospital, 600 N Wolfe Street, Baltimore, MD 21287, USA; [b] Department of Radiology, University of Texas Southwestern, 5323 Harry Hines Blvd, Dallas, TX 75390-9178, USA
* Corresponding author.
E-mail address: jfritz9@jhmi.edu

Neuroimag Clin N Am 24 (2014) 211–234
http://dx.doi.org/10.1016/j.nic.2013.03.028
1052-5149/14/$ – see front matter © 2014 Elsevier Inc. All rights reserved.

pain, with no evidence of an infectious origin and no obvious causative local abnormality.[2] The various causes of chronic pelvic pain syndrome include urologic, gynecologic, gastrointestinal, neurologic, and sexologic causes, and pelvic floor dysfunction. Chronicity may be defined as cyclic and noncyclic pain in women and men for at least 6 months localizing to the anatomic pelvis, anterior abdominal wall at or below the umbilicus, the lumbosacral back, or the buttocks, with associated functional disability, medical care, and negative cognitive, behavioral, sexual, and emotional consequences.[2,6]

Peripheral nerve pain syndromes and pelvic neuropathies constitute an important group of disorders that can cause chronic pelvic pain syndrome.[2] Causes include nerve compression, entrapment, repetitive microtrauma, impact injury, injection injury, surgical incisions, and postoperative scarring. Suggestive symptoms are paresthesia, dysesthesias, allodynia, dysreflexia, dyspareunia, and muscular dysfunction of the anatomic area innervated by the injured nerve. In addition to history, physical examination, and imaging, selective perineural injection with a local anesthetic (nerve block) is a helpful tool in the diagnostic workup of patients in whom a neuropathic origin of pain is suspected (Table 1). Diagnostic nerve blocks are ordered to specifically test the hypothesis that a particular nerve is a source of pain.[7] In cases of unsatisfactory response to conservative therapy, the results of nerve blocks may be used as a tool to help to guide future management. Additionally, locally delivered anti-inflammatory and anesthetic drugs may result in therapeutic benefit by interrupting pathways involved in nociceptor stimulation.[8–10]

MR neurography (MRN)–guided interventional magnetic resonance imaging (MRI) is the combination of limited intraprocedural MRN[11,12] and interventional MRI.[13–15] MRN has the distinct ability to directly visualize and map the course of deep pelvic nerve targets. MRN-guided blocks are typically preceded by high-field MRN, which contributes helpful anatomic information for targeting. With the use of proper technique, the targeted anatomic structure, regional confounding structures, and the location and spread of the injected drug (injectant) can be directly visualized. MRN-guided nerve blocks, therefore, offer exquisite technical accuracy, allowing the interventionalist an objective assessment of the technical validity of the blocks. MRN guidance is especially suited for deeply situated neural targets (pudendal canal, obturator foramen) and small targets (ganglion impar, posterior femoral cutaneous nerve, intrapelvic lateral femoral cutaneous nerve proximal to the inguinal ligament, and neurogenic neoplasms), and where toxic injectants, such as botulinum neurotoxin, are being used. Additionally, MRN guidance is helpful in guiding presurgical planning because of the requirement of a high level of validity.[8]

Ultrasound guidance is frequently adequate for superficial targets; however, deeply situated pelvic nerves are frequently not reliably visualized because of the lack of an acoustic window, limited contrast and spatial resolution, or insufficient penetration depth. Fluoroscopy can guide needle placements using bony landmarks; however,

Table 1
Indications for MRN-guided injections in the pelvis

Diagnostic Nerve Block	Therapeutic Nerve Block
Clinically suspected neuropathy	Adjunct to conservative treatment
Discordance of clinical findings and imaging (false-negative or false-positive results)	Inoperable condition
Presurgical testing (eg, neurolysis and tumor resection in multiple lesions)	Expedite prolonged recovery after surgery
Suspected failed surgery or recurrence	Induce atrophy of the muscle causing nerve compression
Allergy to iodinated contrast agents	Failed nerve surgery or recurrence
	Contraindication or adverse effects to systemic pain medications/steroids and allergy to iodinated contrast agents
	Small piriformis muscle (in a large patient) not adequately visualized or targeted with other techniques

nerves cannot be visualized. Anatomic variants are frequently not seen, which may lead to nerve injury, and confounding spread to adjacent nerves may go unrecognized with fluoroscopy. Computed tomography (CT) guidance has similar limitations and also results in exposure to ionizing radiation. With the exception of the sciatic nerve and piriformis muscle, the low contrast resolution prevents accurate identification of the smaller peripheral nerves without the need for intravenous contrast administration.

MRI guidance obviates procedure-related ionizing radiation exposure of patients and operators, and its related health risks.[16,17] The exact morbidity and mortality related to procedure-related ionizing radiation is not known; however, it was estimated that 1.5% to 2.0% of all U.S. population cancers may be caused by CT radiation exposure.[16] Although the radiation dose of CT can be reduced using intermittent technique and low energy settings, MRN guidance is a preferable technique because of the absence of ionizing radiation. Interventional MRI complies with the ALARA (As Low As Reasonably Achievable) practice mandate in an exemplary fashion and is especially valuable in adolescents, young women of child-bearing age, and pregnant women.[15,17–19] Cumulative radiation doses can be avoided, especially when serial nerve blocks are required.[20] Additional attributes of MRN guidance are the unmatched soft tissue resolution for the differentiation and direct visualization of the target nerve, real-time needle MRI guidance at 1.5 T, easy visualization of the oblique needle paths because of multiplanar imaging capabilities, and real-time monitoring of injections. Because of factors such as cost and time requirements, however, MRN guidance is no substitute for ultrasound and CT guidance, but is rather a tool for selected cases, such as the targeting of and prevention of injury to small and deeply situated nerves for which only MRN guidance can provide the required technical accuracy from direct visualization.

This article discusses the technical background of MRN-guided interventional MRI, reviews important principles of nerve blocks, describes techniques of pelvic injection procedures, and illustrates targets and procedures for the diagnosis and therapy of neurogenic chronic pelvic pain syndrome, in which MRN guidance provides exquisite detail for valid nerve blocks.

MR Imaging Systems

Although MRN-guided interventions may be performed with any MRI system, the introduction of clinical 1.5-T MRI systems with a wide-bore magnet design has greatly improved the utility of MRN-guided injections through obviating the requirement of a dedicated, low-field open magnetic resonance (MR) imaging systems, which were previously used.[8,14,21] The wide bore of the magnet allows improved patient access and needle maneuvering while the patient is in the isocenter of the bore of the magnet, and simultaneous image acquisition and review.[14,15,18] Patient access and the spatial properties are similar to those of current dual-source CT imaging systems.

The use of 1.5-T field-strength magnets, modern coil design and parallel imaging technology can result in less signal averaging and faster image acquisition and display and has advanced the field of MRI-guided and MRN-guided interventions. Because the MR signal increases with the strength of the magnet, MRN-guided injections at 1.5 T provide substantially higher signal-to-noise ratios when compared with low-field MRI systems of 0.2- to 0.5-T strength.[13–15,17–19,22–25] The higher MR signal permits higher spatial resolution and 3-dimensional isotropic MR imaging, which allow direct visualization of small nerves and peripheral branches of the lumbosacral plexus, which is a prerequisite for direct targeting.[26–31] Additionally, higher bandwidths can be used, which are beneficial for accurate needle tip visualization through passive needle artifact creation. Because of proportionally increasing chemical shift, the reliable use of spectral fat saturation techniques is possible, which increases the visibility and detectability of the injected drugs. A field strength of 1.5 T also allows the use of real-time fluoroscopic MR imaging with high spatial and temporal resolution.[15,18,23] MR fluoroscopy describes the continuous acquisition and display of MR images, similar to CT fluoroscopy, which can be used for interactive device handling.[14,15,23]

Safety

The 1.5-T external magnetic field, radiofrequency pulses, and gradients contribute to the environment of an interventional MR suite, similar to diagnostic MRI. Therefore, effective screening procedures are required to guard the safety of MR interventions and avoid accidents.[32] In addition to the general contraindications of MRI, pacemakers and pregnancy require careful consideration.[33] The ferromagnetic devices or equipment traditionally used in interventional radiology must not be brought into the MR environment because they are prone to experience considerable traction forces that may be strong enough to cause serious fatalities, or significant heating that might result in burn injuries to patients and physicians.[34,35] Therefore, conventional stainless steel injection needles cannot be used safely for MRN-guided injections.[14] Today, a variety of MR-compatible needles are commercially available from several vendors for use at 1.5 T.

Needle Visualization

The constant and reliable visualization of the injection needle is a prerequisite for effective and safe percutaneous MR-guided drug delivery. In contrast to conventional radiographic fluoroscopy or CT, which both use attenuation differences of x-rays to visualize the needle, the mechanisms of accurate needle visualization are more complex in interventional MR imaging. In addition to the certified MR compatibility of the needle, spatial misregistration and image distortions must be avoided. The size of the created needle artifact should be large enough to be detectable on MR images but should avoid overlapping with adjacent structures, and the overestimation of the length of the needle should be minimal. With optimized pulse sequences, the passive needle artifact displays the true location of the needle tip with an error margin of only 1 mm at 1.5 T.[36] Of the various techniques for localization and display of the needle tip on MR images, passive visualization has proven to be an easy and effective method because no additional equipment, recalculation, or postprocessing of MR images is needed.[37] The needle artifact is predominantly created by localized spin dephasing, which results from regional field inhomogeneities caused by low magnetic susceptibility alloys of MR-compatible needles and by local gradient disturbances.[38]

Aside from the composition of the needle alloy, needle geometry, and field strength, several variable factors and parameters relevant to the appearance of the needle artifact exist. Familiarity with the practical implications of factors, such as type of pulse sequence, specific parameters (echo time, voxel size, readout and radiofrequency bandwidth), and the relative angle of the needle to the orientation of the external magnetic field influence the needle artifact and enable the operator to optimize the appearance of the needle artifact appearance. In contrast to spin echo and turbo spin echo sequences, gradient echo sequences amplify the needle artifact because of the build-up of field heterogeneities. This effect is more pronounced at 1.5 T.[14] When using gradient echo sequences, minimization of the echo times results in shortening of the time for dephasing and a smaller needle artifact. Although dephasing is less pronounced with turbo spin echo sequences, a similar benefit may result from shortening of echo times and the use of short echo spacing.

Maximizing bandwidths results in similar effects. Maximization of gradient strengths minimizes susceptibility artifacts, which can also be achieved using a small field of view and small slice thickness. The needle artifact is strongest if the needle is perpendicularly oriented to the external magnetic field, whereas it is smallest if oriented parallel.[14] When using an MRI system with a horizontal bore, most injections are performed in the axial plane and therefore the needle is generally oriented 90° to the external magnetic field and parallel to the patient's z-axis.

Visualization of Injectants

Reliable visualization of the deposition and spread of injectants is fundamental to judge the technical adequacy of a nerve block and its validity in terms of patient's pain response.[22] Injectants can be visualized with T1-weighted or T2-weighted MR imaging. The addition of Gadolinium-based contrast to the injectant enables its selective visualization with the use of T1-weighted sequences and fat saturation.[15] The addition of gadolinium-based contrast agent (eg, gadolinium-DTPA) in a ratio of 1:300 results in high contrast-to-noise ratios between the injectant and the surrounding tissues. Injectants may also be visualized with short tau inversion recovery (STIR) imaging or T2-weighted sequences with optional fat saturation, based on the intrinsically long T2 of the water-based injectant.[14,19,23,24,39] In our experience, both techniques can be equally effective. Gadolinium-enhanced injectants are useful for real-time MR fluoroscopic monitoring of the injection and detection of perineural spread when using T1-weighted MR fluoroscopy sequences (**Fig. 1**). The safety of perineural injection of gadolinium-based contrast material with the combination of anesthetic and steroids has been confirmed by several investigations.[40,41] T2-weighted visualization may be preferred because it obviates the addition of gadolinium-based contrast. Either approach can be advantageous in treating patients with hypersensitivity to iodine, for whom iodine-based contrast agents, such as those used in CT and radiographic fluoroscopy are contraindicated.[40,41]

MR Fluoroscopy

MR fluoroscopy is useful for interactive determination of the skin entry site, needle advancement navigation, and real-time monitoring of injections, which can be viewed on an MR-compatible in-room display (see **Fig. 1**).[15,23] The required high temporal resolution results in a trade-off between spatial and contrast resolution. However, both spoiled and balanced gradient echo sequences achieve frame rates of less than 1 second with sufficient spatial and contrast resolution.[15,19]

Protocol

Parallel imaging with the use of surface coils and the table coil elements achieves rapid image acquisition and can increase the signal-to-noise ratio of the target region, as opposed to the use of the body coil, which is installed in the bore of the magnet. In each procedure, limited MRN images are acquired first to map the target nerve. A multichannel surface coil placed over the interventional site is advantageous to achieve the highest resolution. For the needle placement, the multichannel surface coil may be exchanged for a surface loop coil, which facilitates free access to the interventional site and sterile coverage.

All procedures discussed in this article were performed with a clinical, open-bore 1.5-T MRI system (Magnetom Espree, Siemens Healthcare, Erlangen, Germany) following a 6-step algorithm (**Table 2**). Depending on the target, patients are placed either prone or supine on the MR table, depending on the location the target (**Table 3**). T1-weighted MRN images are obtained immediately before the needle placement phase using a multichannel body coil placed over the pelvis (**Table 4**, sequence 1). On these images, the operator maps the target structure from the level of its origin to the periphery, and the needle path is planned on the work station depending on the indication for injection. The coil is then exchanged with a flexible loop-shaped radiofrequency coil with a diameter of 16 cm (Siemens Healthcare). The skin entry point is determined interactively using MR fluoroscopy (see **Table 4**, sequence 2) using a water-filled syringe as a pointing device or the operator's fingertip with the MR fluoroscopy sequence prescribed to the slice position of the selected injection site. The interventional site is then prepped and draped in standard fashion. Conscious sedation may be initiated at this point

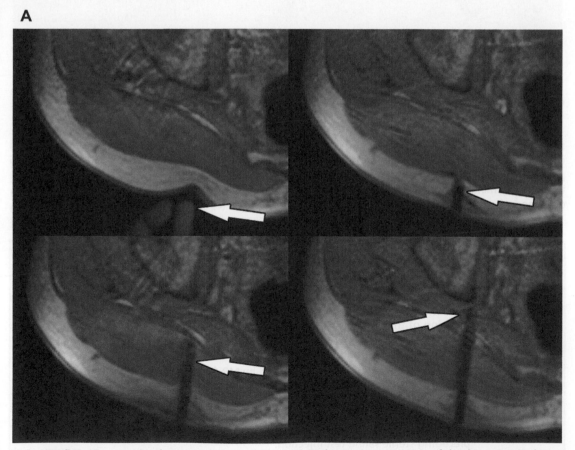

Fig. 1. MR fluoroscopy with a frame rate of 0.8 seconds. (*A*) Real-time determination of the skin entry site by use of a water-filled syringe (*A, left upper frame, arrow*) and subsequent interactive needle placement (*arrows*) to the right infrapiriformis foramen.

B

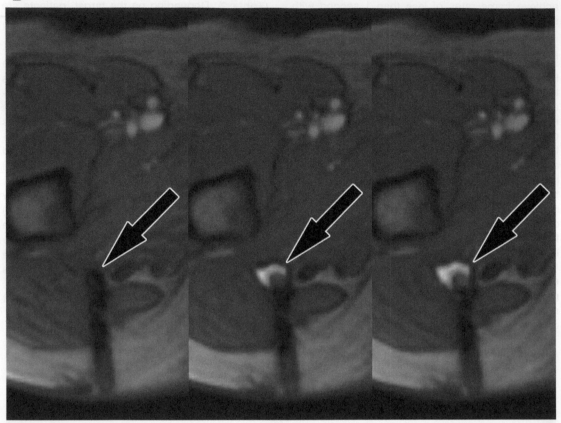

Fig. 1. (*B*) Real-time monitoring of a perineural injection (3 mL) of the right posterior femoral cutaneous nerve.

according to the patient's preference and the procedure type. However, because the described procedures are simple, with an average procedure time of 30 minutes, the authors prefer not to give sedation in order to not confound the pain response. Local anesthesia is administered superficially using 1% lidocaine through a 25-G hypodermic needle. MR-compatible 22- or 20-G injection needles of 10- or 15-cm lengths (MReye, G11583, Cook Medical, Bloomington, IN, USA),

Table 2
A 6-step protocol for MRN-guided MR intervention

Step	Action
1	Limited MRN visualization of the target muscle or nerve, mapping of its course, and planning of the needle path.
2	MR fluoroscopy for the determination of a suitable skin entry point using the tip of a syringe as the pointing device or the operator's finger.
3	Needle placement to the target navigated by MR fluoroscopy or intermittent MR imaging.
4	Confirmation of the adequacy of the location of the needle tip using fast intermediate-weighted MR imaging.
5	Monitoring of the injection by MR fluoroscopy or intermittent MR imaging with optional preceding sterile saline test injection.
6	Final MR imaging for visualizing the injectant, determining the spatial relationship to the target structure, and detecting potential spread to adjacent structures.

Table 3	
Approach to targets	
Anterior	**Posterior**
Lateral femoral cutaneous nerve	Posterior femoral cutaneous nerve
Femoral nerve	Sciatic nerve
Obturator nerve	Pudendal nerve
	Ganglion impar
	Piriformis injection
	Hypogastric plexus
	Sacral foraminal injection

depending on the skin-to-target distance, are then interactively navigated to the target under MR fluoroscopy guidance. Intermittent axial turbo spin echo MR images (see **Table 4**, sequence 3) are acquired for visual assessment of the adequacy of the needle tip location. The administration of gadolinium-enhanced injectant is monitored using T1-weighted MR fluoroscopy, whereas nonenhanced injections are monitored with a fast STIR sequence (see **Table 4**, sequence 4). The location of the delivered injectant is finally visualized using a fat-saturated T1-weighted turbo spin echo MR sequence (see **Table 4**, sequence 5) or an isotropic

3-dimensional T2-weighted MR imaging sequence with or without fat saturation (see **Table 4**, sequence 6).

PRINCIPLES OF DIAGNOSTIC AND THERAPEUTIC PELVIC NERVE BLOCKS

The concept validity of diagnostic and therapeutic use of pelvic injections is based on the theories of pain causation.[7] The selective perineural delivery of a local anesthetic in clinically appropriate concentration to the pain-generating structure results in reversible inhibition of neural conduction through blocking sodium channels located on internal neuronal membranes.[42] In practice, unmyelinated C-fibers (eg, afferent, somatosensory fibers of peripheral nerves), autonomic fibers, and myelinated A-delta fibers (pain, pressure, and temperature) are frequently more sensitive to local anesthetics than larger myelinated A-fibers (motor function, proprioception, touch, and pressure).[43] Temporary blocking of the activity of stimulated nociceptors results in relief of the patient's typical pain. Locally delivered corticosteroids may result in a therapeutic benefit through decreasing the release of local inflammatory mediators, induction of a membrane-stabilizing effect leading to decreased afferent ectopic discharges at the site of nerve injury, and modulation of nociceptive input from peripheral neurons.[9,10] The

Table 4						
MRI protocol for MRN-guided nerve blocks and injections						
	Sequence					
	1	**2**	**3**	**4**	**5**	**6**
Type	Turbo spin echo	FLASH2D	Turbo spin echo	STIR	Turbo spin echo	SPACE
Weighting	T1	T1/T2*	Intermediate	STIR	T1	T2
Fat-saturation	No	No	No	Yes	Yes	Optional
Dimensionality	2D	2D	2D	2D	2D	3D
Orientation	Axial	Axial	Axial	Axial	Axial	Coronal
Repetition time (ms)	691.0	9.3	1200.0	1200.0	500.0	1500.0
Echo time (ms)	20.0	3.5	12.0	29.0	20.0	138.0
Echo train length	5	NA	17	5	6	8
Slice thickness (mm)	4	5	5	5	4	1
Field of view (mm)	360 × 253	256 × 224	256 × 224	256 × 224	200 × 200	300 × 207
Base resolution (pixels)	384	256	320	192	384	384
Phase resolution (%)	70	56	100	45	50	74
Receiver bandwidth (Hz)	102	180	252	542	102	751
Acquisition time	3.6 min	1 s/frame	12 s	32 s	5.1 min	6–7 min

Abbreviations: 2D, 2-dimensional; 3D, 3-dimensional; FLASH2D, two-dimensional fast low angle shot; SPACE, sampling perfection with application optimized contrasts using variable flip angle evolutions; STIR, short tau inversion recovery.

authors use a combination of 1% lidocaine, 0.5% bupivacaine, and 10 mg/mL of dexamethasone in various volumes depending on the target and risk of spread to confounding structure.

Face validity is based on the technical effectiveness of a nerve block in that the locally delivered anesthetic results in temporary anesthesia of the area innervated by the nerve. Because of anatomic variations and overlap of areas of innervation, accurate drug delivery to the target structure is a paramount prerequisite for the face validity of a pelvic nerve block. Face validity is required for a true-positive test result. Small volumes of injectant help safeguard the exclusive anesthesia of the targeted nerve and help avoid spread of the injectant to potential pain generators nearby, which may confound the response (false-positive result). MRN-guided injection is an excellent technique to directly assess face validity in every individual, because it allows direct visualization of the nerve and injectant. Additionally, clinical assessment after the block showing anesthesia of the expected area of innervation adds face validity to the block. In therapeutic injections, the delivery of a sufficient drug quantity to the target site through larger volumes receives priority over exclusivity of the injection, because ideally the pain generator is known at this point of the clinical workup and the intent is treatment (pain relief).

Pain responses may be assessed 30 to 60 minutes after the injection. The assessment may be obtained while the patient is at rest or performing maneuvers that produce the typical pain or discomfort. Pain rating scales may be used for quantification. A positive nerve block maybe defined as substantial pain relief ($\geq$50%) after a technically effective nerve block, and recurrence of the patient's typical pain after the expected action time of injected anesthetic. A positive nerve block confirms that the blocked nerve substantially contributes to the chronic pelvic pain syndrome.

Because comparison of the pain response after a block versus a reference standard is usually not feasible, the significance of a single pain response carries a lower validity. Therefore, the reliability of a pain response should be confirmed with a second block, and optionally a third. Different protocols can be used, including injection of the same anesthetic (confirmatory blocks), a longer-acting anesthetic (comparative blocks), a placebo (placebo-controlled blocks), injection to a different target (target-controlled block), or combinations thereof (Table 5).[22] In confirmatory blocks, the second injection should confirm the test result of the initial injection through reproducing either a similar or expected modification of the pain response, depending on the protocol. With comparative blocks, prolonged pain relief is expected after injection of the longer-acting anesthetic. With placebo-controlled blocks, no pharmacologically induced pain relief is expected at the site of a placebo (eg, sterile saline or no injection). Because the first block requires the use of an anesthetic, this protocol requires 2 additional blocks (total of 3 blocks) to avoid prediction of the second injectant. Target-controlled blocks require a suitable target nearby to keep the needle approach constant and avoid detection by the patient, and should also consist of 3 blocks to avoid predictability of the second block. Controlled blocks may be considered unethical, because no anesthetic effect is expected from one injection. A positive pain response after placebo administration may occur because of a placebo response (almost one-third of cases in some studies) or a psychogenic mechanism. These testing protocols should be especially considered if nerve blocks are obtained to help guide surgical management. If multiple levels are tested, the most objective results may be obtained by testing each implicated level during a separate session.

Table 5 Protocols of repetitive blocks	
Type	**Injectants**
Confirmatory block	The same anesthetic twice (eg, preservative-free lidocaine)
Comparative injections	One block with a short-acting anesthetic (eg, preservative-free lidocaine) and the other block with a long-acting anesthetic (eg, preservative-free ropivacaine)
Placebo-controlled block	One block with a placebo (sterile saline) and 2 blocks with an anesthetic (eg, preservative-free lidocaine and ropivacaine)
Target-controlled block	The same anesthetic 3 times (eg, preservative-free lidocaine), but different anatomic targets

Face validity and reliability of test results build the foundation for obtaining conclusive test results. Face validity, however, is most important, because reliability is a necessary but insufficient condition for face validity. Practically, if no appropriate drug delivery was achieved, either the target nerve was not anesthetized (false-negative result) or results were confounded by anesthesia of a nontargeted nerve (false-positive). These results may still be reproducible, and reliability therefore may be judged acceptable; however, the test results are false. If a block lacks sufficient validity, the defined pain generator will be incorrect, leading to an erroneous diagnosis, ineffective treatment, and increased cost. The importance of face validity is the authors' rationale for using MRN-guided injections. Commitment to general testing principles, the use of repetitive testing protocols, and meticulous technique help maximize the accuracy of pelvic injection procedures.

PROCEDURES
Obturator Nerve

The obturator nerve is formed by the posterior divisions of L2–L4 and descends inside the psoas muscle to emerge from its medial border at the level of the sacroiliac joint.[26,44] The nerve follows the lateral pelvic wall to enter the fibro-osseous obturator canal and exits the pelvis through the obturator foramen (**Fig. 2**).[45] At this level, the nerve then divides into the anterior branches, which provide sensory innervation to the hip joint, motor branches to the superficial hip adductors, and a cutaneous branch that descends in the adductor canal to innervate the skin and fascia of the distal two-thirds of the medial thigh.[44–47] After a technically adequate obturator block, the patient should feel anesthesia of this area. The posterior branch provides motor innervation to the deep hip adductors and an articular branch to the posterior knee joint.

Chronic obturator neuropathy is a complex clinical syndrome that frequently presents as exercise-related groin pain, hip pain, and pain in the adductor region.[48] Symptoms further include medial thigh weakness with leg adduction, and sensory loss in the distal two-thirds of the medial thigh of the affected side. Obturator neuropathy in athletes may be caused by repetitive microtrauma and fascial entrapment.[46] Surgical neurolysis may provide better results than conservative therapy.[46]

Selective obturator nerve blocks are useful to identify the obturator nerve as the pain generator, support the diagnosis of obturator neuropathy in the absence of imaging findings, predict the benefit of surgical neurolysis, and support postoperative recovery by treating subsequent hip pain, and for palliation of chronic hip pain.[46,49,50] Because of the deep location and narrow access of the obturator foramen, selective obturator blocks usually require image guidance. Non-selective obturator blocks performed based on anatomic landmarks and without the use of image guidance result in inconsistent blockage to the obturator nerve,[51] or potential injury. Improved rates have been reported with ultrasound

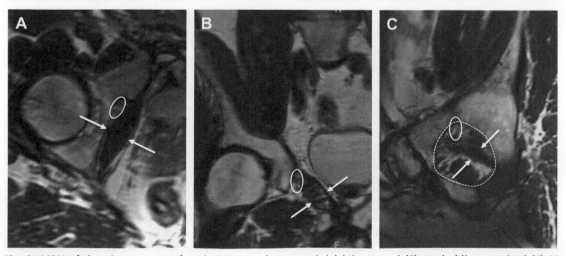

Fig. 2. MRN of the obturator canal and obturator foramen. Axial (*A*), coronal (*B*), and oblique sagittal (*C*) T2 SPACE (sampling perfection with application optimized contrasts using variable flip angle evolutions) MR images at 3 T show the obturator neurovascular bundle (*oval*) entering the obturator canal, at the superior aspect of the obturator foramen (*dotted area*), passing above and superficial to the obturator internus muscle (*arrows*).

guidance, fluoroscopy, and CT guidance.[49,52–54] Pertinent MRN anatomy and the technique of MRN-guided obturator blocks are detailed in **Figs. 2** and **3**.

Pudendal Nerve Entrapment Syndrome

The pudendal nerve descends between piriformis and coccygeal muscles, exits the pelvis through lower part of greater sciatic foramen, passes around the medial portion of the ischial spine between the sacrotuberous and sacrospinous ligaments, and travels in the pudendal (Alcock) canal anteriorly, where it terminates into the perineal nerves and the dorsal nerve of the penis or clitoris (**Fig. 4**).[26] The nerve provides sensation of the scrotum, perineum, and anus, and motor supply to the bulbospongiosus and ischiocavernosus muscles, playing a major role in ejaculation, orgasm, and control of the external anal sphincter.

The perineal branch corresponds with the perineal branch of the posterior femoral cutaneous nerve.

Pudendal nerve entrapment can cause perineal pain syndrome.[55] The Nantes criteria have been developed to increase the clinical diagnostic accuracy of pudendal neuralgia.[56] Key components are (1) pain in the anatomic territory of the pudendal nerve, (2) pain that is worsened by sitting, (3) pain that does not awaken the patient at night, (4) no objective sensory loss on clinical examination, and (5) positive diagnostic pudendal nerve block. Proposed exclusion criteria are purely coccygeal, gluteal, or hypogastric pain; exclusively paroxysmal pain; exclusive pruritus; and the presence of imaging abnormalities able to explain the symptoms.

Together with the history and clinical examination, diagnostic blocks play an important role in the identification of symptomatic pudendal neuropathy and the diagnosis of pudendal

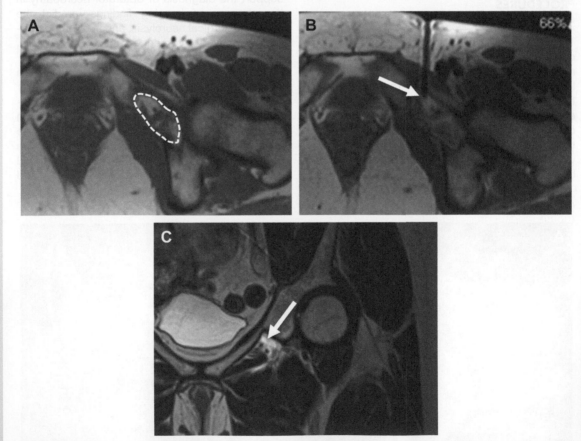

Fig. 3. MRN-guided perineural injection of the left obturator nerve at 1.5 T in a patient with obturator neuropathy. (*A*) T1 turbo spin echo (TSE) MR image at level below the superior pubic rami shows the left obturator canal (*dotted area*). (*B*) TSE MR image confirms the needle tip (*arrow*) location near the neurovascular bundle of the left obturator foramen. (*C*) Coronal T2 SPACE (sampling perfection with application optimized contrasts using variable flip angle evolutions) MR image demonstrates the adequate distribution of the T2 hyperintense injectant (3 mL) around the neurovascular bundle (*arrow*) of the obturator foramen.

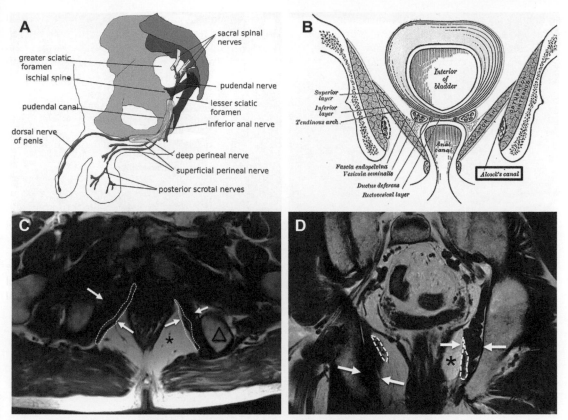

Fig. 4. Anatomy of the pudendal nerve. (*A*) Illustration shows the course and branches of the pudendal nerve (source: Wikipedia, public domain). (*B*) Illustration shows the location of Alcock's (pudendal) canal (public domain[44]). (*C, D*) 3-T axial and coronal T1 turbo spin echo (TSE) MR images show ischial tuberosity (*triangle*), the pudendal neurovascular bundle (*dotted line*) inside the pudendal canal coursing anteriorly along the deep aspect of obturator internus (*arrows*) lateral to the ischiorectal fossa (*asterisk*). ([*A*] *Courtesy of* Mikael Häggström, MD; [*B*] *From* Gray H, Lewis WH. Anatomy of the human body. 20th edition. New York: Bartleby.com; 2000.)

neuralgia.[8,56] Electroneuromyography may contribute helpful information, but was found to have limited sensitivity and specificity in diagnosing pudendal nerve entrapment syndrome.[57] The pudendal nerve may be entrapped at the level of the greater sciatic foramen, ischial spine, inside the pudendal canal, or at the level of distal branches of the pudendal nerve.[8] Depending on the clinically suspected level of the entrapment, the pudendal nerve should be blocked proximally to that location, such as at the greater sciatic foramen, at the iliac spine, and inside the pudendal canal. Techniques for pudendal nerve blocks include non–image-guided blocks and image-guided blocks with fluoroscopy, ultrasound, CT, and MRI.[8,58–61] Selective pudendal blocks may not be possible at the greater sciatic foramen and are difficult to achieve at the ischial spine because of the proximity and spread of the injectant to sympathetic nerves and to the posterior femoral cutaneous nerve, which share sensory perineal innervation and may cause a false-

positive test result. Exclusive anesthesia of the pudendal nerve is best achieved inside the pudendal canal, because its boundaries provide a natural barrier to other neural structures, which helps to avoid a false possible block. Care should be taken to not overfill the pudendal canal to avoid back-spill along the proximal pudendal nerve to the greater sciatic foramen. MRN-guided blocks can be performed at any location, depending on the symptoms (**Fig. 5**). Postinjection MRI at 1.5 T is exquisitely sensitive for determining whether the injection occurred inside the canal where the nerve resides, or medial to the canal where the nerve is shielded by the fascia of the canal and the injectant is likely ineffective (see **Fig. 5**).

Posterior Femoral Cutaneous Nerve

The posterior femoral cutaneous nerve is a sensory nerve of the lumbosacral plexus.[44] It descends through the greater sciatic foramen with

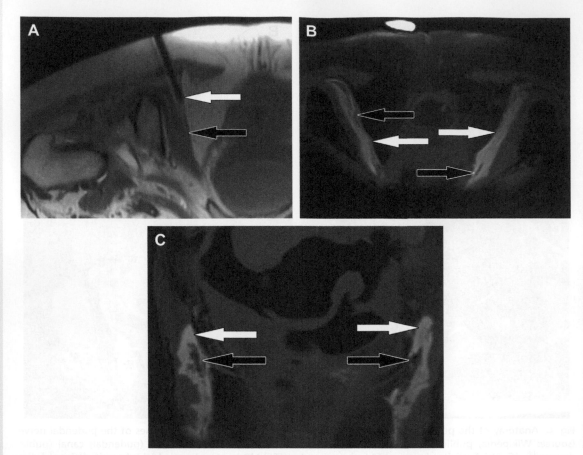

Fig. 5. MRN-guided injection of the left and right pudendal canal at 1.5 T. (*A*) Axial turbo spin echo (TSE) MR image at level below the ischial tuberosity demonstrates the needle tip (*white arrow*) inside the pudendal canal containing the pudendal neurovascular bundle (*black arrows*). (*B, C*) Axial and coronal fat-suppressed T2 SPACE (sampling perfection with application optimized contrasts using variable flip angle evolutions) MR images show the adequate distribution of the T2 hyperintense injectant (4 mL, *white arrows*), which outlines the entirety of the pudendal canal, around the neurovascular bundle (*black arrows*).

the sciatic and pudendal nerves. The nerve travels anterior to the piriformis muscle inferiorly and exits the pelvis under the piriformis muscle (**Fig. 6**). The posterior femoral cutaneous nerve and the sciatic nerve then descend laterally under the gluteus maximus muscle, whereas the pudendal nerve curves around the iliac spine and travels into the pudendal canal. At the level of the inferior edge of the gluteus maximus muscle, the posterior femoral cutaneous nerve gives rise to the inferior cluneal branches, which supply the inferior lateral buttock area. Approximately 4 cm (range, 3.0–5.5 cm) inferior to the termination of the sacrotuberous ligament onto the ischial tuberosity, the perineal branches arise, which innervate the posterolateral perineum, the proximal medial thigh, the posterolateral aspect of the scrotum/labium majus, and a portion of the penis/clitoris. Then the posterior femoral cutaneous nerve

separates from the sciatic nerve and travels posteriorly down the leg under the fascia lata, over the long head of the biceps femoris, and to the back of the knee where it pierces the deep fascia (see **Fig. 6**).

Causes of chronic pain syndromes related to the posterior femoral cutaneous nerve neuropathy include compression, entrapment, repetitive trauma from cycling, impact injury, and injection injury, but in many cases, no origin may be identified. The clinical manifestations of posterior femoral cutaneous nerve neuropathy vary, which is thought to be influenced by the location of the abnormality.[62,63] Posterior femoral cutaneous nerve neuropathy affecting the perineal branch may causes chronic perineal pain, which represents a major differential diagnosis of pudendal neuralgia because of substantial overlap of innervation in the perineal area.[62] Involvement of the

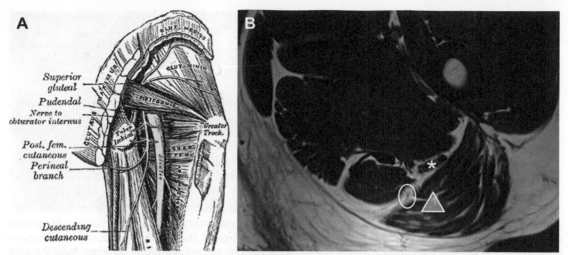

Fig. 6. Anatomy of the posterior femoral cutaneous nerve. (*A*) Illustration shows the course and branches of the posterior femoral cutaneous nerve (public domain[44]). The areas of innervation include the gluteal region, perineum, and back of the thigh and leg. (*B*) Axial T1 MR images at the level of the inferior edge of the gluteus maximus. Posterior femoral cutaneous neurovascular bundle (*oval*) coursing at the deep margin of gluteus maximus (*triangle*), posterior to the sciatic nerve (*asterisk*). ([A] *From* Gray H, Lewis WH. Anatomy of the human body. 20th edition. New York: Bartleby.com; 2000.)

cluneal nerves may cause pain and paresthesia referred to the inferior lateral buttock area (clunealgia),[63] and involvement of the more distal posterior femoral cutaneous nerve may manifest as pain and paresthesia of the posterior thigh.

In cases of unsatisfactory results of conservative therapy or failed selective regional blocks of other nerves (eg, pudendal nerve), selective diagnostic nerve blocks of the posterior femoral cutaneous nerve can be a valuable tool to assess the nerve's contribution to the patient's symptoms and to identify potential surgical targets.[63,64] Previously

described techniques relied on anatomic landmarks, and therefore selective anesthesia of the posterior femoral cutaneous nerve may not have been achieved with certainty.[64–67] High-field MRN reliably displays the course of the posterior femoral cutaneous nerve,[11,26] which can then be used for accurate targeting and selective drug delivery (**Fig. 7**).

Sciatic Nerve

The sciatic nerve is the largest nerve of the human body and supplies a large territory of the skin of the

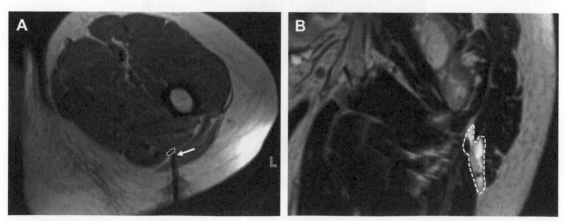

Fig. 7. Diagnostic MRN-guided injection of the distal right posterior femoral cutaneous nerve at 1.5 T in a patient with chronic paresthesia of the posterior thigh. (*A*) Axial MR image shows the needle tip (*arrow*) posterior to the posterior femoral cutaneous nerve (*dotted area*). (*B*) Sagittal high-resolution T2-weighted SPACE (sampling perfection with application optimized contrasts using variable flip angle evolutions) MR image shows the injectant (3 mL, *dotted area*) outlining the posterior femoral cutaneous neurovascular bundle.

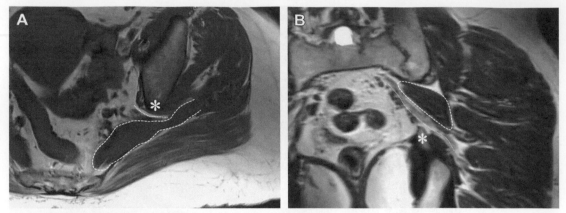

Fig. 8. 3-T axial (*A*) T1-weighted and coronal oblique (*B*) T2-weighted SPACE (sampling perfection with application optimized contrasts using variable flip angle evolutions) MR images. The sciatic nerve (*dotted line*) exits the pelvis under the fan-shaped piriformis muscle (*dotted area*) through the infrapiriformis foramen. Note the proximity of the ischial spine (*asterisk*) at the inferior margin of the sciatic nerve.

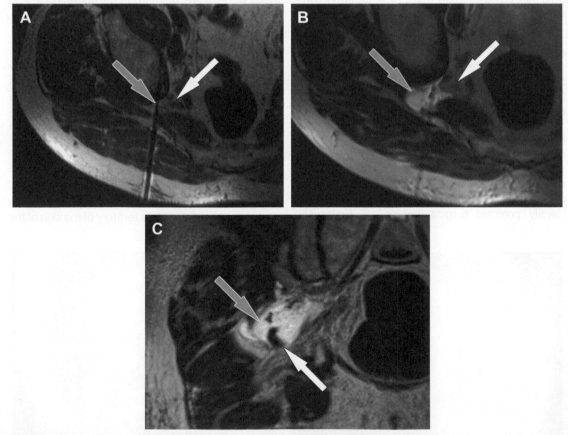

Fig. 9. MRN-guided perineural injection of the left sciatic nerve at level of the infrapiriformis foramen at 1.5 T. (*A*) Axial TSE MR image at the level of the sciatic notch demonstrates the needle tip (*gray arrow*) next to the neurovascular bundle containing the sciatic nerve (*white arrows*). (*B*) Axial T2-weighted turbo spin echo (TSE) MR image demonstrates the injectant (*gray arrow*) in the greater sciatic foramen next to the neurovascular bundle containing the sciatic nerve (*white arrow*). (*C*) Axial T2-weighted SPACE (sampling perfection with application optimized contrasts using variable flip angle evolutions) MR image demonstrates the adequate distribution of the T2 hyperintense injectant (5 mL, *gray arrow*) surrounding the neurovascular bundle and the sciatic nerve (*white arrow*).

leg and the muscles of the back of the thigh, leg, and foot.[44] In most cases, the nerve exits the pelvis between the gemellus superior and piriformis muscles through the greater sciatic foramen, together with the pudendal nerve and the posterior femoral cutaneous nerve to descend posterior to the adductor magnus and anterior to the gluteus maximus muscle (**Fig. 8**).[68] However, up to 35% of cases (average, 16.9%) present with variant anatomy, of which 63.6% are bilateral.[68,69]

Many causes of sciatic neuropathy exist, including diabetic amyotrophy, plexitis, iatrogenic injury, intramuscular injection, trauma, radiation therapy, piriformis syndrome, benign and malignant neurogenic and adjacent neoplasms, endometriosis, vascular malformations, and anatomic variants, such as a prominent lesser trochanter.[27,31]

Diagnostic and therapeutic sciatic blocks may be performed in patients with chronic pain.

The level of the perineural injection depends on the level of the lesion. Distal to the piriformis muscle where the sciatic nerve courses superficially, landmark and ultrasound guidance are frequently successful.[70] MRN guidance is useful for deep sciatic perineural injections at the level of the sciatic foramen (**Fig. 9**) and in the presence of masses affecting the deeply situated portion of the sciatic nerve (**Fig. 10**). The detailed MRN visualization helps ensure safe needle placement into the immediate vicinity of the abnormality, and avoid nerve contact and injury.

Piriformis Muscle

The piriformis muscle is a fan- or pear-shaped muscle that originates from the anterior border of the second to fourth sacral segments, the superior margin of the greater sciatic foramen,

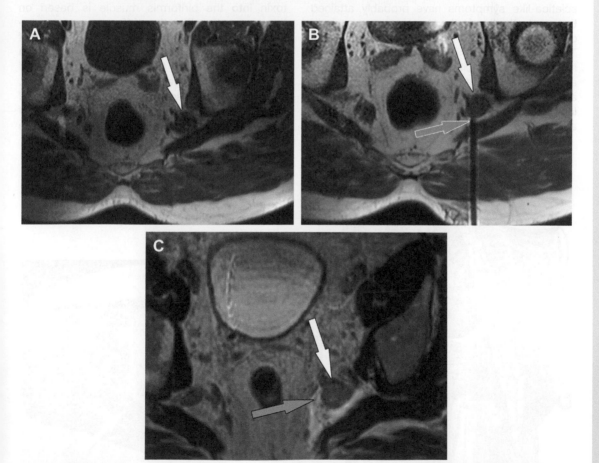

Fig. 10. MRN-guided perineural injection of a deeply situated left sciatic schwannoma before surgery at 1.5 T. (*A*) Axial turbo spin echo (TSE) MR image at the level above the infrapiriformis foramen demonstrates a deeply situated schwannoma of the proximal sciatic nerve (*white arrows*). (*B*) Axial TSE MR image demonstrates the needle tip (*gray arrow*) in the immediate vicinity of the schwannoma (*white arrow*). (*C*) Axial T2-weighted SPACE (sampling perfection with application optimized contrasts using variable flip angle evolutions) MR image demonstrates the T2 hyperintense injectant (5 mL, *gray arrow*) spreading around the sciatic schwannoma (*white arrow*).

and the sacrotuberous ligament as multiple slips (**Fig. 11**).[69] Normally, the lumbosacral plexus is formed anterior to the piriformis muscle. The muscle courses inferolaterally through the greater sciatic foramen with an intimate relationship to the underlying neurovascular bundles, and inserts at the greater trochanter of the femur. The piriformis muscle divides the greater sciatic foramen into the suprapiriformis foramen, which contains the superior gluteal nerve and vessels, and into the infrapiriformis foramen, which contains the inferior gluteal and internal pudendal vessels; inferior gluteal, pudendal, sciatic, and posterior femoral cutaneous nerves; and sympathetic fibers and nerves to the obturator internus and quadratus femoris.[71]

The piriformis syndrome is a controversial entity, which is thought to be a cause of chronic pelvic pain syndrome.[72] Principally, any nerve of the infrapiriformis foramen can be affected, although sciatica-like symptoms have probably attained the most attention in the literature, perhaps indicating that the sciatic nerve is most often affected. The pathophysiology is unclear; however, inflammation and spasticity of the piriformis muscle and compression of the underlying sciatic nerve against the bony pelvis have been postulated.[21,72,73] The syndrome is not well defined and no consensus criteria exit, although hip pain, buttock pain, dyspareunia in women, sciatica, and intolerance to sitting are some of the common symptoms.[74] Variant sciatic anatomy has been described in patients diagnosed with piriformis syndrome; however, the prevalence may not be a lot different compared with that among the normal population.[69] The significance of asymmetry of the piriformis muscles is similarly unclear,[21,75] and the diagnosis of piriformis syndrome frequently remains one of exclusion.[74] 3-T MRN is useful in identifying the coexistent sciatic nerve size and signal changes, apart from the variant anatomy, thereby confirming the diagnosis of sciatic irritation/entrapment from piriformis syndrome.

Therapeutic perineurovascular injections at the level of the sciatic foramen can provide temporary pain relief (see **Fig. 9**) and may be combined with intramuscular injection of steroids and anesthetics.[76] The rationale behind injecting botulinum toxin into the piriformis muscle is based on the assumption that the piriformis muscle produces mechanical irritation or compression of the underlying neurovascular bundle. Botulinum neurotoxin A inhibits the presynaptic release of acetylcholine at the neuromuscular junction, which leads to muscle paralysis and wasting of the muscle belly.[77] Intramuscular injection of 100 or 200 U of botulinum neurotoxin A into the

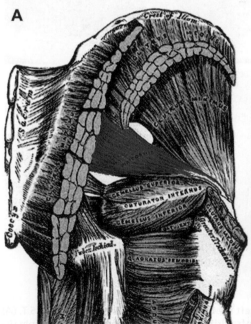

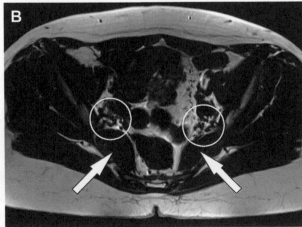

Fig. 11. Anatomy of the piriformis muscle. (*A*) Anatomic illustration shows the location and course of the piriformis muscle (*red area*) (public domain[44]). (*B*) 3-T axial T1-weighted MR image shows the left and right piriformis muscle (*white arrows*) and the proximal neurovascular bundles (*circles*) containing the sciatic nerve. ([*A*] *From* Gray H, Lewis WH. Anatomy of the human body. 20th edition. New York: Bartleby.com; 2000.)

piriformis muscle leads to muscle weakness and atrophy, and potentially reverses the presumed nerve compression.[73,78] A randomized controlled trial showed better efficacy with botulinum toxin A compared with placebo and corticosteroid plus lidocaine.[73,78]

Piriformis muscle injections may be performed under fluoroscopy, ultrasound, CT, and MRI guidance.[21,76,79,80] MRI may be selectively used to improve targeting in cases involving a thin piriformis muscle, a larger patient, or repeat botulinum neurotoxin injection to paralyze the remaining muscle (**Fig. 12**), and when the procedure is combined with a deep therapeutic injection of the infrapiriformis foramen (see **Fig. 9**).

Lateral Femoral Cutaneous Nerve

The lateral femoral cutaneous nerve is a sensory nerve originating from the L2 and L3 spinal nerves and provides sensation to the anterior lateral thigh above the knee.[26,44] It passes through the psoas major muscle and runs obliquely over the iliacus muscle. The nerve most often exits the pelvis under the inguinal ligament, 0.1 to 7.3 cm medial the anterior superior iliac spine.[81,82] However, a variant course occurs in up to 25% of patients.[83] In up to 18.8% to 22.9% patients, the nerve passes lateral to or above the anterior superior iliac spine and iliac crest.[82,84–86] The nerve may pierce through the inguinal ligament in 13.9%.[86] Anatomic variants also exist in the region of the thigh.[86]

Meralgia paresthetica syndrome is typically caused by injury or entrapment of the lateral femoral cutaneous nerve. Burning, tingling, numbness, and pain in the proximal and anterolateral thigh are typical symptoms, which are often aggravated by weight-bearing, hip extension, or the prone position.[87] Although no obvious cause may be identified, high-impact trauma, repetitive

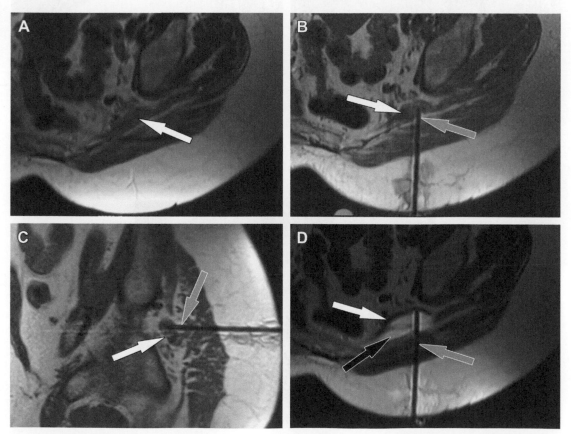

Fig. 12. MR-guided injection of the left piriformis muscle at 1.5 T in a patient with piriformis syndrome and partial response to a previous piriformis injection with botulinum neurotoxin. (*A*) Axial, T1 MR image shows the partially atrophied, thin piriformis muscle (*white arrow*). (*B, C*) Axial and sagittal proton-density TSE images confirm the needle tip (*gray arrows*) inside the piriformis muscle (*white arrow*). (*D*) Axial T2 turbo spin echo (TSE) MR image demonstrates intramuscular accumulation of the injectant (5 mL, *black arrow*) containing botulinum neurotoxin A. The gray arrow shows the needle. The white arrow shows the piriformis muscle containing the injectant.

microtrauma, fascial entrapment, previous surgery and scar encasement, pregnancy, diabetes, and neoplasm have been linked to meralgia paresthetica.[88] The lateral femoral cutaneous nerve can be subject to compression throughout its entire course; however, the typical location of entrapment or compression is under the inguinal ligament where the nerve exits the pelvis.[89]

In addition to nerve conduction studies, which are often of limited use, nerve blocks play an important role when the diagnosis of meralgia paresthetica is uncertain.[90] Superficial blocks targeting the lateral femoral cutaneous nerve at its assumed exit under the inguinal ligaments in the groin and thigh region may be successfully performed without image guidance; however, because of the variable anatomy of the lateral femoral cutaneous nerve, the success rate may be as low as 40%.[91] Ultrasound increases

accuracy of distal lateral femoral cutaneous nerve blocks.[92] MRN-guided blocks are especially helpful for intrapelvic, extraperitoneal blocks of the lateral femoral cutaneous nerve before it exits under the inguinal ligament (**Fig. 13**), because this portion of the nerve may not be identified with certainty on ultrasound images.[93] Because meralgia paresthetica often regresses spontaneously, conservative treatment and therapeutic blocks play an important role in bridging the time to resolution.[88] Therapeutic blocks can achieve high success rates and may be used in addition to conservative therapy with only few patients requiring surgery.[89]

Ganglion Impar

The solitary ganglion impar (also known as the *ganglion of Walther*) is the most inferior

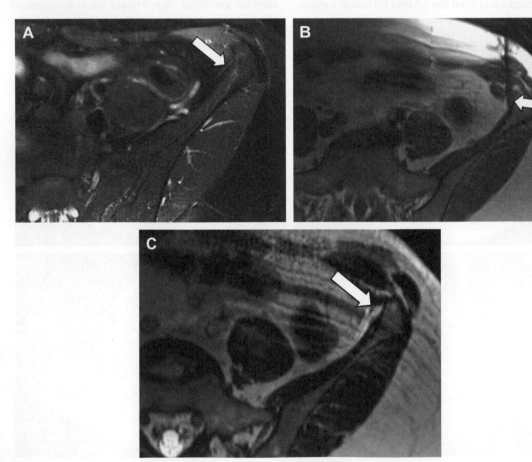

Fig. 13. MRN-guided diagnostic block of the proximal left lateral femoral cutaneous nerve at 1.5 T in a patient with meralgia paresthetica syndrome. (*A*) T2 Spectral Adiabatic Inversion Recovery MR image shows hyperintense, thickened nerve (*arrow*) proximal to its course under the inguinal ligament. (*B*) turbo spin echo (TSE) MR image shows adequate needle placement with the needle tip (*arrow*) located in the immediate vicinity of the nerve. (*C*) Axial oblique T2-weighted SPACE (sampling perfection with application optimized contrasts using variable flip angle evolutions) image confirms that the nerve (4 mL, *arrow*) is completely surrounded by the injectant, indicating a technically adequate block.

sympathetic ganglion.[44] It forms the convergence of the sympathetic chain bilaterally at the anterior aspect of the coccyx. The ganglion impar is often located just anterior to the sacrococcygeal joint in the midline; however, it has been variably reported to be lying anterior to the coccyx or at the tip of the coccyx (Fig. 14). The ganglion measures between 1.1 and 4.2 mm.[94] The average distances of the ganglion impar to the midpoint of the sacrococcygeal joint and to the tip of the coccyx are 8.6° and 25.0 mm, respectively.[94] The ganglion receives nociceptive and sympathetic fibers from the pelvis and is thought to play a major role in coccyx pain syndrome. *Coccyx pain syndrome* is defined as the occurrence of chronic or recurrent episodic pain perceived in the region of the coccyx in the absence of proven infection or other obvious local abnormality.[2] The term *coccydynia* was previously used to describe the same entity.

Blockade and neurolysis of the ganglion impar relieve pain from visceral and/or sympathetic pain syndromes of the perineal region.[95–97] The success rate of this method depends on the anatomic variability of the ganglion location.[98] A transsacrococcygeal technique has been described,[99] which requires forceful needle penetration of the sacrococcygeal disc, which is associated with the risk of discitis and hemorrhage.[98] Fluoroscopy may be successfully used for guidance by landmarks, but cannot visualize the ganglion impar nor the pelvic soft tissues.[97] Direct visualization of the presacral pelvic soft tissues and, ideally, of the ganglion impar is preferable to avoid complications such as needle injury of the colon or bladder, sciatic nerve injury, and inadvertent injection into other organs. Lateral CT-guided approaches with a straight needle have been described and successfully used for ganglion impar block, but have the drawback of exposing the pelvic tissues to ionizing radiation and potential ganglion injury.[96,100,101] MRN can frequently demonstrate the location of the ganglion impar, and enables direct targeting under MR guidance (see Fig. 14; Fig. 15).

Sacral Spinal Nerves

In addition to abnormalities affecting the pelvic nerves originating of the sacral plexus, the contributing sacral spinal nerves may be targeted. In cases involving a high clinical suspicion of a specific pelvic nerve generating the patient's symptoms, but negative selective nerve blocks or unsuccessful therapeutic injection, perineural sacral injections can achieve selective and more-proximal blockage. The dorsal root ganglion and the dorsal horn are considered important structure in the genesis of neuropathic pain, and are thought

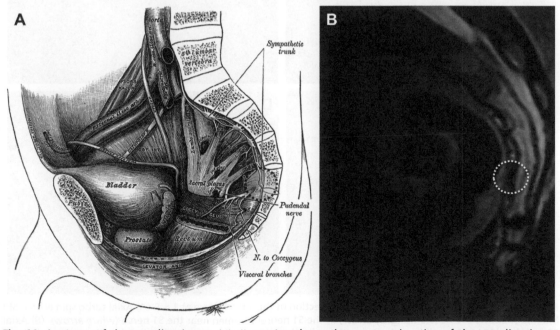

Fig. 14. Anatomy of the ganglion impar. (*A*) Illustration shows the common location of the ganglion impar (*dashed circle*) (public domain[44]). (*B*) 3-T sagittal T2 SPACE (sampling perfection with application optimized contrasts using variable flip angle evolutions) MR image showing the ganglion impar (*dashed circle*) anterior to the sacrococcygeal junction. ([A] *From* Gray H, Lewis WH. Anatomy of the human body. 20th edition. New York: Bartleby.com; 2000.)

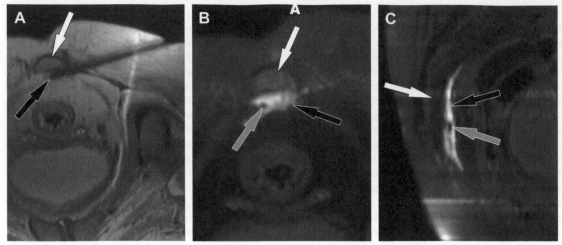

Fig. 15. MRN-guided perineural injection of the ganglion impar at 1.5 T. (*A*) Axial turbo spin echo (TSE) MR image at level of the sacrococcygeal junction (*white arrow*) shows the needle tip (*black arrow*) in the presacral location near the ganglion impar (not shown). (*B, C*) Axial and sagittal T1-weighted TSE MR image with spectral fat saturation shows ganglion impar (*gray arrow*) surrounded by the hyperintense injectant (5 mL, *black arrow*) anterior to the sacrococcygeal junction (*white arrow*).

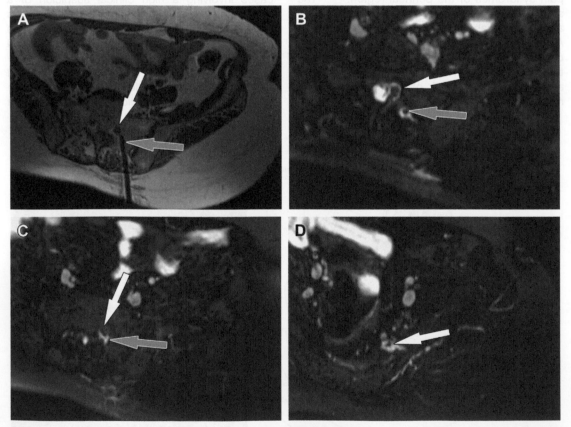

Fig. 16. MR-guided transforaminal perineural injection of the left S1 nerve at 1.5 T. (*A*) Axial turbo spin echo (TSE) MR image shows the needle tip (*gray arrow*) in the S1 neural foramen near the S1 nerve (*white arrow*). (*B*) Axial T2-weighted SPACE (sampling perfection with application optimized contrasts using variable flip angle evolutions) MR image shows the hyperintense injectant surrounding the dorsal root ganglion (*white arrow*) and S1 nerve root (*gray arrow*). (*C*) Axial T2-weighted SPACE MR image shows the hyperintense injectant (*gray arrow*) surrounding the S1 nerve (*white arrow*). (*D*) Axial T2-weighted SPACE MR image with spectral fat saturation shows the hyperintense injectant (5 mL) surrounding the S1 nerve (*white arrow*) distal to the anterior S1 neural foramen.

to play an important role in the setting of peripheral nerve injury and chronic pain.[102,103] Selective spinal nerve root injections can identify pain-mediating spinal nerves and can provide valuable prognostic information about the possible outcome of future surgery.[104]

Therapeutic local anesthetic and steroid injections of nerve roots of the lumbar spine are effective for the nonsurgical treatment of chronic low back pain and have produced encouraging long-term results.[105] Drug delivery may be achieved with a transforaminal approach during fluoroscopy, CT, or MRI.[22] MRN guidance is useful for avoiding damage to the nerve root and monitoring the distribution of the injectant, and has been shown to be superior to CT imaging in these areas (**Fig. 16**).

To conclude, MRN-guided interventional MRI for diagnosing and treating pelvic pain syndrome is a safe and technically valid technique to map and target deeply situated pelvic nerves or muscles, navigate needles to the target, visualize the injected drug, and detect spread to confounding structures.

REFERENCES

1. Latthe P, Mignini L, Gray R, et al. Factors predisposing women to chronic pelvic pain: systematic review. BMJ 2006;332(7544):749–55.

2. Fall M, Baranowski AP, Elneil S, et al. EAU guidelines on chronic pelvic pain. Eur Urol 2010;57(1): 35–48.

3. Mathias SD, Kuppermann M, Liberman RF, et al. Chronic pelvic pain: prevalence, health-related quality of life, and economic correlates. Obstet Gynecol 1996;87(3):321–7.

4. Harris RD, Holtzman SR, Poppe AM. Clinical outcome in female patients with pelvic pain and normal pelvic US findings. Radiology 2000; 216(2):440–3.

5. Reiter RC, Gambone JC. Demographic and historic variables in women with idiopathic chronic pelvic pain. Obstet Gynecol 1990;75(3 Pt 1):428–32.

6. ACOG Committee on Practice Bulletins—Gynecology. ACOG Practice Bulletin No. 51. Chronic pelvic pain. Obstet Gynecol 2004;103(3):589–605.

7. Bogduk N. International Spinal Injection Society guidelines for the performance of spinal injection procedures. Part 1: zygapophysial joint blocks. Clin J Pain 1997;13(4):285–302.

8. Filler AG. Diagnosis and treatment of pudendal nerve entrapment syndrome subtypes: imaging, injections, and minimal access surgery. Neurosurg Focus 2009;26(2):E9.

9. Lee HM, Weinstein JN, Meller ST, et al. The role of steroids and their effects on phospholipase A2. An animal model of radiculopathy. Spine (Phila Pa 1976) 1998;23(11):1191–6.

10. Losel R, Wehling M. Nongenomic actions of steroid hormones. Nat Rev Mol Cell Biol 2003;4(1):46–56.

11. Chhabra A, Lee PP, Bizzell C, et al. 3 Tesla MR neurography–technique, interpretation, and pitfalls. Skeletal Radiol 2011;40(10):1249–60.

12. Howe FA, Filler AG, Bell BA, et al. Magnetic resonance neurography. Magn Reson Med 1992; 28(2):328–38.

13. Carrino JA, Blanco R. Magnetic resonance–guided musculoskeletal interventional radiology. Semin Musculoskelet Radiol 2006;10(2):159–74.

14. Fritz J, Pereira PL. MR-Guided pain therapy: principles and clinical applications. Rofo 2007;179(9): 914–24 [in German].

15. Fritz J, Thomas C, Clasen S, et al. Freehand real-time MRI-guided lumbar spinal injection procedures at 1.5 T: feasibility, accuracy, and safety. AJR Am J Roentgenol 2009;192(4): W161–7.

16. Brenner DJ, Hall EJ. Computed tomography–an increasing source of radiation exposure. N Engl J Med 2007;357(22):2277–84.

17. Fritz J, Thomas C, Tzaribachev N, et al. MRI-guided injection procedures of the temporomandibular joints in children and adults: technique, accuracy, and safety. AJR Am J Roentgenol 2009;193(4):1148–54.

18. Fritz J, Henes JC, Thomas C, et al. Diagnostic and interventional MRI of the sacroiliac joints using a 1.5-T open-bore magnet: a one-stop-shopping approach. AJR Am J Roentgenol 2008;191(6): 1717–24.

19. Fritz J, Tzaribachev N, Thomas C, et al. Evaluation of MR imaging guided steroid injection of the sacroiliac joints for the treatment of children with refractory enthesitis-related arthritis. Eur Radiol 2011; 21(5):1050–7.

20. Sodickson A, Baeyens PF, Andriole KP, et al. Recurrent CT, cumulative radiation exposure, and associated radiation-induced cancer risks from CT of adults. Radiology 2009;251(1):175–84.

21. Filler AG, Haynes J, Jordan SE, et al. Sciatica of nondisc origin and piriformis syndrome: diagnosis by magnetic resonance neurography and interventional magnetic resonance imaging with outcome study of resulting treatment. J Neurosurg Spine 2005;2(2):99–115.

22. Fritz J, Niemeyer T, Clasen S, et al. Management of chronic low back pain: rationales, principles, and targets of imaging-guided spinal injections. Radiographics 2007;27(6):1751–71.

23. Fritz J, Clasen S, Boss A, et al. Real-time MR fluoroscopy-navigated lumbar facet joint injections: feasibility and technical properties. Eur Radiol 2008;18(7):1513–8.

24. Sequeiros RB, Ojala RO, Klemola R, et al. MRI-guided periradicular nerve root infiltration therapy in low-field (0.23-T) MRI system using optical instrument tracking. Eur Radiol 2002;12(6):1331–7.

25. Smith KA, Carrino J. MRI-guided interventions of the musculoskeletal system. J Magn Reson Imaging 2008;27(2):339–46.

26. Chhabra A, Soldatos T, Andreisek G. Lumbosacral plexus. In: Chhabra A, Andreisek G, editors. Magnetic resonance neurography. New Delhi (India): Jaypee Brothers Medical Publishers; 2012. p. 161–81.

27. Chhabra A, Chalian M, Andreisek G. Magnetic resonance neurography of tunnels - Part II: lower extremity nerves. In: Chhabra A, Andreisek G, editors. Magnetic resonance neurography. New Delhi (India): Jaypee Brothers Medical Publishers; 2012. p. 73–111.

28. Chhabra A, Williams EH, Wang KC, et al. MR neurography of neuromas related to nerve injury and entrapment with surgical correlation. AJNR Am J Neuroradiol 2010;31(8):1363–8.

29. Thawait SK, Chaudhry V, Thawait GK, et al. High-resolution MR neurography of diffuse peripheral nerve lesions. AJNR Am J Neuroradiol 2011; 32(8):1365–72.

30. Thawait SK, Wang K, Subhawong TK, et al. Peripheral nerve surgery: the role of high-resolution MR neurography. AJNR Am J Neuroradiol 2012;33(2): 203–10.

31. Wadhwa V, Thakkar RS, Maragakis N, et al. Sciatic nerve tumor and tumor-like lesions-uncommon pathologies. Skeletal Radiol 2012;41(7):763–74.

32. Kanal E, Borgstede JP, Barkovich AJ, et al. American College of Radiology White Paper on MR Safety: 2004 update and revisions. AJR Am J Roentgenol 2004;182(5):1111–4.

33. Shellock FG, Kanal E. Guidelines and recommendations for MR imaging safety and patient management. III. Questionnaire for screening patients before MR procedures. The SMRI Safety Committee. J Magn Reson Imaging 1994;4(5):749–51.

34. Shellock FG, Crues JV. MR procedures: biologic effects, safety, and patient care. Radiology 2004; 232(3):635–52.

35. Dempsey MF, Condon B, Hadley DM. Investigation of the factors responsible for burns during MRI. J Magn Reson Imaging 2001;13(4):627–31.

36. Lewin JS, Duerk JL, Jain VR, et al. Needle localization in MR-guided biopsy and aspiration: effects of field strength, sequence design, and magnetic field orientation. AJR Am J Roentgenol 1996; 166(6):1337–45.

37. Lufkin R, Teresi L, Chiu L, et al. A technique for MR-guided needle placement. AJR Am J Roentgenol 1988;151(1):193–6.

38. Ludeke KM, Roschmann P, Tischler R. Susceptibility artefacts in NMR imaging. Magn Reson Imaging 1985;3(4):329–43.

39. Ojala R, Vahala E, Karppinen J, et al. Nerve root infiltration of the first sacral root with MRI guidance. J Magn Reson Imaging 2000;12(4):556–61.

40. Safriel Y, Ali M, Hayt M, et al. Gadolinium use in spine procedures for patients with allergy to iodinated contrast—experience of 127 procedures. AJNR Am J Neuroradiol 2006;27(6):1194–7.

41. Shetty SK, Nelson EN, Lawrimore TM, et al. Use of gadolinium chelate to confirm epidural needle placement in patients with an iodinated contrast reaction. Skeletal Radiol 2007;36(4):301–7.

42. Butterworth JF, Strichartz GR. Molecular mechanisms of local anesthesia: a review. Anesthesiology 1990;72(4):711–34.

43. Craig AD. How do you feel? Interoception: the sense of the physiological condition of the body. Nat Rev Neurosci 2002;3(8):655–66.

44. Gray H, Lewis WH. Anatomy of the human body. 20th edition. New York: Bartleby.com; 2000.

45. Kendir S, Akkaya T, Comert A, et al. The location of the obturator nerve: a three-dimensional description of the obturator canal. Surg Radiol Anat 2008;30(6):495–501.

46. Bradshaw C, McCrory P. Obturator nerve entrapment. Clin J Sport Med 1997;7(3):217–9.

47. Birnbaum K, Prescher A, Hessler S, et al. The sensory innervation of the hip joint—an anatomical study. Surg Radiol Anat 1997;19(6):371–5.

48. Tipton JS. Obturator neuropathy. Curr Rev Musculoskelet Med 2008;1(3–4):234–7.

49. House CV, Ali KE, Bradshaw C, et al. CT-guided obturator nerve block via the posterior approach. Skeletal Radiol 2006;35(4):227–32.

50. Macalou D, Trueck S, Meuret P, et al. Postoperative analgesia after total knee replacement: the effect of an obturator nerve block added to the femoral 3-in-1 nerve block. Anesth Analg 2004;99(1):251–4.

51. Wassef MR. Interadductor approach to obturator nerve blockade for spastic conditions of adductor thigh muscles. Reg Anesth 1993;18(1):13–7.

52. Akkaya T, Ozturk E, Comert A, et al. Ultrasound-guided obturator nerve block: a sonoanatomic study of a new methodologic approach. Anesth Analg 2009;108(3):1037–41.

53. Viel EJ, Perennou D, Ripart J, et al. Neurolytic blockade of the obturator nerve for intractable spasticity of adductor thigh muscles. Eur J Pain 2002;6(2):97–104.

54. Heywang-Kobrunner SH, Amaya B, Okoniewski M, et al. CT-guided obturator nerve block for diagnosis and treatment of painful conditions of the hip. Eur Radiol 2001;11(6):1047–53.

55. Stav K, Dwyer PL, Roberts L. Pudendal neuralgia. Fact or fiction? Obstet Gynecol Surv 2009;64(3): 190–9.

56. Labat JJ, Riant T, Robert R, et al. Diagnostic criteria for pudendal neuralgia by pudendal nerve

entrapment (Nantes criteria). Neurourol Urodyn 2008;27(4):306–10.

57. Lefaucheur JP, Labat JJ, Amarenco G, et al. What is the place of electroneuromyographic studies in the diagnosis and management of pudendal neuralgia related to entrapment syndrome? Neurophysiol Clin 2007;37(4):223–8.

58. Filippiadis DK, Velonakis G, Mazioti A, et al. CT-guided percutaneous infiltration for the treatment of Alcock's neuralgia. Pain Physician 2011; 14(2):211–5.

59. Romanzi L. Techniques of pudendal nerve block. J Sex Med 2010;7(5):1716–9.

60. Thoumas D, Leroi AM, Mauillon J, et al. Pudendal neuralgia: CT-guided pudendal nerve block technique. Abdom Imaging 1999;24(3):309–12.

61. Rofaeel A, Peng P, Louis I, et al. Feasibility of real-time ultrasound for pudendal nerve block in patients with chronic perineal pain. Reg Anesth Pain Med 2008;33(2):139–45.

62. Tubbs RS, Miller J, Loukas M, et al. Surgical and anatomical landmarks for the perineal branch of the posterior femoral cutaneous nerve: implications in perineal pain syndromes. Laboratory investigation. J Neurosurg 2009;111(2):332–5.

63. Darnis B, Robert R, Labat JJ, et al. Perineal pain and inferior cluneal nerves: anatomy and surgery. Surg Radiol Anat 2008;30(3):177–83.

64. Hughes PJ, Brown TC. An approach to posterior femoral cutaneous nerve block. Anaesth Intensive Care 1986;14(4):350–1.

65. Barbero C, Fuzier R, Samii K. Anterior approach to the sciatic nerve block: adaptation to the patient's height. Anesth Analg 2004;98(6):1785–8.

66. Chelly JE, Delaunay L. A new anterior approach to the sciatic nerve block. Anesthesiology 1999;91(6): 1655–60.

67. De Tran QH, Clemente A, Finlayson RJ. A review of approaches and techniques for lower extremity nerve blocks. Can J Anaesth 2007;54(11):922–34.

68. Beason L, Anson B. The relation of the sciatic nerve and its subdivisions to the piriformis muscle. Anat Rec 1937;70:1–5.

69. Smoll NR. Variations of the piriformis and sciatic nerve with clinical consequence: a review. Clin Anat 2010;23(1):8–17.

70. Gelfand HJ, Ouanes JP, Lesley MR, et al. Analgesic efficacy of ultrasound-guided regional anesthesia: a meta-analysis. J Clin Anesth 2011;23(2):90–6.

71. Rohen JW, Yokochi C, Ltjen-Drecoll E. Color atlas of anatomy a photographic study of the human body. 5th edition. Philadelphia: Lippincott Williams & Wilkins; 2002.

72. Robinson D. Piriformis syndrome in relation to sciatic pain. Am J Surg 1947;73:355–8.

73. Fishman LM, Anderson C, Rosner B. BOTOX and physical therapy in the treatment of piriformis syndrome. Am J Phys Med Rehabil 2002;81(12): 936–42.

74. Halpin RJ, Ganju A. Piriformis syndrome: a real pain in the buttock? Neurosurgery 2009;65(Suppl 4): A197–202.

75. Russell JM, Kransdorf MJ, Bancroft LW, et al. Magnetic resonance imaging of the sacral plexus and piriformis muscles. Skeletal Radiol 2008;37(8): 709–13.

76. Benzon HT, Katz JA, Benzon HA, et al. Piriformis syndrome: anatomic considerations, a new injection technique, and a review of the literature. Anesthesiology 2003;98(6):1442–8.

77. Blasi J, Chapman ER, Link E, et al. Botulinum neurotoxin A selectively cleaves the synaptic protein SNAP-25. Nature 1993;365(6442):160–3.

78. Childers MK, Wilson DJ, Gnatz SM, et al. Botulinum toxin type A use in piriformis muscle syndrome: a pilot study. Am J Phys Med Rehabil 2002;81(10): 751–9.

79. Broadhurst NA, Simmons DN, Bond MJ. Piriformis syndrome: correlation of muscle morphology with symptoms and signs. Arch Phys Med Rehabil 2004;85(12):2036–9.

80. Porta M. A comparative trial of botulinum toxin type A and methylprednisolone for the treatment of myofascial pain syndrome and pain from chronic muscle spasm. Pain 2000;85(1–2):101–5.

81. Grothaus MC, Holt M, Mekhail AO, et al. Lateral femoral cutaneous nerve: an anatomic study. Clin Orthop Relat Res 2005;(437):164–8.

82. Kosiyatrakul A, Nuansalee N, Luenam S, et al. The anatomical variation of the lateral femoral cutaneous nerve in relation to the anterior superior iliac spine and the iliac crest. Musculoskelet Surg 2010; 94(1):17–20.

83. de Ridder VA, de LS, Popta JV. Anatomical variations of the lateral femoral cutaneous nerve and the consequences for surgery. J Orthop Trauma 1999;13(3):207–11.

84. Aszmann OC, Dellon ES, Dellon AL. Anatomical course of the lateral femoral cutaneous nerve and its susceptibility to compression and injury. Plast Reconstr Surg 1997;100(3):600–4.

85. Murata Y, Takahashi K, Yamagata M, et al. The anatomy of the lateral femoral cutaneous nerve, with special reference to the harvesting of iliac bone graft. J Bone Joint Surg Am 2000;82(5):746–7.

86. Ray B, D'Souza AS, Kumar B, et al. Variations in the course and microanatomical study of the lateral femoral cutaneous nerve and its clinical importance. Clin Anat 2010;23(8):978–84.

87. Roth V. Meralgia paresthetica. Med Radiol (Mosk) 1895;43:678.

88. Hui GK, Peng PW. Meralgia paresthetica: what an anesthesiologist needs to know. Reg Anesth Pain Med 2011;36(2):156–61.

89. Alberti O, Wickboldt J, Becker R. Suprainguinal retroperitoneal approach for the successful surgical treatment of meralgia paresthetica. J Neurosurg 2009;110(4):768–74.

90. Russo MJ, Firestone LB, Mandler RN, et al. Nerve conduction studies of the lateral femoral cutaneous nerve. Implications in the diagnosis of meralgia paresthetica. Am J Electroneurodiagn Technol 2005;45(3):180–5.

91. Shannon J, Lang SA, Yip RW, et al. Lateral femoral cutaneous nerve block revisited. A nerve stimulator technique. Reg Anesth 1995;20(2):100–4.

92. Ng I, Vaghadia H, Choi PT, et al. Ultrasound imaging accurately identifies the lateral femoral cutaneous nerve. Anesth Analg 2008;107(3):1070–4.

93. Aravindakannan T, Wilder-Smith EP. High-resolution ultrasonography in the assessment of meralgia paresthetica. Muscle Nerve 2012;45(3):434–5.

94. Oh CS, Chung IH, Ji HJ, et al. Clinical implications of topographic anatomy on the ganglion impar. Anesthesiology 2004;101(1):249–50.

95. Plancarte R, Amescua C, Patt R. Presacral neurectomy of the ganglion impar (Ganglion of Walther). Anesthesiology 1990;73:A751.

96. Agarwal-Kozlowski K, Lorke DE, Habermann CR. CT-guided blocks and neuroablation of the ganglion impar (Walther) in perineal pain: anatomy, technique, safety, and efficacy. Clin J Pain 2009; 25(7):570–6.

97. Toshniwal GR, Dureja GP, Prashanth SM. Transsacrococcygeal approach to ganglion impar block for management of chronic perineal pain: a prospective observational study. Pain Physician 2007;10(5):661–6.

98. Loev MA, Varklet VL, Wilsey BL, et al. Cryoablation: a novel approach to neurolysis of the ganglion impar. Anesthesiology 1998;88(5):1391–3.

99. Wemm K Jr, Saberski L. Modified approach to block the ganglion impar (ganglion of Walther). Reg Anesth 1995;20(6):544–5.

100. Datir A, Connell D. CT-guided injection for ganglion impar blockade: a radiological approach to the management of coccydynia. Clin Radiol 2010; 65(1):21–5.

101. Ho KY, Nagi PA, Gray L, et al. An alternative approach to ganglion impar neurolysis under computed tomography guidance for recurrent vulva cancer. Anesthesiology 2006;105(4): 861–2.

102. Wall PD, Devor M. Sensory afferent impulses originate from dorsal root ganglia as well as from the periphery in normal and nerve injured rats. Pain 1983;17(4):321–39.

103. Woolf CJ, Shortland P, Coggeshall RE. Peripheral nerve injury triggers central sprouting of myelinated afferents. Nature 1992;355(6355):75–8.

104. North RB, Kidd DH, Zahurak M, et al. Specificity of diagnostic nerve blocks: a prospective, randomized study of sciatica due to lumbosacral spine disease. Pain 1996;65(1):77–85.

105. Riew KD, Park JB, Cho YS, et al. Nerve root blocks in the treatment of lumbar radicular pain. A minimum five-year follow-up. J Bone Joint Surg Am 2006; 88(8):1722–5.

The Role of Magnetic Resonance Neurography in the Postoperative Management of Peripheral Nerve Injuries

Pablo A. Baltodano, MD[a], Anne J.W. Tong, MBBS[a],
Avneesh Chhabra, MD[b], Gedge D. Rosson, MD[a,*]

KEYWORDS

- Peripheral nerve • Nerve injuries • Nerve repair • Postoperative management
- Magnetic resonance neurography

KEY POINTS

- Nerve injuries may significantly affect patients' life, and timely surgical treatment can improve outcomes.
- Diagnostic limitations exist with current methods of postoperative evaluation, and newer techniques that may play useful role in adequately following up nerve repairs are actively sought.
- Emerging imaging techniques, such as high-resolution magnetic resonance neurography may play an important role in the postoperative follow-up of nerve repairs.
- A multidisciplinary approach entailing active discussion of findings among radiologists, electrophysiologists, and peripheral nerve surgeons can be helpful in planning surgical treatment and follow-up of patients.

INTRODUCTION TO PERIPHERAL NERVE REPAIR

Nerve injuries can significantly impair patients' quality of life. Motor and sensory functional loss may result in substantial debilitation of these patients and may even have psychosocial repercussions.[1] Thus, the physicians or surgeons dealing with such patients should have a good understanding of the principles behind optimal nerve injury management to enhance outcomes.

Although different types and indications of nerve repairs exist,[2] the postoperative imaging of nerve repairs remains a new and thus poorly defined field.

High-field (3-T) and high-resolution magnetic resonance neurography (MRN) imaging holds promise in both diagnostic and prognostic realms. In this article, the nerve injury grading, various types of nerve repair techniques, and approaches available for postoperative follow-up are discussed.

PERIPHERAL NERVE ANATOMY AND PATHOPHYSIOLOGY

Knowledge of normal nerve anatomy is essential in understanding and managing peripheral nerve injuries; thus we briefly outline some pertinent anatomy here. Each nerve contains neural tissue and

Potential Conflicts of Interest. P. Baltodano, A.J.W. Tong, G.D. Rosson: None. A. Chhabra: Grant support-Siemens, Integra Life Sciences, Siemens. MSK CAD consultant: Siemens.

[a] Department of Plastic and Reconstructive Surgery, The Johns Hopkins Hospital, 601 North Caroline Street, Baltimore, MD 21287, USA; [b] Department of Radiology and Orthopedic Surgery, University of Texas South Western Medical Center, Dallas, TX 75390, USA
* Corresponding author. Department of Plastic and Reconstructive Surgery, The Johns Hopkins University School of Medicine, Suite 8161, JHOC eighth Floor, 601 North Caroline Street, Baltimore, MD 21287.
E-mail address: gedge@jhmi.edu

connective tissue. The basic unit of a nerve is the axon. A sheath of connective tissue called the endoneurium surrounds each axon. A bundle of axons are surrounded by the perineurium, forming a fascicle. The fascicles may convey pure motor, sensory, or autonomic functions, or a mixture of these. The connective tissue stroma that surrounds a group of fascicles is called the epineurium.[3] The nerves can be injured by a variety of systemic causes or local mechanisms. The local injuries are typically divided into compression or penetrating injuries. Seddon[4] and Sunderland[5] have classified the basic management strategies of peripheral nerve injuries (Table 1). Each degree corresponds to a more severe level of functional compromise that may increase the need for surgical exploration (eg, fourth-degree, fifth-degree, and sixth-degree injuries warrant surgical repair).[6] Although diverse methods exist for treatment of these injuries, in general, several factors related to nerve injury or patient demographics influence the outcome of surgical treatment (Table 2).[7–12]

TYPES OF NERVE REPAIRS

The available options for the treatment of peripheral nerve injuries include neurolysis, direct nerve repair, nerve graft, nerve transfer, tendon/muscle transfer, and bone/joint procedures.[13–15]

Neurolysis

Neurolysis is a surgical procedure performed to release the injured nerve from the surrounding scar tissue. It is categorized into internal and external neurolysis. External neurolysis involves exposing the entire nerve diameter and releasing it from its sheath and surrounding scar tissue. Internal neurolysis implies excision and release of scar tissue between the nerve fascicles in the intraepineural space. External neurolysis is more commonly performed, because the results of internal neurolysis are not encouraging.[16,17]

MRN can prudently guide the surgical treatment by identifying the perineural scarring, nerve hyperintensity, or entanglement by focal fibrosis or thickened fascia as well as internal heterogeneity of the nerve, reflecting scar tissue with irregular/disrupted fascicles, as commonly seen with neuroma in continuity (Figs. 1 and 2).[18,19]

With successful neurolysis, the nerve T2 signal intensity should diminish over 4 to 6 weeks and size should become near normal. Failed neurolysis cases may show a combination of findings, such as worsening nerve T2 signal intensity, fascicular swelling, increasing nerve size, increasing perineural fibrosis, worsening regional muscle denervation changes, altered nerve course, or flattening due to encasement by fibrosis (Fig. 3A–C).

Direct Repair

Most peripheral nerve surgeons pursue an end-to-end direct nerve repair whenever a tensionless coaptation is possible. This setting is ideal because tension between repaired ends can compromise recovery by interrupting vascular flow, subsequently leading to nerve scarring at both ends.[20] Large nerve gaps (≥2 cm) can give rise to tension in anastomosis. This situation requires other alternatives, such as the use of nerve grafts.[21] In our preliminary experience, MRN has proved useful to follow up nerve coaptations. The study should show homogeneous bright nerve signal intensity with current techniques, and over time, fascicular definitions should become perceptible as the axonal growth fills up the connections. The regional muscle denervation changes should also regress with time, observed as decreased signal intensity on fluid-sensitive fat-suppressed T2-weighted images and increased muscle bulk on T1-weighted images.[22]

In surgical failures, the nerve signal changes from bright to black to bright at the site of coaptation as the nerve is followed on sequential scans from proximal to distal, because of interval scarring and formation of proximal neuroma (Fig. 4). The regional muscle denervation changes also worsen, with progressive edema-like signal and atrophy.

Nerve Graft

When nerve damage leaves a gap that is not amenable to repair by primary tensionless anastomosis, the gold standard is the use of autologous grafts. Various types and designs of nerve grafts are used. Examples of commonly used nerve grafts include the medial antebrachial cutaneous nerve in the forearm and the sural nerve in the leg. Vascularized nerve grafts are commonly applied, with the hypothesis that their added blood supply may improve regeneration. These grafts have produced mixed outcomes in the surgical setting.[23–25] The harvest of a nerve graft is complicated, with donor-site morbidity. Although expected, this loss should be balanced with the extra gain of functional outcome in the repaired nerve (eg, in the case of sural nerve harvested as a graft, the patients are advised to expect some degree of permanent sensory loss in the lateral leg and foot).

With recent advances and application of biomaterials, artificial conduits have emerged as promising alternatives to autologous grafts, to limit donor-site morbidity. Commonly used products

Table 1
Classification and expected recovery of nerve injuries

Classification		Nerve Component Injured						Expected Recovery			Surgery Indicated
Seddon	Sunderland Degree (Modified)	Myelin	Axon	Endoneurium	Perineurium	Epineurium		Extent	Rate		
Neurapraxia	First	Yes	No	No	No	No		Complete	Fast		None
Axonotmesis	Second	Yes	Yes	No	No	No		Good	Slow		None
Axonotmesis	Third	Yes	Yes	Yes	No	No		Variable	Slow		None or neurolysis
Axonotmesis	Fourth	Yes	Yes	Yes	Yes	No		None	None		Nerve repair
Neurotmesis	Fifth	Yes	Yes	Yes	Yes	Yes		None	None		Nerve repair
Neurotmesis	Sixth	Combination of injury						Variable	Variable		Variable

Data from Baltodano P, Rosson G. Nerve injury and repair. In: Cameron JL, Cameron AM, editors. Current surgical treatment. 11th edition. Amsterdam: Mosby Elsevier.

Table 2
Factors reported to influence nerve repair outcomes

Relevant Factors	Functional Outcomes
Patient's age	Younger patient > Older patient
Level of injury	Distal > Proximal
Type of nerve injured	Pure nerves > Mixed nerves
Injured nerve	Radial nerve > Median nerve > Ulnar nerve Nerves C5 and C6 and those of the upper trunk > Nerves C8 to T1 and those of the lower trunk Tibial nerve > Peroneal nerve
Injury mechanism	Lacerations > Low-velocity gunshot injuries > High-velocity gunshot injuries Transections > Crush or avulsion injuries Stretch injuries > Ruptures > Avulsions
Time frame between injury and repair	The "earlier the better", Waiting 2–3 weeks might be reasonable in some instances (blunt or ragged transections or injuries with significant crush or avulsion component) to allow time for better definition of the zone of injury
Type of repair	Neurolysis alone in lesions with (+) nerve action potential has good results 90% of the time Direct end-to-end nerve repair > Interpositional nerve grafting Distal nerve transfer > Proximal nerve grafts Direct nerve transfers > Nerve transfers with interpositional grafts
Cognitive capacity	Higher verbal learning and visuo-spatial logic correlates with improved sensibility outcomes
Early psychological stress	Early psychological stress hampers functional outcome and work resumption

Data from Refs.[7–12]; and *Modified from* Baltodano P, Rosson G. Nerve injury and repair. In: Cameron JL, Cameron AM, editors. Current surgical treatment. XI edition. Amsterdam: Mosby Elsevier.

include synthetic nerve tube and acellular cadaver nerve graft. Success has been reported in the use of nerve tube for repair of sensory nerves and for bridging short gaps (<3 cm) of nerve defects.[26,27] A few of the cases that have used MRN have been studied.[28]

Nerve regeneration through these small tubes can be challenging if careful attention is not paid to the surgical site during image protocol and interpretation. The nerve tube margin may be detected as a hypointense serrated or uniform lining, and show increasing fascicular definition in the expected location of the tube over time. Functional return occurs when the axons successfully reach their distal motor or sensory targets. Careful clinical evaluation, including attention to advancing Tinel sign and magnetic resonance evidence of regression of muscle denervation changes on

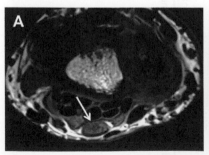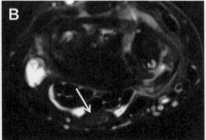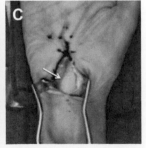

Fig. 1. 65-year-old woman with remote history of injury and presenting with symptoms of carpal tunnel syndrome. Axial T1-weighted (*A*) and T2-weighted spectral attenuated inversion recovery (*B*) images show enlarged median nerve with heterogeneous signal intensity and diminished fascicular definition (*arrows*), in keeping with a neuroma in continuity. Intraoperative image (*C*) confirms the findings of neuroma in continuity (*arrow*). Epineurectomy and minimal interfascicular dissection was performed. ([*C*] *Courtesy of* Dr Damon S. Cooney, MD, PhD, The Johns Hopkins University School of Medicine, Baltimore, MD.)

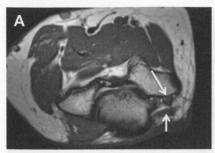
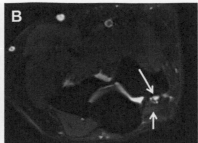
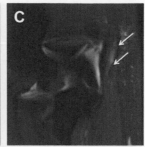

Fig. 2. 52-year-old woman presenting with symptoms of ulnar neuropathy. Axial T1-weighted (*A*) and T2 spectral attenuated inversion recovery (*B*) images show enlarged ulnar nerve (*large arrow*) with prominent hyperintense fascicles. Notice minimal perineural scarring and muscular insertion of medial head of triceps with extension into the cubital tunnel (*small arrows*). Coronal three-dimensional maximum intensity projection fat-suppressed T2-weighted image (*C*) delineates the longitudinal extent of neuropathy (*arrows*).

serial imaging, aids in accurate diagnosis of successful nerve repairs. On the other hand, failure of successful growth is seen as formation of end-bulb neuroma and worsening muscle denervation (**Fig. 5**).

Nerve Transfers

Nerve transfer (also known as neurotization) involves taking a healthy, less important donor nerve and transferring it to the distal stump of an avulsed nerve. This treatment is indicated when the damaged nerve is irreparable by end-to-end anastomosis or interpositioning of a nerve graft.[15,29]

Although the aim is to restore the motor/sensory function of the recipient nerve, it should be cautiously weighed against the morbidity of the donor nerve sacrifice. Nerve transfer holds a unique role in the microsurgical repair of peripheral

nerve injuries and its use has been pioneered since the late nineteenth century. Spinal accessory nerve transfer to repair facial nerve paralysis was first performed by Drobnik in 1895.[30] Yeoman and Seddon[31] described the use of intercostal nerves for the repair of brachial plexus injuries. These techniques have been refined over many decades and are still used in surgical practice.

Nerve transfers are divided into 2 categories: intraplexal and extraplexal. Intraplexal, as the name implies, refers to using functional nerves from the same plexus to neurotize the avulsed counterparts. An example is the transfer of the long thoracic nerve to the suprascapular nerve in an attempt to regain shoulder abduction.[32] In extraplexal transfer, the source of donor nerve is obtained from outside the nerve plexus to neurotize the damaged nerve. The use of the phrenic nerve for brachial plexus injury is one such example.[33]

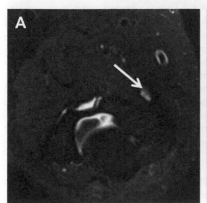
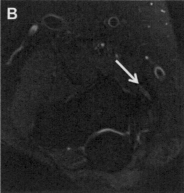
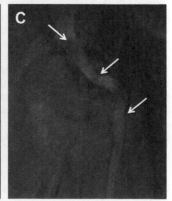

Fig. 3. 52-year-old woman presenting with recurrent symptoms of ulnar neuropathy after failed anterior submuscular transposition. Axial T1-weighted (*A*) and T2 spectral attenuated inversion recovery (*B*) images show the enlarged and hyperintense anteriorly transposed ulnar nerve (*arrow in A*) with abnormal flattening under the thickened pronator teres fascial edge and perineural scarring (*arrow in B*). Coronal oblique three-dimensional weighted reversed fast imaging with steady state free precession (PSIF) image (*C*) delineates the longitudinal extent of neuropathy and abnormal angulations caused by recurrent entrapment (*arrows*).

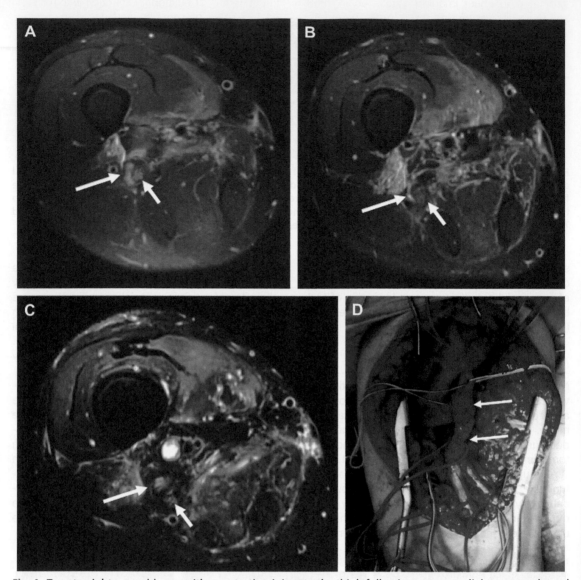

Fig. 4. Twenty-eight-year-old man with penetrating injury to the thigh following anteromedial to posterolateral trajectory. The vascular injury to the superficial femoral vessels was repaired during the debridement, and additional sciatic nerve coaptation was performed in the same setting. Patient presented with persistent sciatic neuropathy symptoms 2 months after the injury. Sequential axial T2 SPAIR (*A–C*) images from proximal to distal show the enlarged and hyperintense tibial nerve (TN, *small arrow* in A) and common peroneal nerve (CPN) with disrupted fascicles of CPN (*large arrow* in A). (*B*) Abrupt signal alteration of the sciatic nerve to hypointensity (*arrows*) followed by increased signal in the more distal image with return of fascicular appearance in the TN and CPN (*arrows* in C). Intraoperative image (*D*) confirms scarring at the coaptation site (*arrows* in D), which was immediately repaired by scar resection and co-axial cable grafting of the freshened nerve edges. ([D] *Courtesy of Dr Eric H. Williams, MD, The Dellon Institutes for Peripheral Nerve Surgery.*)

There are situations in which nerve transfers can yield superior results compared with primary nerve graft repair. In the upper extremity, nerve transfer is commonly indicated for sensory restoration in injuries of the hand and brachial plexus. Another example of its use is when nerve roots have been avulsed from the spinal cord (known as preganglionic injury). Nerve transfer allows repair to be performed closer to the end-muscle target. Reinnervation can be expected to occur and complete earlier. Theoretically, this technique presents a distinct advantage to the other types of repair.[34] MRN is commonly used to detect preganglionic avulsions or differentiate Sunderland grade 4 and 5 injuries from stretch injuries, where the nerve is in continuity. It thereby helps plan the type of

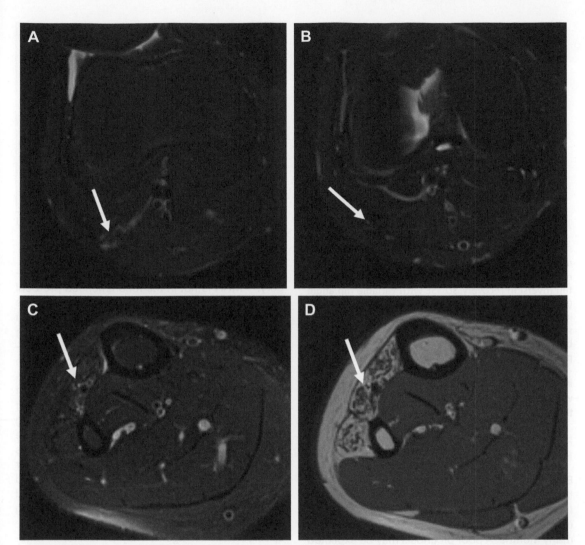

Fig. 5. 16-year-old boy with previous common peroneal nerve (CPN) repair after cadaver nerve grafting and resection of a benign tumor from the CPN. Sequential axial T2 spectral attenuated inversion recovery images of the lower leg from proximal to distal (*A–C*) show end-bulb neuroma with thickened nerve sprouts at the proximal aspect of the repair site (*arrow* in *A*) and distally nonconnected hyperintense CPN (*arrow* in *B*). Also note muscle denervation edemalike hyperintense signal in the extensor and peroneal muscles (*arrow* in *C*) and complete fatty replacement in axial T1-weighted image (*arrow* in *D*), consistent with failed nerve grafting.

surgical repair (**Fig. 6**).[35] However, after nerve transfer, MRN cannot be used in the detection of nerve regeneration, because the resolution is not adequate to detect axonal growth in these small nerves, located in anatomically complex or surgically distorted fields.

Muscle/Tendon Transfers

Similar to nerve transfer, muscle or tendon transfers involve using a functioning muscle/tendon to restore the functional loss of a denervated muscle. In situations in which nerve repair does not readily restore muscle function, muscle or tendon

transfers are sought for palliative purposes.[36,37] Although partial function restoration is the goal, cosmetic deformity should be expected.

Bone/Joint Procedures

Bone and joint procedures, such as osteotomy and arthrodesis (joint fusion), are also performed to augment the functional outcomes of nerve repair. A combination of procedures is sometimes sought to maximize these aims. Arthrodesis, in conjunction with tendon transfers, is performed to stabilize the shoulder function when there is refractory damage from repair of brachial plexus

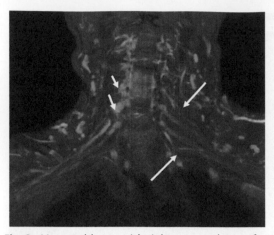

Fig. 6. 44-year-old man with right arm weakness after motor vehicle accident. Maximum intensity projection reconstruction form coronal three-dimensional short-tau inversion recovery 3D TSE with variable flip angle (SPACE) sequence shows postganglionic Sunderland V injuries of C5 and C6 nerves (*small arrows*) and stretch-related hyperintensity to the remaining right brachial plexus nerves. Notice normal left brachial plexus (*large arrows*).

injuries. This procedure should be complemented with physical therapy to train muscles to regain the best possible function over time.

POSTOPERATIVE MANAGEMENT AND FOLLOW-UP

Because recovery from nerve repair invariably takes time, a standardized protocol of careful focused clinical evaluation and tests should be used on each patient over serial intervals lasting many months. A poor prognosis may be expected in the elderly individual, complex soft tissue injuries or fractures, contaminated wounds, or systemic and immune problems, which can interfere with nerve regeneration.

A commonly used clinical test is the advancing Tinel sign, which is elicited to determine the level of nerve regeneration. In many cases of nerve lesions, electromyography and nerve conduction studies are scheduled at monthly intervals to record the progress of nerve regeneration; however, electrical activity may be delayed for many months after surgery, reflecting significant limitation with these techniques. The Medical Research Council (MRC) scale is a commonly used clinical tool to grade muscle power after nerve surgeries, such as testing for elbow flexion after nerve transfer in brachial plexus injuries (Table 3).[38]

Physical therapy should be scheduled in the early stage of follow-up to maintain joint mobility and to prevent joint contractures. Reeducation of nerve transfers, especially of sensory nerves, is

Table 3
The MRC muscle power grading scale

Grade	Description
0	No contraction
1	Flicker or trace of contraction
2	Active movement, with gravity eliminated
3	Active movement, against gravity
4	Active movement, against gravity and resistance
5	Normal power

Data from Gelberman RH. Operative nerve repair and reconstruction. J Pediatr Orthop 1992;12:550.

crucial to maintain the good outcomes of the surgery.[39] MRN is not in the recommended protocol for the follow-up of these patients, because the nerves may remain hyperintense for prolonged periods after surgery. However, MRN is being increasingly ordered by referring physicians because it has multiple advantages: noninvasive technique, objective showing of nerve and perineural tissues, fascicular depiction as a result of high-resolution capabilities, objective showing of successful treatment on serial interval imaging (nerve size normalization, decreased T2 nerve signal intensity and muscle denervation changes over time), depiction of neuroma in continuity or end-bulb neuroma in surgical failures, and showing increasing nerve signal changes and regional muscle denervation changes in worsening cases. In future, diffusion tensor imaging or nerve-specific contrast agents may be useful in functional evaluation of the nerve regeneration.[40–44]

PATHOPHYSIOLOGY OF FAILED NERVE REPAIRS

Nerve repairs are one of the most challenging surgical problems, because the outcomes are variable and recovery is slow. Several studies have analyzed the pathophysiology and identified factors that influence the outcome of nerve repairs (see Table 2).[7–12] The interaction between these factors determines the final outcome of the reconstruction. In addition, several causes of failed nerve repairs have been identified (Box 1).[12,45–51] Tension over the reconstruction site is considered one of the most important causes of nerve reconstruction failures.[49–51] Research has shown that tension causes connective tissue proliferation and scar formation, which obstructs axonal regeneration.[47–51] Thus, tensionless nerve repairs should be the first goal of any nerve reconstructive strategy. The nerve repair salvage or reintervention should be carefully planned between the peripheral nerve surgeon and the radiologist, taking into account all the factors that relate to outcomes.

Close communication and collaboration between the referring physician and the radiologist are essential for early diagnosis and clarification of abnormal MRN findings after failed nerve repairs.

SUMMARY

Peripheral nerve surgery involves a variety of techniques and high-resolution MRN is a useful adjunct to clinical examination and electrophysiologic studies in preoperative planning of patients being considered for prospective surgery and during follow-up of failed nerve repairs.

REFERENCES

1. Dolan RT, Butler JS, Murphy SM, et al. Health-related quality of life and functional outcomes following nerve transfers for traumatic upper brachial plexus injuries. J Hand Surg 2012;37:642–51.
2. Boyd KU, Nimigan AS, Mackinnon SE. Nerve reconstruction in the hand and upper extremity. Clin Plast Surg 2011;38:643–60.
3. Thomas M. New atlas of human anatomy. China: Metro Books; 1999. p. 96–7.
4. Seddon HJ. Three types of nerve injuries. Brain 1943;66:237–88.
5. Sunderland S. A classification of peripheral nerve injuries producing loss of function. Brain 1951;74:491–516.
6. Pabari A, Yang SY, Seifalian AM, et al. Modern surgical management of peripheral nerve gap. J Plast Reconstr Aesthet Surg 2010;63:1941–8.
7. Scholz T, Krichevsky A, Sumarto A, et al. Peripheral nerve injuries: an international survey of current treatments and future perspectives. J Reconstr Microsurg 2009;25:339–44.
8. Ruijs AC, Jaquet JB, Kalmijn S, et al. Median and ulnar nerve injuries: a meta-analysis of predictors of motor and sensory recovery after modern microsurgical nerve repair. Plast Reconstr Surg 2005;116:484–94.
9. Siemionow M, Brzezicki G. Current techniques and concepts in peripheral nerve repair. Int Rev Neurobiol 2009;87:141–72.
10. Jaquet JB, Luijsterburg AJ, Kalmijn S, et al. Median, ulnar, and combined median-ulnar nerve injuries: functional outcome and return to productivity. J Trauma 2001;51:687–92.
11. Mackenzie IG, Woods CG. Causes of failure after repair of the median nerve. J Bone Joint Surg Br 1961;43:465–73.
12. Schoeller T, Otto A, Wechselberger G, et al. Distal nerve entrapment following nerve repair. Br J Plast Surg 1998;51:227–9.
13. Gelberman RH. Operative nerve repair and reconstruction. J Pediatr Orthop 1992;12:550.
14. Seddon HJ. Nerve grafting. J Bone Joint Surg Br 1963;43:447–61.
15. Tung TH, Mackinnon SE. Nerve reconstruction in the hand and upper extremity nerve transfers: indications, techniques, and outcomes. J Hand Surg Am 2010;35:332–41.
16. Mackinnon SE, McCabe S, Murray JF, et al. Internal neurolysis fails to improve the results of primary carpal tunnel decompression. J Hand Surg Am 1991;16:211–8.
17. Holmgren-Larsson H, Leszniewski W, Lindén U, et al. Internal neurolysis or ligament division only in carpal tunnel syndrome–results of a randomized study. Acta Neurochir 1985;74:118–21.
18. Filler AG, Maravilla KR, Tsuruda JS. MR neurography and muscle MR imaging for image diagnosis of disorders affecting the peripheral nerves and musculature. Neurol Clin 2004;22:643–82.
19. Thawait SK, Chaudhry V, Thawait GK, et al. High-resolution MR neurography of diffuse peripheral nerve lesions. AJNR Am J Neuroradiol 2011;32:1365–72.
20. Driscoll PJ, Glasby MA, Lawson GM. An in vivo study of peripheral nerves in continuity: biomechanical and physiological responses to elongation. J Orthop Res 2002;20:370–5.
21. Millesi H. Microsurgery of peripheral nerves. Hand 1973;5:157–60.
22. Kikuchi Y, Nakamura T, Takayama S, et al. MR imaging in the diagnosis of denervated and

reinnervated skeletal muscles: experimental study in rats. Radiology 2003;229(3):861–7.

23. Merle M, Dautel G. Vascularized nerve grafts. J Hand Surg Br 1991;16:483–8.

24. Terzis JK, Kostopoulos VK. Vascularized nerve grafts for lower extremity nerve reconstruction. Ann Plast Surg 2010;64:169–76.

25. Birch R, Dunkerton M, Bonney G, et al. Experience with the free vascularized ulnar nerve graft in repair of supraclavicular lesions of the brachial plexus. Clin Orthop Relat Res 1988;237:96–104.

26. Mackinnon SE, Dellon AL. Clinical nerve reconstruction with a bioabsorbable polyglycolic acid tube. Plast Reconstr Surg 1990;85:419–24.

27. Weber RA, Breidenbach WC, Brown RE, et al. A randomized prospective study of polyglycolic acid conduits for digital nerve reconstruction in humans. Plast Reconstr Surg 2000;106:1036–45.

28. Thawait SK, Wang K, Subhawong TK, et al. Peripheral nerve surgery: the role of high-resolution MR neurography. AJNR Am J Neuroradiol 2012;33: 203–10.

29. Lee SK, Wolfe SW. Nerve transfers for the upper extremity: new horizons in nerve reconstruction. J Am Acad Orthop Surg 2012;20:506–17.

30. Narozny W, Kuczkowski J, Mikaszewski B. Thomasz Drobnik: great Polish surgeon and patriot. Otol Neurotol 2005;26:551.

31. Yeoman PM, Seddon HJ. Brachial plexus injuries: treatment of the flail arm. J Bone Joint Surg 1961; 43:493–500.

32. Lurje A. Concerning surgical treatment of traumatic injury of the upper division of the brachial plexus (Erb's-type). Ann Surg 1948;127:317–26.

33. Gu Y-D, Wu MM, Zhen YL. Phrenic nerve transfer for brachial plexus motor neurotization. Microsurgery 1989;10:287–9.

34. Brown JM, Shah MN, Mackinnon SE. Distal nerve transfers: a biology-based rationale. Neurosurg Focus 2009;26:E12.

35. Chhabra A, Thawait GK, Soldatos T, et al. High-resolution 3T MR neurography of the brachial plexus and its branches, with emphasis on 3D imaging. AJNR Am J Neuroradiol 2013;34(3):486–97.

36. Bourrel P. Transplantation of the m. tibialis posterior on the m. tibialis anterior and of the common flexor of the toes on the m. extensor hallucis longus and the common extensor of the toes in external popliteal sciatic paralysis. Apropos of 27 cases. Ann Chir 1967;21:1451–60 [in French].

37. Wiesseman GJ. Tendon transfers for peripheral nerve injuries of the lower extremity. Orthop Clin North Am 1981;12:459–67.

38. O'Brien M. Aids to the investigation of peripheral nerve injuries. Medical Research Council: Nerve Injuries Research Committee. His Majesty's Stationery Office: 1942; pp. 48 (iii) and 74 figures and 7 diagrams; with aids to the examination of the peripheral nervous system. Brain 2010;133:2838–44.

39. Brunelli GA. Sensory nerves transfers. J Hand Surg Br 2004;29:557–62.

40. Takagi T, Nakamura M, Yamada M, et al. Visualization of peripheral nerve degeneration and regeneration: monitoring with diffusion tensor tractography. Neuroimage 2009;44:884–92.

41. Puckett CL, Meyer VH. Results of treatment of extensive volar wrist lacerations: the spaghetti wrist. Plast Reconstr Surg 1985;75:714–21.

42. MacKenzie EJ, Shapiro S, Smith RT, et al. Factors influencing return to work following hospitalization for traumatic injury. Am J Public Health 1987;77: 329–34.

43. Dellon AL, Curtis RM, Edgerton MT. Reeducation of sensation in the hand after nerve injury and repair. Plast Reconstr Surg 1974;53:297–305.

44. Oud T, Beelen A, Eijffinger E, et al. Sensory reeducation after nerve injury of the upper limb: a systematic review. Clin Rehabil 2007;21:483–94.

45. Kalomiri DE, Soucacos PN, Beris AE. Nerve grafting in peripheral nerve microsurgery of the upper extremity. Microsurgery 1994;15:506–11.

46. Dellon AL, Mackinnon SE. Selection of the appropriate parameter to measure neural regeneration. Ann Plast Surg 1989;23:197–202.

47. Berger A, Millesi H. Nerve grafting. Clin Orthop 1978;133:49–55.

48. Millesi H. Interfascicular nerve grafting. Orthop Clin North Am 1981;12:287–301.

49. Millesi H. The nerve gap: theory and clinical practice. Hand Clin 1986;2:651–63.

50. Sunderland IR, Brenner MJ, Singham J, et al. Effect of tension on nerve regeneration in rat sciatic nerve transection model. Ann Plast Surg 2004;53:382–7.

51. Schmidhammer R, Zandieh S, Hopf R, et al. Alleviated tension at the repair site enhances functional regeneration: the effect of full range of motion mobilization on the regeneration of peripheral nerves–histologic, electrophysiologic, and functional results in a rat model. J Trauma 2004;56: 571–84.

Magnetic Resonance Neurography
Diffusion Tensor Imaging and Future Directions

Patrick Eppenberger, MD[a], Gustav Andreisek, MD[a],*,
Avneesh Chhabra, MD[b]

KEYWORDS

- MR neurography (MRN) • Three-dimensional (3D) • Whole-body MR
- Diffusion-weighted imaging (DWI) • Diffusion tensor imaging (DTI) • Magnetization transfer imaging
- MR contrast

KEY POINTS

- Magnetic resonance (MR) neurography is an excellent technique for axial and multiplanar depiction of peripheral nerve anatomy and disorders.
- Three-dimensional isotropic spin-echo–type imaging is currently being used on high-field scanners for longitudinal demonstration of nerve disorders for the benefit of referring physicians.
- Whole-body MR imaging is being widely used to image tumors. Whole-body MR neurography holds promise in the depiction of diffuse peripheral nerve disorders and neurocutaneous syndromes.
- Diffusion-weighted imaging and diffusion tensor imaging permit functional imaging of nerves and related lesions, and allow tractography for presurgical planning and postsurgical follow-up.
- Magnetization transfer imaging and nerve-specific MR contrast agents are under development and in feasibility stages for the assessment of nerve degeneration and regeneration, which is beyond the scope of anatomic pulse sequences.

INTRODUCTION

Magnetic resonance (MR) neurography (MRN) is a noninvasive technique using high-resolution magnetic resonance (MR) imaging to diagnose peripheral nerve disorders and their underlying causes, such as indirect or direct penetrating injury, compression, stretch, friction, and iatrogenic insult, as well as to monitor processes of peripheral nerve degeneration and regeneration. At present, anatomic MRN is being widely used for a variety of nerve disorders.[1–9] Because of the continuous technological advancements, MRN diagnostic capabilities have improved in

the last 2 decades, and MRN is therefore likely to play an important role in the diagnostic algorithm of peripheral nerve disorders.[1,10–16] This article reviews evolving novel MRN technologies currently used and under development with regard to their potential to meet the requirements for noninvasive imaging of peripheral nerves in both clinical and research settings.

NERVE ANATOMY AND PERIPHERAL NEUROPATHY

To understand the new MRN technologies, as well as related normal and abnormal appearances of

a Department of Radiology, University Hospital Zurich, Ramistrasse 100, Zurich CH – 8091, Switzerland; b The University of Texas Southwestern, 5323 Harry Hines Blvd, Dallas, TX 75390-9178, USA
* Corresponding author.
E-mail address: gustav@andreisek.de

Neuroimag Clin N Am 24 (2014) 245–256
http://dx.doi.org/10.1016/j.nic.2013.03.031

the peripheral nervous system (PNS) using these techniques, an understanding of the peripheral nerve structure, composition of its different tissues, and knowledge of the widely used classification of peripheral neuropathy is important.

The axon is the functional unit of the peripheral nerve, supported by surrounding Schwann cells and myelin layers. A layer of loose connective tissue, the endoneurium, surrounds each axon and its Schwann cells, to form a nerve fiber. Multiple nerve fibers are enclosed in robust connective tissue, the perineurium, to form a nerve fascicle. All nerve fascicles are surrounded by the epineurium, to form a peripheral nerve.[2,7] Overall, peripheral nerve morphology shows a strong longitudinal order of its different compositional tissues. As a consequence, the axoplasmatic flow within peripheral nerves and, at a molecular level, the diffusion of water protons is aligned along these longitudinal structures.

Peripheral neuropathy is a general term. Three subtypes might be distinguished, namely mononeuropathy, mononeuropathy multiplex, or polyneuropathy. In peripheral neuropathies, it is essential to also determine whether the primary pathophysiology is of demyelinating or axonal type.[17,18] Nerve injuries are traditionally classified according to the Seddon and Sunderland grading systems. The Seddon classification divides nerve injuries based on their severity into neurapraxia, axonotmesis, and neurotmesis. Neurapraxia, the mildest type of injury, involves only pathologic changes in the myelin sheath around the axon resulting in a conduction block and transient functional loss. It is associated with a good prognosis. In axonotmesis, the axon suffers injury resulting in wallerian degeneration of its distal segment; however, the supporting structures, including the perineurium and epineurium, remain intact. The prognosis for recovery remains good, but time is required for axonal regeneration (~ 1 mm per day) from the point of injury to the target tissue. Neurotmesis is the most severe type of injury and refers to complete severance of the nerve. The functional loss is complete, and unless early surgical intervention is performed clinical recovery is not expected.

Sunderland proposed a 5-degree classification system with first-degree and second-degree injuries corresponding with neurapraxia and axonotmesis and third, fourth, and fifth degrees corresponding with endoneural, perineural, and epineural injuries, respectively.[1,19,20]

LIMITATIONS OF CURRENT DIAGNOSTIC TESTS AND IMAGING

In addition to the clinical examination, nerve conduction and electromyography (EMG) studies and quantitative neurosensory testing are most commonly used to assess peripheral neuropathies and nerve injuries. Although these techniques remain the reference standard, there are limitations. First, the information about the exact location, extent, and cause of nerve disorders is often limited.[21] In addition, electrodiagnostic studies depend on operative and interpretative skills of the examiner and are not practical in patients with, for example, skin disorders or bleeding diathesis. In some studies, the positive predictive values are in the 30%–40% range and asymptomatic slowing of nerves is common. Nerve biopsy is often too invasive and may lead to considerable morbidity.[2,8,22–25] Another fundamental issue is the evaluation of stage-specific interventions, to improve nerve regeneration. Key to this is the ability to follow the growth state of the neuron and associated axonal elongation/regeneration in the nerve (pathway) before its reconnection with target tissues.[8,26–31] Current anatomic MRN techniques using fat-suppressed T2-weighted sequences are not able to sufficiently show nerve function and recovery.[32,33] Therefore, further development of functional MRN technologies are of foremost interest if they can provide useful information not only on gross nerve morphology but also on microstructure, collagen integrity, demyelination, and, if possible, nerve function.

HIGH-RESOLUTION MRN AND NEW THREE-DIMENSIONAL SEQUENCES

The increasing use of 3-T MR scanners, new phased-array surface coils, and parallel imaging techniques allow the acquisition of high-resolution and high-contrast images in short imaging times. Current state-of-the-art MRN provides detailed anatomic depiction of peripheral nerves and improved characterization of pathologic states (**Figs. 1** and **2**).[1,27,29,30]

Axial T1-weighted and fluid-sensitive fat-suppressed T2-weighted images serve as the mainstay in MRN interpretation for prudent assessment of peripheral nerve imaging characteristics, such as signal intensity evaluation, course, caliber, fascicular pattern, size, and perineural fibrosis, or mass lesions.[1,10] Normal nerves show intermediate signal intensity (similar to muscle) on T1-weighted images and intermediate to minimally increased signal intensity on T2-weighted images, depending on the amount of endoneural fluid and background fat suppression (see **Fig. 1**).[34] MRN is a highly sensitive technique and may show abnormalities not revealed with electrophysiologic tests (**Fig. 3**).

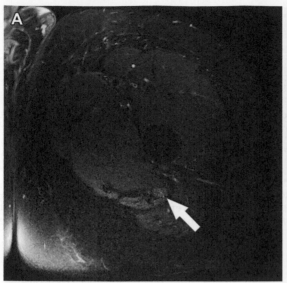
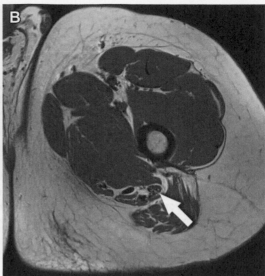

Fig. 1. Axial T2 spectral adiabatic inversion recovery (SPAIR) (*A*) and T2-weighted (T2 W) (*B*) images show normal sciatic nerve fascicular appearance (*arrows*).

However, the imaging abnormality may not recede immediately and completely despite patient improvement following treatment (**Fig. 4**). Serial evaluation is nonetheless helpful to assess increase in size and signal abnormality in worsening cases. Focal alterations in nerve contour, course, and caliber are best depicted on longitudinal images reconstructed along the course of the nerve on dedicated imaging workstations using various techniques, such as multiplanar reconstruction, curved-planar reconstruction, and maximum intensity projection (MIP).[10,35] For such reconstructions, imaging sequences should be

acquired as near isotropic as possible (eg, 0.6–1 mm resolution). Only isotropic voxel sizes allow smooth reconstructions in any desired plane. Therefore, preferably three-dimensional (3D) sequences such as 3D fast (turbo) spin-echo (TSE) or 3D gradient-echo sequences should be used. The advantages of 3D TSE sequences (acronyms include VISTA [Phillips, Best, the Netherlands], SPACE [Siemens, Erlangen, Germany], CUBE [GE, Waukeesha, WI]) are that they combine high spatial resolution and, in theory, pure T2 contrast, if needed. The latter is important for the superior spatial depiction of the nerves coursing obliquely

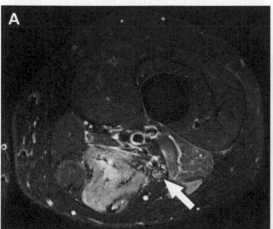
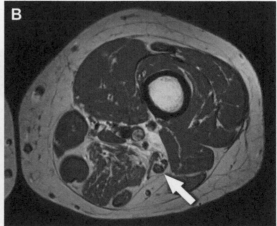

Fig. 2. Axial T2 SPAIR (*A*) and T2 W (*B*) images in a 51-year-old man presenting with foot drop following motor vehicle accident. Notice abnormal vessel-like hyperintensity of the nerve, mild nerve enlargement (*arrows*), and muscle denervation changes in the hamstrings in keeping with a stretch injury with axonotmesis.

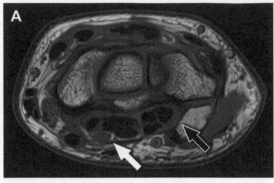
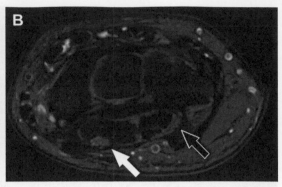

Fig. 3. A 31-year-old woman with wrist pain and symptoms of carpal tunnel syndrome and normal nerve conduction study. Axial proton density-weighted (*A*) and T2 SPAIR (*B*) images show effacement of deep carpal tunnel fat and moderate hyperintensity of the median nerve (*white arrows*) with normal appearance of the ulnar nerve (*black arrows*).

and for the interpretation of mild T2 because this could be an isolated sign of neuropathy.[34,36] To enhance contrast/noise ratio between abnormal nerves with increased signal intensity and surrounding tissue, good fat-suppression techniques using spectral adiabatic inversion recovery (SPAIR) or short tau inversion recovery (STIR) techniques are frequently applied to those MRN sequences (**Fig. 5**). Some vendors even allow the use of different strengths of fat saturation (eg, Phillips), which eases detection of abnormalities of thin nerves. In addition, 3D TSE sequences provide a familiar T2-weighted type of contrast.[37] 3D TSE is useful for longitudinal depiction of nerve disorders, for the benefit of referring physicians and radiologists not reading MRN images on a routine basis.

Another new category of sequences to image peripheral nerves in the extremities are 3D diffusion-weighted (DW) reversed fast imaging with steady-state precession (3D DW-PSIF) sequences. This imaging technique has previously been used for the evaluation of cranial nerves and the lumbar plexus with good vascular suppression and has recently been applied to MR imaging of peripheral nerves.[9,10,35,37–40] Besides retaining all the advantages of a traditional 3D sequence, 3D DW-PSIF provides a selective suppression of moving structures, including vascular flow, leading to an improved identification of nerves compared with standard two-dimensional T2-weighted images (**Fig. 6**). It should therefore be incorporated in the MRN protocol whenever accurate nerve localization and/or presurgical evaluation are required.[38]

In general, all new high-resolution and 3D sequences benefit from high field strength because of the significant increase in signal/noise ratio. If available, MRN studies should therefore be performed on MR units with 3.0 T or higher.

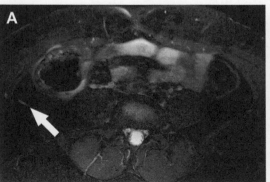
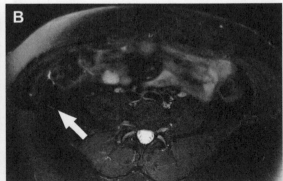

Fig. 4. A 38-year-old woman who underwent neurolysis of the ilioinguinal nerve at the anterolateral abdominal wall. The scans show the limitation of MRN. The nerve is abnormally bright on both scans (*arrows*), although less intense on the later scan (*B*) obtained many months after the first scan (*A*).

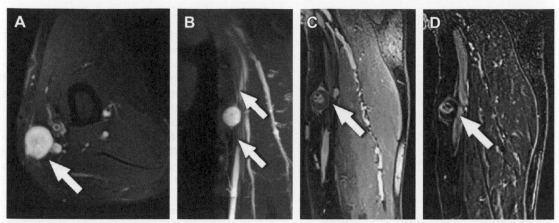

Fig. 5. A 44-year-old man with clinically suspected medial antebrachial cutaneous nerve mass. Axial T2 SPAIR (*A*) image shows the peripheral nerve sheath tumor with a classic target sign (*arrow*). Corresponding 3D STIR SPACE coronal MIP (*B*) image shows the relationship of the mass with the antebrachial cutaneous nerve (*arrows*). Postcontrast T1 VIBE (volume-interpolated breath-hold examination) (*C*) and subtraction (*D*) images show peripheral and central enhancing components of the lesion (*arrows*).

WHOLE-BODY MRN

Multimodality scanners which are able to acquire coregistered structural and functional information, such as single-photon emission computed tomography (SPECT)/computed tomography (CT) and positron emission tomography (PET)/CT, play an increasingly important role in the evaluation of human disease. However, disadvantages of SPECT/CT and PET/CT are a long preparation time for the examination, exposure to ionizing radiation, and possible mismatch between anatomic and functional data sets caused by the patient repositioning.[41] MR imaging is able to provide both

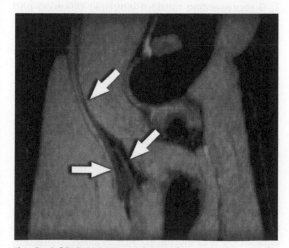

Fig. 6. A 3D DW-PSIF MIP image in a volunteer at the level of the elbow shows the normal median nerve and its muscular branch as well as the anterior interosseus nerve (*arrows*).

anatomic and functional information within a single examination without these disadvantages. Whole-body MR imaging and whole-body DW imaging (DWI) can be performed in the same scanner, without patient repositioning. Furthermore, whole-body DWI does not require any contrast agent administration. In 2004, Takahara and colleagues[3,32,42,43] showed the feasibility of whole-body DWI under free breathing. This concept is also known as DW whole-body imaging with background body signal suppression (DWIBS). Whole-body DWI, using the concept of DWIBS, may be a powerful adjunct to anatomic whole-body MR imaging, by detecting subtle lesions and pathologic changes in normal-sized structures, thanks to its high contrast/noise ratio (CNR). Feasibility studies showed the potential of DWI in visualizing the brachial plexus and the sacral plexus.[3,32,42,43] Whole-body MR imaging also has a significant potential in assessing disease load and treatment response in cases of neurocutaneous syndromes (**Fig. 7**). However, for any disorders, whole-body DWI should always be evaluated together with other (anatomic) whole-body MR imaging sequences, to avoid false-positive results.[42,44–47] In addition, whole-body MRN is becoming feasible using DWI (**Fig. 8**).[3] These technical developments will likely play an important role in the assessment of disease burden in neurocutaneous syndromes, such as neurofibromatosis and schwannomatosis, and in diffuse polyneuropathy conditions such as Charcot-Marie-Tooth disease and chronic inflammatory demyelinating polyneuropathy (CIDP).

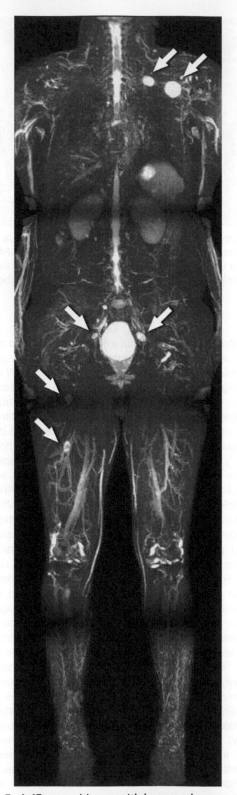

Fig. 7. A 47–year-old man with known schwannomatosis. Whole-body 3D STIR SPACE MIP MR image shows multiple nerve sheath tumors (*arrows*).

DIFFUSION TENSOR IMAGING/DWI

DWI and diffusion tensor imaging (DTI) in particular are MR imaging techniques based on the thermally driven random motion (diffusion) of water molecules within biologic tissues. Tissues have distinct structural properties which hinder diffusion in some directions and facilitate it in other directions.

DTI shows great potential as a noninvasive technology to detect axonal injury in the central nervous system (CNS), which has been shown by a large number of studies; data in CNS studies indicate that DTI parameters are sensitive and specific imaging biomarkers for detection of myelinated axons and nerve fiber loss.[35] As mentioned earlier, there is also a substantial clinical need for reliable measures to assess the PNS, especially regarding regeneration after traumatic injuries or nerve surgery. For these applications, DTI is currently the most promising technology with immediate availability.[37,48–51]

Neural tissues are densely packed with nerve fibers and tracts and water molecules therefore tend to diffuse in a preferential orientation along these nerve fibers and tracts; this is called anisotropic diffusion.[52,53] To characterize the amount and principal direction of diffusion, image sets from 6 or more different DW acquisitions are usually acquired. In DTI, the main diffusion direction is indicated by the tensor's main eigenvector. In color-coded maps, the directional component is assigned to different colors (typically red, green, and blue). The resulting image is weighted with the fractional anisotropy (FA) map to exclude tissues with isotropic diffusion. FA is an anisotropy index describing the degree of anisotropy in a tissue. It is a scalar parameter, scaled between 0 and 1; 0 representing random isotropic diffusion and 1 representing complete anisotropy. Mean diffusivity, also called anisotropic diffusion coefficient (ADC), is a measure of diffusion magnitude along a given direction, or averaged over several directions. In addition, tractography can be used to visualize the 3D course of nerve fibers and bundles and the fiber density.[54–56]

DTI has recently been applied to the study of peripheral nerves, to show the feasibility of the method[56–58] and to study nerve regeneration after median-nerve injury and fascicular repair,[56,59] as well as nerve entrapment in carpal tunnel syndrome.[56,60–62] Various nerve abnormalities and injuries, such as trauma, entrapment, tumor, and inflammation, may lead to decreased fractional anisotropy and increased ADC values; therefore, these findings should be taken in the context of morphologic nerve findings on MRN studies along with the available clinical information.[63] In general,

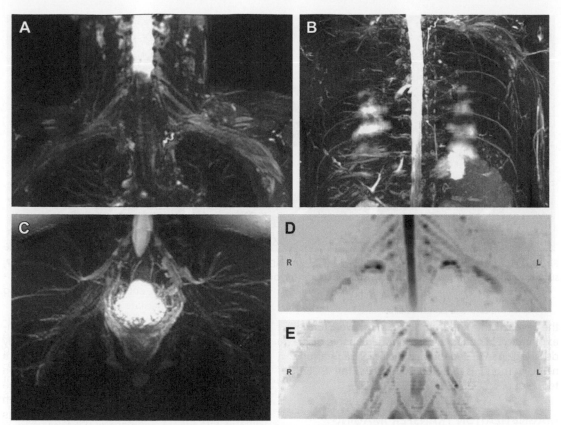

Fig. 8. A 28-year-old healthy volunteer. Whole-body high-resolution MRN with diffusion tensor imaging (DTI). Note the normal symmetric appearance of the brachial plexus (*A*), intercostal nerves (*B*), and sciatic plexus (*C*) on anatomic sequences as well as on DTI maps (*D, E*).

increased mean diffusivity may reflect inflammation or edema, whereas decreased FA may reflect damaged tissue microstructure, demyelination, axonal loss, or increase in isotropic water volume.[56] Increasing FA values within peripheral nerves have also been observed in animal models correlating with functional motor and sensory recovery and may depict nerve regeneration after successful entrapment release.[50,56–60,62] In peripheral nerve sheath tumors, high diffusivity values are seen within benign lesions (1.1–2.0), whereas low diffusivity values (0.7–1.0) are seen in malignant lesions in early studies by the authors (**Fig. 9**). However, single measurements have limited value in any lesion and interval measurements over time have significant potential usefulness in follow-up of these lesions upon medical treatment. In addition, tractography provides another insight into the pathophysiologic mechanisms of these lesions. With future research, DWI and DTI will likely play an important role in the evaluation and further understanding of neuromuscular diseases and are expected to be an important adjunct to the currently established, mostly anatomy-based, MRN protocols.

Subtraction of unidirectionally encoded images for suppression of heavily isotropic objects (SUSHI) is a recently proposed MR technique for selective peripheral nerve imaging that is related to DTI. Given that, in DWI, many structures surrounding a nerve, such as lymph nodes, bone marrow, veins with slow blood flow, and articular fluids, in contrast with the nerve itself, show a high signal intensity regardless of the direction of the applied diffusion-sensitizing gradients, a DWI data set acquired with a first pair of diffusion-sensitizing gradients with a direction parallel to the course of the peripheral nerve to be imaged is subtracted from another DWI data set acquired with a second pair of diffusion-sensitizing gradients in a perpendicular direction to the first data set. This technique results in a selective representation of the peripheral nerve of interest. This method has been surveyed with 6 volunteers on the brachial plexus, and with 7 volunteers on the sciatic, common peroneal, and tibial nerves at

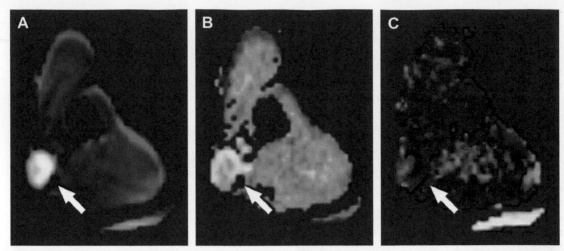

Fig. 9. DTI of the same case as in Fig. 5. Trace image (*A*), ADC image (*B*), and FA image (*C*). The ADC value was 1.7, suggesting a benign peripheral nerve sheath tumor (*arrows*).

the level of the knee, at 1.5 T. However, further exploration in patients with peripheral nerve disorders (eg, nerve degeneration, nerve trauma, and nerve tumors) is needed to assess the SUSHI technique.[42,64]

MAGNETIZATION TRANSFER IMAGING

On conventional MR imaging, tissue contrast is generated from variations in proton density and relaxation times of water protons. Longitudinal and transverse components of the magnetization in homogeneous samples relax monoexponentially with characteristic decay times T1 and T2. In biologic tissues there are protons with free mobility (water protons) and protons with restricted mobility because of bonds to macromolecules or membranes. These restricted protons have a T2 relaxation time too short to be detected by conventional proton MR imaging techniques. Magnetization transfer (MT) imaging generates tissue contrast depending on the magnetization exchange between free and restricted protons. MT effects in tissues are usually assessed by measuring the MT ratio (MTR), which yields a contrast sensitive to the protons associated with the bound proton pool. The MTR is a semiquantitative parameter, and its value depends on the type of MR sequence, as well as the sequence parameters.[7,65]

MT imaging thus offers a characterization of the macromolecular protons invisible in standard MR imaging. Besides improving the contrast, MT provides quantitative information about tissue structure and pathologic changes beyond conventional T1, T2, and T2* contrast.[65] Off-resonance

radiofrequency pulses are the most popular technique to perform MT imaging. They are usually Gaussian or sync pulses with a bandwidth of a few hundred Hertz at frequency offsets between 50 Hz and 50 kHz from the free proton resonance frequency. The pulses are applied before each excitation. High-energy deposition in tissue, as measured by the specific absorption rate, may be a problem during application of this technique.

In present clinical settings, MT imaging is predominantly used to suppress background signals from tissues in MR angiography. Regarding the potential application of MT imaging to peripheral nerve disorders, the tissue content and structure of the PNS must be considered in order to understand the origin of MT contrast in nerves. The bound protons in peripheral nerves are represented by collagen tissue, myelin, and the proteins contained in the nerve fibers, all possibly contributing to the observed MTR. Thus, MT imaging could be advantageous in peripheral neuropathy studies because it may provide information on nerve damage, collagen integrity, and demyelination. In studies of CNS disorders, such as multiple sclerosis, MT contrast has shown its feasibility to detect plaques based on their altered macromolecular content.[7,66] In the musculoskeletal system, MT imaging was used to assess muscle atrophy in patients with diabetic foot neuropathy and CIDP.[7,67–69] To our knowledge, there is only 1 report on MT imaging of peripheral nerves in which MTR was used for high-resolution tracking of thin forefoot nerves.[7] Overall, MT imaging might offer an alternative to the commonly used T2-weighted sequences, in which higher signal intensity, originating from prolonged T2 relaxation, indicates nerve abnormality. Although MTR is a semiquantitative index, the MTR approach has potential advantage compared with T2-weighted nerve imaging because it permits longitudinal studies when a change in MTR may be more useful than T2 signal intensity.[7,65]

CONTRAST AGENTS AND NON-MR IMAGING TECHNIQUES

Because the current mainstay of MRN is T1-weighted and T2-weighted imaging, use of extracellular contrast agents in peripheral neuropathy is clinically often limited to inflammatory or infectious and tumorous conditions. It may also be used postoperatively to assess scar tissue and in diffuse peripheral neuropathies. As a consequence, any new contrast agents to be introduced for peripheral nerve imaging must have a significant advantage compared with current extracellular contrast agents to overcome their limitations. One possible new MR contrast agent is gadofluorine M, which accumulates selectively in nerve fibers undergoing wallerian degeneration and disappears with remyelination. Thus, gadofluorine M has the potential to show demyelination and remyelination processes in peripheral nerves. However, many clinical studies with, for example, histopathologic correlation are needed to prove this theory for a variety of pathologic conditions before any US Food and Drug Administration (FDA) approval or widespread clinical use.

The most commonly applied contrast agents for cellular and molecular MR imaging purposes are superparamagnetic iron oxide particles, which come in a wide range of sizes and a variety of coatings. The popularity of these agents is predominantly based on their biocompatibility and their capacity to efficiently disturb local magnetic fields, thereby generating localized hypointense areas on T2-weighted and T2*-weighted MR images.[70–73] The second important class of contrast agents is formed by the FDA-approved and European Medicines Evaluation Agency–approved low-molecular-weight paramagnetic gadolinium (Gd) polyaminocarboxylate chelates (eg, Gd-diethylenetriamine pentaacetic acid and Gd-tetraazacyclododecane tetraacetic acid), which are applied to induce hyperintense signals on T1-weighted MR images. Another established platform for contrast enhancement is available in the form of lipid-based nanoparticles. Lipid-based nanoparticles, such as micelles, emulsions, or liposomes, are composed of a biocompatible lipid monolayer or bilayer coating that encapsulates either an aqueous or hydrophilic core,

offering a versatile and tunable compound for a wide variety of applications.[73–76] At present, molecular labeling and fluorescent imaging is only applicable to transgenic mice/animals labeled with specific fluorescent proteins and not applicable for clinical use. Future studies in animal models and human subjects, including adequate assessment of safety issues associated with nanoparticle injection, will provide further details on the usefulness of cellular and molecular MR imaging in preclinical and clinical settings.[73,77]

SUMMARY

MRN has progressed greatly in the past 2 decades. Excellent depiction of 3D nerve anatomy and disorders is currently possible using state-of-the-art MR imaging techniques. Further developments in the years to come will include the use of high-resolution 3D and diffusion-based imaging and potentially nerve-specific MR contrast agents as well as molecular imaging.

REFERENCES

1. Chhabra A, Andreisek G, Soldatos T, et al. MR neurography: past, present, and future. AJR Am J Roentgenol 2011;197:583–91.
2. Chhabra A, Lee PP, Bizzell C, et al. 3 Tesla MR neurography–technique, interpretation, and pitfalls. Skeletal Radiol 2011;40:1249–60.
3. Yamashita T, Kwee TC, Takahara T. Whole-body magnetic resonance neurography. N Engl J Med 2009;361:538–9.
4. Dailey AT, Tsuruda JS, Filler AG, et al. Magnetic resonance neurography of peripheral nerve degeneration and regeneration. Lancet 1997;350:1221–2.
5. Grant GA, Britz GW, Goodkin R, et al. The utility of magnetic resonance imaging in evaluating peripheral nerve disorders. Muscle Nerve 2002; 25:314–31.
6. Filler AG, Howe FA, Hayes CE, et al. Magnetic resonance neurography. Lancet 1993;341:659–61.
7. Gambarota G, Krueger G, Theumann N, et al. Magnetic resonance imaging of peripheral nerves: differences in magnetization transfer. Muscle Nerve 2012;45:13–7.
8. Sheikh KA. Non-invasive imaging of nerve regeneration. Exp Neurol 2010;223:72–6.
9. Filler AG, Maravilla KR, Tsuruda JS. MR neurography and muscle MR imaging for image diagnosis of disorders affecting the peripheral nerves and musculature. Neurol Clin 2004;22:643–82, vi–vii.
10. Chhabra A, Williams EH, Wang KC, et al. MR neurography of neuromas related to nerve injury and entrapment with surgical correlation. AJNR Am J Neuroradiol 2010;31:1363–8.

11. Kim JY, Ihn YK, Kim JS, et al. Non-traumatic peroneal nerve palsy: MRI findings. Clin Radiol 2007; 62:58–64.

12. Hof JJ, Kliot M, Slimp J, et al. What's new in MRI of peripheral nerve entrapment? Neurosurg Clin North Am 2008;19:583–95, vi.

13. Martinoli C, Bianchi S, Gandolfo N, et al. US of nerve entrapments in osteofibrous tunnels of the upper and lower limbs. Radiographics 2000;20: S199–213 [discussion: S213–7].

14. Visser LH. High-resolution sonography of the common peroneal nerve: detection of intraneural ganglia. Neurology 2006;67:1473–5.

15. Gruber H, Peer S, Meirer R, et al. Peroneal nerve palsy associated with knee luxation: evaluation by sonography–initial experiences. AJR Am J Roentgenol 2005;185:1119–25.

16. Kim S, Choi JY, Huh YM, et al. Role of magnetic resonance imaging in entrapment and compressive neuropathy - what, where, and how to see the peripheral nerves on the musculoskeletal magnetic resonance image: part 1. Overview and lower extremity. Eur Radiol 2007;17:139–49.

17. Narayan KM, Boyle JP, Thompson TJ, et al. Lifetime risk for diabetes mellitus in the United States. JAMA 2003;290:1884–90.

18. England JD, Asbury AK. Peripheral neuropathy. Lancet 2004;363:2151–61.

19. Seddon HJ, Medawar PB, Smith H. Rate of regeneration of peripheral nerves in man. J Physiol 1943; 102:191–215.

20. Sunderland S. A classification of peripheral nerve injuries producing loss of function. Brain 1951;74: 491–516.

21. Andreisek G, Crook DW, Burg D, et al. Peripheral neuropathies of the median, radial, and ulnar nerves: MR imaging features. Radiographics 2006;26:1267–87.

22. Dellon AL. Management of peripheral nerve problems in the upper and lower extremity using quantitative sensory testing. Hand Clin 1999;15: 697–715, x.

23. Filler AG, Kliot M, Howe FA, et al. Application of magnetic resonance neurography in the evaluation of patients with peripheral nerve pathology. J Neurosurg 1996;85:299–309.

24. Jablecki CK, Andary MT, So YT, et al. Literature review of the usefulness of nerve conduction studies and electromyography for the evaluation of patients with carpal tunnel syndrome. AAEM Quality Assurance Committee. Muscle Nerve 1993; 16:1392–414.

25. Kuntz CT, Blake L, Britz G, et al. Magnetic resonance neurography of peripheral nerve lesions in the lower extremity. Neurosurgery 1996;39:750–6 [discussion: 756–7].

26. Britz GW, Haynor DR, Kuntz C, et al. Ulnar nerve entrapment at the elbow: correlation of magnetic resonance imaging, clinical, electrodiagnostic, and intraoperative findings. Neurosurgery 1996; 38:458–65 [discussion: 465].

27. Freund W, Brinkmann A, Wagner F, et al. MR neurography with multiplanar reconstruction of 3D MRI datasets: an anatomical study and clinical applications. Neuroradiology 2007;49:335–41.

28. Jarvik JG, Yuen E, Haynor DR, et al. MR nerve imaging in a prospective cohort of patients with suspected carpal tunnel syndrome. Neurology 2002; 58:1597–602.

29. Vargas MI, Viallon M, Nguyen D, et al. New approaches in imaging of the brachial plexus. Eur J Radiol 2010;74:403–10.

30. Viallon M, Vargas MI, Jlassi H, et al. High-resolution and functional magnetic resonance imaging of the brachial plexus using an isotropic 3D T2 STIR (short term inversion recovery) SPACE sequence and diffusion tensor imaging. Eur Radiol 2008;18: 1018–23.

31. Zhang H, Xiao B, Zou T. Clinical application of magnetic resonance neurography in peripheral nerve disorders. Neurosci Bull 2006;22:361–7.

32. Takahara T, Imai Y, Yamashita T, et al. Diffusion weighted whole body imaging with background body signal suppression (DWIBS): technical improvement using free breathing, STIR and high resolution 3D display. Radiat Med 2004;22:275–82.

33. Aagaard BD, Maravilla KR, Kliot M. MR neurography. MR imaging of peripheral nerves. Magn Reson Imaging Clin North Am 1998;6:179–94.

34. Husarik DB, Saupe N, Pfirrmann CW, et al. Elbow nerves: MR findings in 60 asymptomatic subjects–normal anatomy, variants, and pitfalls. Radiology 2009;252:148–56.

35. Zhang Z, Song L, Meng Q, et al. Morphological analysis in patients with sciatica: a magnetic resonance imaging study using three-dimensional high-resolution diffusion-weighted magnetic resonance neurography techniques. Spine (Phila Pa 1976) 2009;34:E245–50.

36. Chappell KE, Robson MD, Stonebridge-Foster A, et al. Magic angle effects in MR neurography. AJNR Am J Neuroradiol 2004;25:431–40.

37. Andreisek G, Burg D, Studer A, et al. Upper extremity peripheral neuropathies: role and impact of MR imaging on patient management. Eur Radiol 2008;18:1953–61.

38. Chhabra A, Subhawong TK, Bizzell C, et al. 3T MR neurography using three-dimensional diffusion-weighted PSIF: technical issues and advantages. Skeletal Radiol 2011;40:1355–60.

39. Zhang Z, Meng Q, Chen Y, et al. 3-T imaging of the cranial nerves using three-dimensional reversed

FISP with diffusion-weighted MR sequence. J Magn Reson Imaging 2008;27:454–8.

40. Zhang ZW, Song LJ, Meng QF, et al. High-resolution diffusion-weighted MR imaging of the human lumbosacral plexus and its branches based on a steady-state free precession imaging technique at 3T. AJNR Am J Neuroradiol 2008;29:1092–4.

41. Townsend DW. Multimodality imaging of structure and function. Phys Med Biol 2008;53:R1–39.

42. Takahara T, Hendrikse J, Kwee TC, et al. Diffusion-weighted MR neurography of the sacral plexus with unidirectional motion probing gradients. Eur Radiol 2010;20:1221–6.

43. Takahara T, Hendrikse J, Yamashita T, et al. Diffusion-weighted MR neurography of the brachial plexus: feasibility study. Radiology 2008; 249:653–60.

44. Kwee TC, Takahara T, Ochiai R, et al. Whole-body diffusion-weighted magnetic resonance imaging. Eur J Radiol 2009;70:409–17.

45. Kwee TC, Takahara T, Ochiai R, et al. Diffusion-weighted whole-body imaging with background body signal suppression (DWIBS): features and potential applications in oncology. Eur Radiol 2008;18:1937–52.

46. Ohno Y, Koyama H, Onishi Y, et al. Non-small cell lung cancer: whole-body MR examination for M-stage assessment–utility for whole-body diffusion-weighted imaging compared with integrated FDG PET/CT. Radiology 2008;248:643–54.

47. Chhabra A, Blakely J. Whole-body imaging in schwannomatosis. Neurology 2011;76:2035.

48. Andreisek G, White LM, Kassner A, et al. Evaluation of diffusion tensor imaging and fiber tractography of the median nerve: preliminary results on intrasubject variability and precision of measurements. AJR Am J Roentgenol 2010;194:W65–72.

49. Andreisek G, White LM, Kassner A, et al. Diffusion tensor imaging and fiber tractography of the median nerve at 1.5T: optimization of b value. Skeletal Radiol 2009;38:51–9.

50. Ringleb SI, Bensamoun SF, Chen Q, et al. Applications of magnetic resonance elastography to healthy and pathologic skeletal muscle. J Magn Reson Imaging 2007;25:301–9.

51. Khalil C, Budzik JF, Kermarrec E, et al. Tractography of peripheral nerves and skeletal muscles. Eur J Radiol 2010;76:391–7.

52. Basser PJ, Mattiello J, LeBihan D. MR diffusion tensor spectroscopy and imaging. Biophys J 1994;66:259–67.

53. Stieltjes B, Kaufmann WE, van Zijl PC, et al. Diffusion tensor imaging and axonal tracking in the human brainstem. Neuroimage 2001;14:723–35.

54. Mori S, Kaneda T, Fujita Y, et al. Diffusion tensor tractography for the inferior alveolar nerve (V3):

initial experiment. Oral Surg Oral Med Oral Pathol Oral Radiol Endod 2008;106:270–4.

55. Mori S, Zhang J. Principles of diffusion tensor imaging and its applications to basic neuroscience research. Neuron 2006;51:527–39.

56. Hiltunen J, Kirveskari E, Numminen J, et al. Pre- and post-operative diffusion tensor imaging of the median nerve in carpal tunnel syndrome. Eur Radiol 2012;22(6):1310–9.

57. Hiltunen J, Suortti T, Arvela S, et al. Diffusion tensor imaging and tractography of distal peripheral nerves at 3 T. Clin Neurophysiol 2005;116:2315–23.

58. Skorpil M, Karlsson M, Nordell A. Peripheral nerve diffusion tensor imaging. Magn Reson Imaging 2004;22:743–5.

59. Meek MF, Stenekes MW, Hoogduin HM, et al. In vivo three-dimensional reconstruction of human median nerves by diffusion tensor imaging. Exp Neurol 2006;198:479–82.

60. Kabakci N, Gurses B, Firat Z, et al. Diffusion tensor imaging and tractography of median nerve: normative diffusion values. AJR Am J Roentgenol 2007; 189:923–7.

61. Stein D, Neufeld A, Pasternak O, et al. Diffusion tensor imaging of the median nerve in healthy and carpal tunnel syndrome subjects. J Magn Reson Imaging 2009;29:657–62.

62. Khalil C, Hancart C, Le Thuc V, et al. Diffusion tensor imaging and tractography of the median nerve in carpal tunnel syndrome: preliminary results. Eur Radiol 2008;18:2283–91.

63. Takagi T, Nakamura M, Yamada M, et al. Visualization of peripheral nerve degeneration and regeneration: monitoring with diffusion tensor tractography. Neuroimage 2009;44:884–92.

64. Takahara T, Kwee TC, Hendrikse J, et al. Subtraction of unidirectionally encoded images for suppression of heavily isotropic objects (SUSHI) for selective visualization of peripheral nerves. Neuroradiology 2011;53:109–16.

65. Gloor M, Scheffler K, Bieri O. Quantitative magnetization transfer imaging using balanced SSFP. Magn Reson Med 2008;60:691–700.

66. Dousset V, Grossman RI, Ramer KN, et al. Experimental allergic encephalomyelitis and multiple sclerosis: lesion characterization with magnetization transfer imaging. Radiology 1992;182: 483–91.

67. Bus SA, Yang QX, Wang JH, et al. Intrinsic muscle atrophy and toe deformity in the diabetic neuropathic foot: a magnetic resonance imaging study. Diabetes Care 2002;25:1444–50.

68. Greenman RL, Khaodhiar L, Lima C, et al. Foot small muscle atrophy is present before the detection of clinical neuropathy. Diabetes Care 2005; 28:1425–30.

69. Brash PD, Foster J, Vennart W, et al. Magnetic resonance imaging techniques demonstrate soft tissue damage in the diabetic foot. Diabet Med 1999;16:55–61.

70. Gossuin Y, Gillis P, Hocq A, et al. Magnetic resonance relaxation properties of superparamagnetic particles. Wiley Interdiscip Rev Nanomed Nanobiotechnol 2009;1:299–310.

71. Weissleder R, Stark DD, Engelstad BL, et al. Superparamagnetic iron oxide: pharmacokinetics and toxicity. AJR Am J Roentgenol 1989;152: 167–73.

72. Bulte JW, Vymazal J, Brooks RA, et al. Frequency dependence of MR relaxation times. II. Iron oxides. J Magn Reson Imaging 1993;3:641–8.

73. Deddens LH, Van Tilborg GA, Mulder WJ, et al. Imaging neuroinflammation after stroke: current status of cellular and molecular MRI strategies. Cerebrovasc Dis 2012;33:392–402.

74. Mulder WJ, Strijkers GJ, van Tilborg GA, et al. Nanoparticulate assemblies of amphiphiles and diagnostically active materials for multimodality imaging. Acc Chem Res 2009;42:904–14.

75. Klibanov AL, Maruyama K, Torchilin VP, et al. Amphipathic polyethyleneglycols effectively prolong the circulation time of liposomes. FEBS Lett 1990;268:235–7.

76. van Tilborg GA, Strijkers GJ, Pouget EM, et al. Kinetics of avidin-induced clearance of biotinylated bimodal liposomes for improved MR molecular imaging. Magn Reson Med 2008;60:1444–56.

77. Witzel C, Rohde C, Brushart TM. Pathway sampling by regenerating peripheral axons. J Comp Neurol 2005;485:183–90.

Magnetic Resonance Neurography Research
Evaluation of Its Effectiveness

Gaurav K. Thawait, MD[a], Avneesh Chhabra, MD[b],
John A. Carrino, MD[a], John Eng, MD[c],*

KEYWORDS

* MR neurography * Research * Clinical outcome * Nerve surgery

KEY POINTS

* Radiologists involved in magnetic resonance neurography (MRN) research should use appropriate methodology to evaluate the effectiveness of this imaging technique.
* Clinical research involving MRN has focused on establishing technical and diagnostic accuracy efficacy. Future research is needed to evaluate MRN with respect to the higher levels in the efficacy hierarchy: therapeutic, patient outcome, and societal.
* Data collection from the treating physician is necessary to address the higher levels in the efficacy hierarchy.

INTRODUCTION

The rapid advent of new diagnostic techniques in radiology has led to the notion that these new technologies should be evaluated not only for optimal image quality and diagnostic accuracy but also for cost-effectiveness and ultimate improvement in patient care. In addition, in order for a modality to be considered appropriate, its value compared with current methods of diagnosis should be established. Taking these factors into consideration, the evaluation of a diagnostic technology can be complicated and, for a new technology to become a viable option for incorporation in a diagnostic algorithm, it should excel in multiple categories of diagnostic technology assessment.

Extensive work has been done in the methodology of technology assessment. Fineberg and

colleagues,[1] in 1977, described 4 levels of efficacy to evaluate the clinical effectiveness of a diagnostic procedure. Fryback and Thornbury,[2] and later Thornbury,[3] revised it to a 6-tiered model for efficacy. These models incorporate evaluation of both efficacy and effectiveness. The term efficacy defines the probability of benefit from the technology under ideal conditions of use, whereas the term effectiveness is used to reflect the performance in everyday clinical practice.[4] Hunink and Krestin[5] have argued that evaluation of a new diagnostic test on the 6-tier model might be challenging because of time and economic constraints.

Magnetic resonance neurography (MRN) is a specialized technique that is rapidly becoming part of the diagnostic algorithm in the clinical evaluation of peripheral nerve injury. However, in order for this modality to be considered appropriate, its

Disclosures: A. Chhabra received patient research grants from Siemens, Integra Life Sciences and GE-AUR; J.A. Carrino received a patient research grant from Siemens.
[a] Musculoskeletal Radiology Section, The Russell H. Morgan Department of Radiology and Radiological Science, The Johns Hopkins Hospital, 601 North Caroline Street, JHOC 5168, Baltimore, MD 21202, USA; [b] University of Texas Southwestern, 5323 Harry Hines Boulevard, Dallas, Texas 75390, USA; [c] The Russell H. Morgan Department of Radiology and Radiological Science, The Johns Hopkins Hospital, 600 North Wolfe Street, Baltimore, Maryland 21287, USA
* Corresponding author.
E-mail address: jeng@jhmi.edu

value compared with current methods of diagnosis should be established. Therefore, radiologists involved in MRN research should use appropriate methodology to evaluate MRN's effectiveness, ideally with a multidisciplinary approach. This article reviews the classic hierarchical model used in assessing diagnostic technologies along with a discussion of how this model can be applied to MRN. The article also emphasizes how to evaluate the impact of MRN on diagnostic thinking and therapeutic decisions.

SIX TIERS OF DIAGNOSTIC EFFICACY

The classic diagnostic efficacy model approximates the sequence of image generation and its use, so a brief review of the work flow is useful. An image is recorded by the imaging device and stored. This image is then interpreted by the radiologist who generates a report based on various normal and abnormal findings. The clinician uses this information to arrive at the final clinical diagnosis and drives the therapeutic decision-making process. The clinician's treatment decisions affect the patient's health outcome(s) and ultimately contribute to the economic and overall health outcomes at the societal level.

The 6-tiered model of efficacy starts at the level of imaging quality with level 1, defined as technical efficacy; level 2, defined as diagnostic accuracy efficacy, relates to image interpretation; levels 3 and level 4, defined as diagnostic thinking efficacy and therapeutic efficacy, respectively, take into account the clinician's decision making; level 5 is defined as patient outcome efficacy and describes the effect from a patient's perspective; and level 6, societal efficacy, encompasses the effect on the health care system and society as a whole. In this hierarchical model, the relevance of higher levels depends on the proven efficacy at the lower levels. Also, an improvement at the lower levels of efficacy should be justified by a tangible effect on the higher levels. For example, there is no relevance of diagnostic accuracy efficacy until the technical efficacy is proved; in contrast, there may be more scope to improve the technical efficacy but it might not necessarily improve the diagnostic accuracy efficacy. The 6 levels of assessment are discussed in the following sections along with how they apply to the evaluation of MRN.

Level 1: Technical Efficacy

Technical efficacy is under the physicist's purview. It evaluates the technical characteristics of an image like signal, noise, quality, and spatial and contrast resolution. The technical efficacy is tested on phantoms and then on patients. MRN is currently performed at few centers in the country, and every center should optimize the imaging quality to obtain high-resolution and high-contrast two-dimensional and three-dimensional imaging before they use the technique on their patients. The technical efficacy for images obtained by MRN has been successfully studied in some centers, and it continues to improve.[6–9]

Level 2: Diagnostic Accuracy Efficacy

This refers to image interpretation by the radiologist to make a diagnosis. Several descriptive statistics are used for this evaluation, such as sensitivity, specificity, positive and negative predictive values, and receiver operating characteristics (ROC) analysis. The diagnostic accuracy efficacy is a combined function of the image quality and observer interpretation. The observer interpretation is reader dependent. In MRN, the learning curve is steep and readers must learn normal nerve anatomy, anatomic variations, imaging pitfalls, nerve pathophysiology, and the wide spectrum of lesions encountered in a busy neuromuscular practice. To alleviate potential interpretation errors and to attain reasonable diagnostic performance, MRN readers must improve their interpretation skills by reading current articles and regularly participating in multidisciplinary conferences. In the literature, MRN has been shown to correlate with clinical, electrophysiological, and surgical findings, and good to excellent diagnostic accuracy and interobserver reproducibility has been observed in the evaluation of various small and large peripheral nerves.[10–13] Chhabra and colleagues[13] reported the optimal cutoff value of nerve/vessel signal intensity ratio for predicting sciatic neuropathy was 0.89, with sensitivity of 94.1% and specificity of 90.2% (area under the ROC curve, 0.963; 95% confidence interval, 0.886–0.994). Although anatomic MRN is practiced with good accuracy, functional diffusion tensor imaging (DTI) is also gaining acceptance. Andreisek and colleagues[8] reported that there were no side-to-side statistically significant differences on fiber tracking of median nerves in healthy volunteers, reflecting the good precision of DTI. Guggenberger and colleagues[14] showed the fractional anisotropy and apparent diffusion coefficient threshold values of normal and pathologic median nerves.

Level 3: Diagnostic Thinking Efficacy

Diagnostic thinking efficacy measures the ability of a new technology to provide clinically useful information and alter the diagnostic algorithm. A diagnostic test might have high sensitivity and specificity, but it should be able to make a difference in establishing the diagnosis or affecting the diagnostic work-up. Diagnostic thinking efficacy can be evaluated by using questionnaires that are completed by clinicians before and after receiving the image interpretation results. The questionnaire may pertain to certainty of diagnosis or the physician's confidence in certain clinical

findings, before and after imaging results. One such questionnaire used in our practice (**Fig. 1**) uses ordinal scales to simplify completion of the questionnaire. The physician reports on the specific nerve abnormality along with the degree of confidence before and after the imaging results. The change in degree of nerve injury is also

---

Appendix: Survey Questionnaire

1. What type of evidence is available at the time of completing this survey?

☐ Electromyography ☐ Quantitative neurosensory Testing ☐ Magnetic Resonance Neurography

2. Nerve abnormality present?

☐ Yes ☐ No Which nerve?_____

If the answer is No-

a. Degree of confidence in nerve abnormality?

☐1 Low ☐2 Moderate ☐3 High

b. Degree of confidence in no nerve abnormality?

☐1 Low ☐2 Moderate ☐3 High

c. Based on Seddon classification, categorize the nerve injury?

☐ Neuropraxia ☐ Axonotmesis ☐ Neurotmesis

3. Any differential diagnosis : _____

4. Does the patient need surgery- degree of confidence?

☐1 Low ☐2 Moderate ☐3 High

5. Timing of surgery?

☐1 Immediate ☐2 Not sure and follow up in three months ☐3 Surgery not needed

6. Approach to surgery?

Site of incision: _____

Length of incision: _____

7. Degree of confidence in approach to surgery?

☐1 Low ☐2 Moderate ☐3 High

8. Estimated length of surgery?

☐1 <2 hours ☐2 2-4 hours ☐3 4-6 hours ☐4 6-8 hours ☐5 >8 hours

Fig. 1. Survey questionnaire used in our MRN research.

recorded. The ordinal scale provides a semiquantitative approach that reduces the quandary of subjectivity.

Level 4: Therapeutic Efficacy

Therapeutic efficacy assesses the magnitude to which a diagnostic test affects the patient's treatment plan. This efficacy can also be measured by using clinician questionnaires, as shown in **Fig. 1**. The physician records the change in degree of confidence in need for surgery, the anatomic approach to surgery, and the timing and duration of surgery. The questionnaire compares the preliminary treatment options before the diagnostic test result with the treatment plan after the test results are made available to the physician. The new diagnostic test is most efficacious if it completely changes the treatment plan for the patient. However, an argument can be made that, even if the new diagnostic test has no effect on the therapy, it helps in reassuring the clinician or affects the diagnostic certainty (measured by degree of confidence). This reassurance can be considered a beneficial effect. In 2008, Andreisek and colleagues[15] conducted a successful study to show the value of MRN in influencing patient management.

Level 5: Patient Outcome Efficacy

This level of efficacy evaluation is the most important from the individual patient's perspective. It measures the level of patient satisfaction and the change in level of functionality after the treatment. Many questionnaires are available that can be used for estimating the functional capacity/disability and quality of life. These questionnaires can be general or specific to different sites of involvement in the patient. For example, Disabilities of the Arm, Shoulder, and Hand (DASH) can be used for upper extremity neuropathies[16]; Foot and Ankle Ability Measure (FAAM) for foot and ankle neuropathies[17]; and Boston Carpal Tunnel Questionnaire (BCTQ), which is specific for carpal tunnel syndrome[18]. Techniques are also available for measuring less specific health outcomes such as Quality of Life (QOL) and Quality-adjusted Life Years (QALY).[19,20] However, these measures can be difficult to accomplish because it requires the patient's compliance and repeated follow-ups, which might be arduous for a busy radiologist/clinician.

Level 6: Societal Efficacy

This final level of efficacy evaluation assesses the critical question of whether the new diagnostic technology leads to an efficient use of the health care resources and is beneficial to the society as a whole. The value (benefit/cost) is established by cost-effectiveness analyses and modeling methods. A cost-effectiveness study remains to be performed for MRN's societal impact, and the study design could be similar to other diseases/modalities.

SUMMARY

The past and recent literature on MRN has focused on the technical and diagnostic accuracy efficacy, leaving out the other levels in the 6-tier model. This focus has led to an insufficient assessment of this technology, because the clinical usefulness and its effect on patient clinical outcome have not been documented. As more and more institutions use MRN, the challenge is to adequately assess the technique while it is being accommodated into clinical practice. The technical effectiveness and diagnostic accuracy have been established,[21,22] so researchers should now focus on the remaining tiers of efficacy assessment, which can be accomplished by using clinician and patient surveys as described earlier and by studying homogenous populations of specific neuropathy sites or particular causes of neuropathy. Valid clinical studies of the higher levels of efficacy that can be generalized require collaboration between imaging researchers and the clinicians who are directly taking care of these patients.

It is imperative to determine the clinical impact of MRN. The prospective research should focus on the assessment of MRN's effect on clinicians' diagnostic thinking and therapeutic decision making as well as patient outcomes. Institutions currently using MRN as a diagnostic tool should conduct more studies relating to diagnostic, treatment, and societal outcomes.

REFERENCES

1. Fineberg HV, Bauman R, Sosman M. Computerized cranial tomography. Effect on diagnostic and therapeutic plans. JAMA 1977;238(3):224–7.
2. Fryback DG, Thornbury JR. The efficacy of diagnostic imaging. Med Decis Making 1991;11(2):88–94.
3. Thornbury JR. Intermediate outcomes: diagnostic and therapeutic impact. Acad Radiol 1999;6(Suppl 1): S58–65 [discussion: S66–8].
4. Brook RH, Lohr KN. Efficacy, effectiveness, variations, and quality. Boundary-crossing research. Med Care 1985;23(5):710–22.
5. Hunink MG, Krestin GP. Study design for concurrent development, assessment, and implementation of new diagnostic imaging technology. Radiology 2002;222(3):604–14.
6. Howe FA, Filler AG, Bell BA, et al. Magnetic resonance neurography. Magn Reson Med 1992;28(2):328–38.

7. Zhang Z, Meng Q, Chen Y, et al. 3-T imaging of the cranial nerves using three-dimensional reversed FISP with diffusion-weighted MR sequence. J Magn Reson Imaging 2008;27(3):454–8.

8. Andreisek G, White LM, Kassner A, et al. Evaluation of diffusion tensor imaging and fiber tractography of the median nerve: preliminary results on intrasubject variability and precision of measurements. AJR Am J Roentgenol 2010;194(1):W65–72.

9. Chhabra A, Subhawong TK, Bizzell C, et al. 3T MR neurography using three-dimensional diffusion-weighted PSIF: technical issues and advantages. Skeletal Radiol 2011;40(10):1355–60.

10. Thawait SK, Chaudhry V, Thawait GK, et al. High-resolution MR neurography of diffuse peripheral nerve lesions. AJNR Am J Neuroradiol 2011;32(8):1365–72.

11. Viallon M, Vargas MI, Jlassi H, et al. High-resolution and functional magnetic resonance imaging of the brachial plexus using an isotropic 3D T2 STIR (Short Term Inversion Recovery) SPACE sequence and diffusion tensor imaging. Eur Radiol 2008;18(5):1018–23.

12. Vargas MI, Viallon M, Nguyen D, et al. New approaches in imaging of the brachial plexus. Eur J Radiol 2010;74(2):403–10.

13. Chhabra A, Chalian M, Soldatos T, et al. 3-T high-resolution MR neurography of sciatic neuropathy. AJR Am J Roentgenol 2012;198(4):W357–64.

14. Guggenberger R, Markovic D, Eppenberger P, et al. Assessment of median nerve with MR neurography by using diffusion-tensor imaging: normative and pathologic diffusion values. Radiology 2012;265(1):194–203.

15. Andreisek G, Burg D, Studer A, et al. Upper extremity peripheral neuropathies: role and impact of MR imaging on patient management. Eur Radiol 2008;18(9):1953–61.

16. Jester A, Harth A, Wind G, et al. Disabilities of the Arm, Shoulder and Hand (DASH) questionnaire: determining functional activity profiles in patients with upper extremity disorders. J Hand Surg Br 2005;30(1):23–8.

17. Martin RL, Irrgang JJ, Burdett RG, et al. Evidence of validity for the Foot and Ankle Ability Measure (FAAM). Foot Ankle Int 2005;26(11):968–83.

18. Padua L, Padua R, Aprile I, et al. Boston Carpal Tunnel Questionnaire: the influence of diagnosis on patient-oriented results. Neurol Res 2005;27(5):522–4.

19. Bleichrodt H, Johannesson M. The validity of QALYs: an experimental test of constant proportional trade-off and utility independence. Med Decis Making 1997;17(1):21–32.

20. Padilla GV. Validity of health-related quality of life subscales. Prog Cardiovasc Nurs 1992;7(1):13–20.

21. Chhabra A, Subhawong TK, Williams EH, et al. High-resolution MR neurography: evaluation before repeat tarsal tunnel surgery. AJR Am J Roentgenol 2011;197(1):175–83.

22. Bäumer P, Dombert T, Staub F, et al. Ulnar neuropathy at the elbow: MR neurography–nerve T2 signal increase and caliber. Radiology 2011;260(1):199–206.

Index

Note: Page numbers of article titles are in **boldface** type.

Moving?

Make sure your subscription moves with you!

To notify us of your new address, find your **Clinics Account Number** (located on your mailing label above your name), and contact customer service at:

Email: journalscustomerservice-usa@elsevier.com

800-654-2452 (subscribers in the U.S. & Canada)
314-447-8871 (subscribers outside of the U.S. & Canada)

Fax number: 314-447-8029

Elsevier Health Sciences Division
Subscription Customer Service
3251 Riverport Lane
Maryland Heights, MO 63043

*To ensure uninterrupted delivery of your subscription, please notify us at least 4 weeks in advance of move.

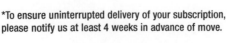

Printed and bound by CPI Group (UK) Ltd, Croydon, CR0 4YY

03/10/2024

01040378-0007